CU00688884

COPYRIGHT

TABLE OF CONTENTS

Introduction

INTRODUCTION

What you are about to read is an unusually large collection of health related gems rarely found in one place. To be clear, this isn't just another hyped-up health book – it's the Swiss army knife of health books, a comprehensive problem solving tool.

Based on six years of meticulous research, this remarkable story quickly unfolds into a step-by-step guide to wellness. Concise, yet oozing with originality, think of these coming chapters as stepping stones to healthier lands; they are your shortcut to a less stressed, more energized, healthier version of you.

A rich vein of insight also comes to the table via the author's own battle with serious illness. As such, a sense of united understanding quietly flows from page to page. At times complex information is broken down and presented like two old friends chatting over a pot of tea. For those already frustrated by illness, this relaxed, easy to follow format becomes a welcome break from the norm.

I know what you're thinking because I've had the same thought: *in a world with so much information swirling around, do we really need another book about health?*

It's true, everything you need to know is already in print *somewhere,* but with so much information, so little time, and so many potential causes of illness, wouldn't it be nice if everything you needed to know could be found in just one book?

Rather than deliver empty promises, here's a book that goes the extra mile, offering quality information that's actually enjoyable to read. Leaving no stone unturned, we'll also explore the role of nutrition and the importance of stress management. As an added bonus, many of the topics covered inside are interactive. At the end of each section, leading health experts come to you in the form of clickable video links. Handpicked with intent, these short clips help to smooth out the learning process as well as bringing insight and balance to the many topics discussed. Whether your goal is to stay well or get well, following these suggested links becomes a real game changer. We'll also look at a wide range of household items that have the potential to make you sick, and how best to avoid them.

Okay, let's cut to the chase. No matter how good the information in a book is, unless it's delivered in an interesting way, the book is destined to collect dust along with all your other half-read health books. *Am I Right?*

Not this book. This emotionally engaging story comes alive from the get-go. Clearly there are some lessons that *only* adversity can teach. Free of complex medical jargon, the route back to wellness is about to take you on some beautifully winding roads. Let this book show you all the shortcuts to take along the way. It's all in here waiting for you – peppered with a delicate hint of British humor,

Here's what we know for sure: a day of illness comes to each and every one of us. In a perfect world, a solution would be quickly found and once again life would be good. But I'm guessing you already know the world we live in is far from perfect. What becomes of those who leave the doctor's office with a set of lingering symptoms or a treatment plan that appears to make things worse? What's your next move if you are told your illness has no solution? *Do you have a plan?*

Come in and close the door behind you, let's set about finding all those elusive answers you crave. In every sense of the word, this is a truly independent book which means there is nothing to fear from telling it like it is. With no slick million-dollar marketing team to pump up sales, it's actually quite remarkable that you even found this unusual book **or perhaps this book found you.**

To get the most out of this journey, it pays to bring along an open mind. If you have no room for such mental flexibility **then better to leave now, empty handed.** While I'd be sorry to lose you so early, there is peace in knowing that neither one of us is wasting our time. For those who stay, I suspect illness unites us, if only in our vulnerability to it.

What follows is sure to be a refreshingly honest read. It's to be enjoyed, debated, and even disagreed with. It's *not* intended to replace mainstream medical advice but rather to be of service and used as a tool to complement it. My willingness to share the disclaimer below is an acknowledgment that *your* health is as important to me as it should be to you.

DISCLAIMER

Ready to come inside?

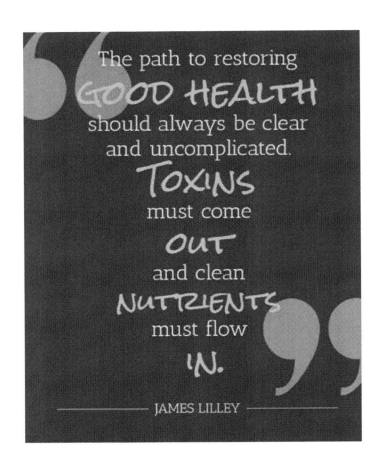

The path to restoring **GOOD HEALTH** should always be clear and uncomplicated. **TOXINS** must come **OUT** and clean **NUTRIENTS** must flow **IN.**

— JAMES LILLEY —

Amazon
Top customer reviews

An interesting read

As a holistic therapist, I have literally read hundreds of "health" books. None have impacted me as strongly or deeply as this one. Not only have I come away with a long list of valuable healing concepts and ideas, but found that the author's open, self-revealing writing style touched both my heart and soul in ways that have stayed with me.

Sandra Kagan, Ph.D.

Top customer reviews

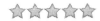

Your roadmap to health is here!!!

I am VERY impressed by the clarity, coherency, and compassion of this book. When you are ready to take personal responsibility for your own health you will find this book to be an invaluable asset. This book features dozens of well-researched, easy to implement health strategies for directing your own personal path to health and happiness. This is a heartfelt and inspiring work. Do yourself a favor and buy it! Your good health is in your hands!

Top customer reviews

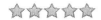

Informative and very helpful, thank you!

I'd recommend this book to absolutely anybody particularly those struggling with regular prescriptions for illnesses and ailments.
It has helped me enormously, I feel reinvigorated and full of life. My kids attitudes towards healthy eating have completely changed and they love fresh healthy food which will stand them in good stead for years to come. Many thanks to the author, genuinely (and for the humour!).

Top customer reviews

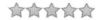

An incredibly insightful book about illness and how we can get well

I found this book incredibly insightful and it's quite amazing how James turned his health around significantly by thinking outside the box and persisting.

This book is great for people who want something simple and groundbreaking that sheds light on why people get ill and what can make them better. It's also a fun read full of lots of humorous and heartbreaking stories and anecdotes.

Top customer reviews

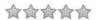

One of the most real and influential books I have read!!!

First let me say I have never read a "health" book before. This was not just a book about someone telling you that you HAVE to live your life a certain way. This book makes you look at everything in a very different perspective. The author brings us into his struggles (which we all have in one way or another) and talks through his book as if he is talking one on one with a friend. This was a fantastic read and I strongly suggest anyone reading it.

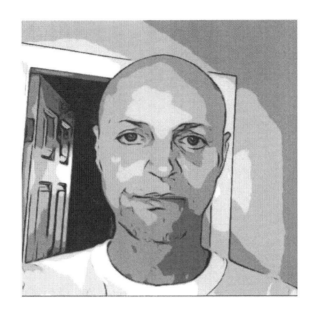

Like an incessant obsession, this book has quietly burned inside me. This wasn't the story I intended to tell, and yet here we are, staring each other firmly in the eye. – Welcome.

Chapter 1

CAUGHT WITHOUT A PLAN

There could be many reasons why you picked up this book. Your goal might be to have more energy, better mental clarity, or you might simply have come in search of tools to help you overcome a stubborn illness. Let's explore that last option first, and then work our way backward.

Illness is a puzzle; to try to solve it we first need to understand it. Typically, there are two ways to do this. The first is to enlist the services of a medical professional. This approach is not without merit, but it often involves taking medications. Perhaps you have already tried this route and did not find a lasting solution.

The second option is to stop what you are doing and listen. Do you hear it? Those annoying symptoms we all complain about are actually a fascinating and effective two-way system of communication. They are your body's way of letting you know that something you are doing sucks. Until now, you may not have been paying close attention. That's okay – you will because your body is sure to soon send you a much clearer signal. And the medical term for that signal is pain.

Symptoms let us know there is a problem in the body, much the same way a vehicle Check Engine light might alert us to a problem under the hood. Symptoms also offer important clues to help us find solutions. Unfortunately, there are times when these clues are suppressed by prescription drugs such as painkillers.

If the prescription drug approach has worked for you in the past, then I suspect you wouldn't be reading this book. For some, drugs do little to address the root cause of the problem and so the underlying health problem rarely goes away. In addition, many drugs cause negative side effects. Now you have two medical problems. Shall we go for three?

In the U.S., taking prescribed drugs has become a leading cause of death. Some estimates put the figure at over 100,000 deaths per year.

That's twice as many Americans dying from prescription drugs than are killed in car accidents. To simplify: you go to the doctor, he or she gives you something for your symptoms, you take it, and you die. *I know, right?* What's up with that?

By comparison, the only side effect of listening to your symptoms is likely to be a rapid improvement in your health. This is how good medicine was practiced for thousands of years before illness became profitable. Make no mistake, serious illness has become a seriously lucrative business. At this point you should be asking, "How the heck did we get here?"

Our modern lives are a cozy and mundane loop of birthdays, holiday celebrations, polite conversation, countless shopping excursions, and not great television and nobody seems to mind. Until we are stripped bare of such impetuous pleasantries, wellness can remain a misunderstood and often fickle destination. But when serious illness strikes, it offers us a unique opportunity to see what's *really* important in this life and does so by sweeping aside the superficial with cold, clinical precision. Then we find ourselves asking, "How did we get so ill, and why?" When we are forced to look through the lens of serious illness, what we see has the potential to either shape us or break us.

So it seems that illness can actually be a beautiful gift, for it is here, in the midst of adversity that we find out who we *really* are. Pain leaves no room for a middle ground in which we can waiver or be wishy-washy. And hidden deep within that necessary intensity we discover our very reason for being here.

Illness is a truly obnoxious intruder and getting rid of it now depends largely on your perception of the problem and your desire to overcome it.

Let's explore this a little.

All illness brings with it two burning questions: *what* do I have, and *how* is it treatable? While these types of questions are justifiable, they can also be thought of as looking at the *outer* layers of the onion. To penetrate the center of the onion we need to ask ourselves a more probing question:

why did we become ill? Once we have the *why,* the *what* and the *how* begin to fall neatly into line.

How do I know this?

In 2011, I became seriously ill and found that the medical profession could not cope with the complexity of my symptoms. With an extremely persistent nature and a diligent mind, six years of *meticulous* research followed. The good news is I eventually succeeded where highly educated people had failed me. Had I known then what I know now, I believe I could have avoided my illness altogether, or, failing that, my recovery would have come much sooner than it did.

Either way, my findings are presented here as a coherent roadmap that will lead you to a place of wellness. You can think of the following chapters as missing pieces of a puzzle and, depending on your situation, you may need some of them or you may need all of them.

You will not be surprised that many of these findings run contrary to what is usual, traditional, or embraced by mainstream medicine. They also fly in the face of what you now believe to be true. They *have to* or quite simply your health would already be thriving.

Because I am unhindered by the corporate greed that is so often part of the medical establishment, my education has always been free to go in any direction that brings results. My gold standard for finding what works is always simple and unassuming: something either works or it does not. My interest is piqued by things that bring progress, and not by out-of-date and inflexible concepts. When the body is in a full- blown crisis, everything has to be done out of pure *necessity* with zero tolerance for a middle road.

To put your health back on the road, there are no shortcuts; it can take a sustained effort to become ill and an equal effort to pull away from it. However, with the right approach, positive results *are* attainable within a relatively short time. With that in mind, it's important not to skip over *any* sections in this book and I strongly urge you to take full advantage of the video gurus offered along the way

Shall we begin?

The anniversaries of our miraculous arrival in this life are celebrated with cake; our departure is more difficult to acknowledge. When faced with the option of cake or death, we assure ourselves with fearful confidence that 80+ years is somehow owed to us, preferring to think of illness as the *other* person's disease. I hate to be the one to break this disheartening news so early on, but that body you live in has an expiration date: there comes a day when we *all* turn to dust. Even you. How we get there, and when, is defined by the choices we make today.

It's a little harsh, I know, but the value of health begins to shift dramatically when it registers that serious illness *already* knows where you live. Like a visitor that's coming but you aren't sure when, illness has little regard for whom it calls on. It flirts indiscriminately with black and white, rich and poor, and even makes a fool of the rich man as he keenly strives to acquire wealth before health. With patient curiosity, illness waits for even the busiest person in the cruel hope of one day stopping them *dead* in their tracks.

A fleeting visit from illness may bring comfort but, unless you take good care of yourself, illness has the power to consume. I wouldn't wish it even on my worst enemy.

Friend, heed this warning: illness knows the names of each and every one of us. Before illness calls us, we are offered this simple choice: **make time for your health *now* or be forced to take time out for sickness later.**

As I write this, I know some will listen and others will resist. Sooner or later we must all come to the understanding that an ounce of prevention clearly outperforms a pound of cure.

It's worth remembering that illness rarely falls from the deep blue sky: there *has* to be a reason. The trick is to find what's stressing the body and then develop an effective strategy to overcome it. Once we have a starting point, the logical progression is to swiftly find an end.

Along the way, symptoms are sent to guide us. Some symptoms are subtle, others are more pronounced. *All are relevant.* For example: a drippy nose, profuse sweating, debilitating migraines, projectile vomiting, intense itching, tremors, unique body odors, intolerable joint pain, along with a silent hankering for sanity are all just a handful of the more *obvious* clues that *must* be matched with solutions in order for illness to subside.

Turning a deaf ear to these important clues (or choosing to suppress them with drugs) will inevitably provoke a stronger reaction. With each warning we choose to ignore, we move a little closer to our appointment with a more serious version of ill health.

And here's the rub ...

If you have already been through the medical system you may have had the misfortune to hear that your suffering is merely genetic, or bad luck, or simply old age. When blame is neatly nudged in your direction, a feeling of helplessness ensues. This damning news suddenly presents a much bigger problem to *you* than it does to the doctor treating you.

A few misplaced words from a well-meaning specialist can leave a person feeling like a rudderless ship left to drift in open water. If they only knew that the human body in which you live is a highly complex marvel with the power to heal itself. We just have to get out of the way and allow it. For now, let's agree to suspend such *wasted* thoughts. If one other person has successfully dealt with the health issue you face, then there are no – as in *zero* – good reasons why you can't overcome it too. Be still, and know that "Everything will be okay in the end. If it's not okay, it's not the end." (John Lennon)

Perhaps we have become a tad too keen to accept less health as inevitable, rather than making a conscious effort to improve it. It really *doesn't* have to be this way; health problems have solutions, just as all doors have keys.

HERE'S THE HOW

The path to restoring good health should always be clear and uncomplicated. Toxins must come out and clean nutrients must flow in. I have seen this principle work in myself and I have seen it work in others. Put simply, give your body what it needs and steer it well away from what it doesn't. To help you do this, this book has all the information you need.

From here, you will be encouraged to take a hard look at the many toxic elements that have become a part of our murky world. Then we will systematically look to eradicate each of those toxic substances one by one. You may choose to ignore these warnings if you wish, but by the time you've finished this book, you will not be able to say you weren't aware of them.

It is with some irony that we sometimes say that good health simply costs too much and at the same time we cram our houses with superficial *things* that please us. Our closets contain expensive shoes we hardly wear, our garden sheds overflow with equipment we do not use, our pockets are stuffed with expensive electronic devices, and yet the mere mention of paying 50 cents more for a clean head of broccoli threatens to bring the household budget crashing down!

We are too quick to quibble with the local farmer over the price of his grass-fed meat, preferring to stand in a line at the supermarket hoping to snag what's on sale. Save money if you must, but first look to cut meaningless waste from your budget and *not* the quality of the food you eat. Do this one thing and you will see that true wealth comes from within. There really is no such thing as cheap food: *either we pay the farmer or we pay the doctor.*

For some, a visit to the doctor brings *immediate* success; for others improvement can be more fleeting. When solutions become elusive, we spend our days sitting in hospital waiting rooms and our nights frantically searching for answers online until finally a self-perpetuating loop of self-doubt develops and we can no longer see the woods for the trees. This path leads to frustration *and I know it well.*

To be clear, in every emergency room around the world doctors can and do perform with *outstanding* efficiency. The skill of these dedicated men and women should be recognized and genuinely applauded. These types of doctors are used to seeing devastating physical injuries and provide a professional service for fixing them. But when symptoms present themselves in a less obvious fashion, we are quickly reminded that doctors are not gods and these same medical experts may even fall short of our expectations.

Today in modern medicine it's fair to say that shades of grey exist: cancer continues to frustrate science, as does the common cold. We could also add to that list devastating chronic fatigue, gut-wrenching anxiety, difficult to manage depression, and the mystery of more than a hundred deeply disturbing autoimmune conditions.

It's a worry that should be commanding front page news but instead we fill our news with the gossip of celebrities we will never meet. Conditioned not to question, and too trusting of those who least deserve it, we face a slick, billion-dollar industry that thinks nothing of offering us both hope and an outlandish variety of dangerous side effects in the same TV commercial. *I know, right? You can't make this stuff up.* Allowing a single group of people to hold a monopoly over your health may seem like a sensible move, but should the results become stagnant, it's absolutely okay to step in and play a bigger role in your own recovery. The goal of this book is to help you do just that.

The good news is that serious illness also brings with it clarity of mind, and that ensures that answers are more likely to be found. You may even find those material "things" are quick to lose their fleeting value. Serious illness reveals that health *is* the most valuable commodity we own. It's *not* a faster car, it's *not* a better house, and it's certainly *not* an elite set of friends.

How so?

Vomiting on the bathroom floor doesn't allow us to drive that fancy car. When strapped to a hospital bed we aren't sitting in our bigger house. As for that new clique of friends ... well, if your illness remains undiagnosed, nobody ever wants to risk getting sick from you.

Keep coming if you must – one misdirected dollar bill at a time – but you should know a day is coming, without warning, when the cost of illness becomes relative and easily trumps celebrity gossip for our attention.

THE WALL

Any unexpected visit from serious illness can be like hitting a brick-wall at 100 mph. I've already discovered this and found that illness is a highly effective teacher, always bringing into focus what is important. Beyond the obvious challenges, there is also a certain beauty to any catalyst that brings about permanent change. For those, like me, who are fortunate enough to recover, the insights gained can change your very understanding of life itself.

For me, the brick-wall I hit was also a place of frustration, fear, and uncompromising pain – and going back is no longer an option. *Now I listen, now I hear.* Unless you have been to this point, such harsh lessons are difficult to comprehend.

What's clear is the majority of health problems *don't* lack solutions. Rather, in this technological age there can be *too much* information to choose from. I'm offering a way to blast through that mass of digital information and open up new paths to allow your health to move forward.

Unfortunately, watching other good people go to the wall can be like watching a slow motion car crash. For those who refuse to listen, the brick-wall can be an enlightening destination. No matter how distressing at the time, it's entirely possible that survivors of the wall will be positively changed by the experience.

The next chapter reveals how I came into contact with my own brick-wall and why this book was written. Before we go there, I'd again like to point out that this is *not* a book for those who have yet to give traditional medicine a chance to succeed, *nor is it a good fit for those who are firm in the belief that mainstream medicine will always prevail.* But for those who have tried the conventional route and have become frustrated by a lack of progress, then this book is for you.

Come if you must with an open mind, or do not come at all.
Only then will you find value.
− James Lilley

Chapter 2

THE TURNING OF A TOXIC WORM

This is not some elaborate program that you need to buy into. I have no expensive pills or products to sell you. The absence of product links in this book is *intentional.* From this point on my affiliation is with you alone.

I am keenly aware that this is a book all about *you* and *your* health and I have that task firmly in my mind. However, before we set off on this journey together, I'd like to take this opportunity to first introduce myself and share with you a brief glimpse of my own destructive collision with ill health. The aim of retelling my story is pure and simple: to convey a clear message that *I get it* – illness can be profoundly devastating *but I learned to navigate my own way out of it.*

It's debatable what the best way to learn is. Some could argue that first-hand experience is most effective; others will argue for formal learning. While both styles have merit, seeking answers out of pure necessity is a little different than paying for medical training as part of a lucrative career choice.

> *Experience without theory is blind,*
> *but theory without experience is mere intellectual play.*
> – Immanuel Kant

Example: ask any qualified veterinarian about the strength of a pit bull's jaw and you are sure to get a detailed reply. But if you want to know how sharp the dog's teeth are, find a mailman who's been bitten by one. When you live it, you'd better understand it. Real life experience absolutely has value—more so when your health depends on it, as mine did.

If you are curious to know how serious illness affected me personally, then keep reading; this is the preferred route. All the techniques I used in my recovery are covered in this book. However, if you are in a rush to get well, feel free to skip these next few chapters and I'll meet you at the beginning of chapter five.

So, my story begins in the north of England. Growing up in a tough working class area, I quickly learned that school could be a repressive and intimidating place. By the time I left school at the age of fifteen it's fair to say I had learned how to write and fight. The relevance of this will become more obvious in later chapters. Leaving home shortly after gave me ample opportunity to run with the wrong crowd; the rules of the street were often harsh and I got to know them all rather well.

Throughout my problem years, *which were many,* my dad never lost faith in me. A man of great patience, he also gave me my gift of unbending persistence. Little did I know at the time that this quality would one day save my life.

It seems my life moves in units of five. A five-year stint in the British military seemed to straighten me out. The local paper even ran a story on me because I had won an award relating to physical training. Thankfully, my entire service was completed in peacetime and the only foreign soil I visited was European and U.S. Fast-forward to the end of my military career and I was right back where I started, moving with ease in bad company.

Against all the odds, *again* I managed to break free of my stale environment and, for the next five years, found myself running a successful business. I employed almost fifty people and in doing so my life went from rags to riches and *that* time a local radio station came.

The day I drove my first Mercedes SL out of the showroom, my dad proudly stood there to see it. For sure this path hadn't always been easy on either one of us. Zip forward *five* more years and the breakup of a long-term relationship found me alone and *without* a business. I felt I needed to get away and found myself standing on American soil.

HERE SHE COMES

When I arrived in the United States I quickly found an unusual ally. In a crowded bar she caught me looking and, when a smile came back, it lit up the room. With a face that wouldn't have been out of place on the cover of a magazine, her natural beauty quickly drew me in.

She was elegant and had a warm intelligent voice. As most Americans do, she enjoyed listening to my heavy British accent, curious opinions, and even my terrible jokes. I mentioned that she looked exactly like my *second* wife. Her eyes widened and she asked me how many wives I'd had?

Without missing a beat, I said, "Just one."

She must have found me as charming as I was trying to be because one year later she really did become my second wife. We decided to move out of the city and found ourselves embracing a much simpler lifestyle than either of us had been accustomed to. Deep in the heart of rural America we purchased an old farmhouse in need of repair; this was to be our American dream.

That summer I worked my ass off. If I wasn't busy fixing something inside, I'd be up on the roof or down in the basement crawling around doing some type of repair. I'd always liked solving problems by working them backward and then re-applying common sense and logic to them. It never occurred to me that one day this type of thinking would help me out of a wheelchair.

My beautiful wife had long suspected that I was a workaholic. For me, peace came from working with a purpose or perhaps I just liked to stay busy. I actually enjoyed being outside in the rain chopping firewood in preparation for a long winter ahead. My parents had been hard workers and a strong work ethic was instilled in me at an early age. I guess I was fortunate to have inherited an intuitive mind and a surplus of energy, seven days a week.

Several happy years of married life breezed past and we remained inseparable best friends. By now I was fully submerged in the local lifestyle and grateful to have found a corner of the world very different from the one I grew up in. Living in a small mountain community in northern New Hampshire gave me the opportunity to see that doing the right thing was more important than doing the easy thing.

Here it was refreshing to find a man's word still had value. I became a product of my new environment and it turned me into an honest and dedicated family man. Together my wife and I raised a small family and grew a garden. Life was good. Up until that point in my life, serious illness was a stranger to me.

HERE "IT" COMES

I'd *always* been one of the lucky ones; as a child I once got chicken pox but bounced right back within a week or so. I'd maybe get a cold every other year but before you could say sick-note I'd be over it and back at work. In short, my immune system was working just as nature intended.

However, by the beginning of 2011 things were about to change beyond anything I could have foreseen or comprehended. A relatively routine visit to a health center found me sitting in front of a female doctor who encouraged me to be *proactive* with my health.
At 10:15 a.m. on the 16th of February my doctor suggested that I protect myself from a list of diseases that, honestly, had not for 47 years been a problem. But like most people, I wanted to do the right thing, and following through with my doctor's advice seemed like the right thing to do. By 10:30 that morning, the ink on my consent form was dry and I'd put my full trust in the medical establishment. By doing so, I had also handed over complete responsibility for my health. And this is where it gets tricky. Here's why.

What had just happened to me was in no way my fault, and it's an area of medicine that has become the source of many heated discussions. Some folks are totally for it, and some folks are totally against it. It doesn't matter to me which group you are in, only that you understand why this wasn't my fault. I simply did what the good doctor suggested, and for whatever reason things went wrong. At this early stage in the book, I don't wish to open up a can of worms or put myself in the center of a polarizing debate. But having lived through this, I know that I'm not the first person this has happened to, and I suspect I won't be the last. Beyond that, I'm going to respectfully refrain from going into more detail. If it makes you feel better, please know that this book has no hidden agenda, this isn't about being pro or anti anything, it's about helping to keep you well. At this moment in my story, it's about to start raining on me, but before too long the sun will once again be coming out to shine. So, shall we just press on?

As I left the health center something didn't quite feel right, but I'd never been seriously ill in my life so I shook it off, confident that whatever had just happened would work itself out, just as it always had.

By the time I got home a few things already felt different: my neck was ultra-tight, as if I had somehow pulled a muscle, and both hamstrings were in a state of tension. By nightfall my head was pounding and I was sensing the *beginning* of an illness I hadn't experienced before.

Over the next few days my body alternated between burning up and shivering violently in a sweat-drenched bed; my teeth actually chattered on occasion and a feeling of uneasiness washed over me. As each new morning broke, I found myself already awake and staring at the ceiling.

Unfortunately, I still had work left to do and I was determined to finish it so that I could go back to bed in peace. While picking up my car keys to leave the house it suddenly felt as if I was carrying a large stone in my pocket. I'd never noticed the weight of a key before, so that was a little strange. As I got into my pickup truck, I clipped the top of my head on the doorframe and then did the exact same thing again when I got out. *What the...?*

I'd only climbed back out of the vehicle to check the deck for lost fluid because, on that day of all days, it seemed that the power steering fluid had sprung a leak. As I scanned the ground for leaked fluid, I felt my shoulders and head drop simultaneously. An utterly dry patch underneath the truck told me that the fault *wasn't* with the power steering; it was with my arms.

These were arms that were used to hard work; they often toiled from sun up to sun down and yet here I was struggling to turn the damned steering wheel on my pickup truck.

As the morning progressed I forced myself to keep moving. I've always prided myself on finishing anything I start but by midday lifting everyday objects simply became too much and I settled for dragging them, and myself, around. By lunchtime my body was under siege and I just needed to go home.

PIN?

This is where things started to get even more bizarre. When I stopped for gas, I suddenly couldn't remember my debit card PIN number. The bank later called to say I had left my card in the ATM machine. I'd always been so diligent with money so this was an *absolute* first for me. Once home, the slightest noise became an irritation: the tick-tick-ticking clock, a ball bouncing outside, the sound of water running; even the clicking on and off of a light switch was magnified to the point where I could no longer think straight.

Now my eyes began to bother me, giving way to a sharp, intense pain, which seemed to come and go at random, particularly in my right eye. Both eyes developed ultra-sensitivity to light and, as nightfall came around again, I lay in the dark awake and alone with my thoughts.

It had long become a habit for my two young children to poke their wee heads around the bedroom door each night to say goodnight. Under the circumstances, I did my very best to smile, but tonight it wasn't my usual smile and it was clear I hadn't even come close to fooling them.

As the weeks progressed, so too did my symptoms. My sleep was impaired by truly harrowing nightmares that leached into my mind with horrific regularity. It honestly felt as if the gates of hell had slammed shut behind me. What worries me to this day is *I didn't even see this coming.*

But it was my legs that were now my biggest concern. I'd always carried a spring in my step – these were legs that enjoyed walking; now they just felt different. They were gripped in a constant state of tension. This feeling was most evident in both hamstrings, even as I lay in bed, they just felt … well … different.

As I tried to make sense of what was happening to me, a torrent of questions flooded my mind. Answers did *not*. Was it the muscles in my legs or could it be the tendons or maybe even the nerves? But *if* this was a form of neuropathy, was it myopathy or polyneuropathy? Maybe this was the start of some new autoimmune condition that had been primed to attack from within? But was it ALS or MS? Around and around and around in endless circles with no answer to be found.

The only thing I knew for sure was my previously robust immune system had been compromised and these alarming sensations weren't leaving my side. I am someone who likes to be productive so I hated being sick. Days soon began to melt into nights with annoying repetition.

After another week of incessant illness, my biggest fear was that I wasn't bouncing back. Up until this point in my life I had rarely seen a doctor, nor had my elderly parents. It had been a successful strategy that had allowed my health to flourish unhindered; now I was paying the price for allowing others to meddle. This wasn't my fault but it was now my problem.

I hated the very thought of going back to the doctor with every fiber in my body. I was actually relieved when the receptionist announced in an upbeat tone, "It will be another week before we can get you back in again."

Each new day presented more problems with no end in sight. I watched in absolute horror as random muscles now began to twitch throughout my body. This unsettled me and, deep down, I knew I was in trouble.

Three, four, maybe even five weeks later (it's hard to be exact when you can't think straight) a string of futile doctors' visits had been the only thing worth dragging myself out of bed for. If anyone had the elusive answers I so desperately needed, they weren't telling.

Throughout this period my elderly parents had been telephoning every day from England just to check in on me. Dad would try to cheer me up with his brand of terrible jokes. (*Why do dads do that?*) Mom wasn't quite so upbeat; it was clear from the crackled tone in her voice that she was

29

suffering right along with me. I can only imagine what she was thinking as her only son lay on a doctor-induced sickbed in a faraway land alternating between hardship and pain.

As time edged forward I could sense that we were already at the back end of winter and spring was approaching. I desperately wanted to be working outside in the cool spring air as I always had, but by the time spring ended I had spent most of it confined to my bedroom. There had been some nights when it felt as if the coldness of death wanted to climb deep inside me. And there were times when I truly wished it had.

Going to the doctors now became my only outdoor activity. It was of little comfort that my blood tests had all come back as "normal." The irony was that the doctor who had propelled me into this shitty mess was now the same one trying to get me out of it.

Her advice to be "proactive" with my health had spectacularly backfired. Unable to figure out what had gone wrong, she then referred me to another doctor, and then another. Maybe you can relate?

Now too weak to work, I again took to my sweat-drenched bed and prayed for this all to go away. Being the independent problem solving type, I'd spent most of my adult life being self-employed and I liked it that way. But I was now in the undesirable position of being too ill to work, but not quite ill enough to die.

Without any type of safety net, another month or so passed. And for my family and me, the marking of time wasn't passing too easily. Without a comprehensive health plan or paycheck coming in we were now slipping into financial decline. The absurdity of the situation was that, even in the grip of serious illness, I still wanted to do the *right* thing and pay my bills on time. Quietly, one by one, the things I had worked so hard for all began creeping out the door.

Despite the hardship that comes from choosing to live a life in rural America, there is also a strong sense of community—maybe more so in the mountains. As our situation continued to go from bad to worse, the news of what was happening to our family trickled through the rest of our small, tight-knit community.

These were *not* people of any great wealth but they were the type of people who pressed hard cash into the hand of anyone in need and refused to accept no for an answer. Get Well Soon cards began to appear in our mailbox with prepaid grocery cards tucked inside them. Another envelope came with *no note,* just a $100 bill inside.

As a fiercely independent person, it's never been easy for me to accept help from anyone. A month or so later I reluctantly sold my pickup truck. Fortunately, we still had my wife's car as a backup. Being driven to and from doctors' appointments by my wife soon had me floundering in my own self-pity.

This is where unhelpful male pride begins to kick in. I remember thinking this isn't how I live; this isn't who I am. *I know, right? A prideful heart that needs to be taught humility; unfortunately, this harsh lesson was only just beginning.*

To help keep us afloat, my wife turned her hand to selling knitting patterns online. How she managed to remain creative under this level of stress is beyond me, but a small flurry of sales always seemed to come in just when we needed them the most. I thanked God that we shared a modest two-bedroom house with small bills. Had it not been for these combining factors I doubt we would have been able to keep the lights on.

OLD SCHOOL

At this point you may be wondering why I didn't try to sue the doctor who had sent me into this unintended tailspin. This is America; everyone sues in America, right? First, you have to understand that I was ill, seriously ill, and just doing the best I could to get through each terrifying day. Also, when you suddenly discover that you are the *only* one standing at the edge of the abyss, the *last thing* on your mind is fighting over money in court.

I'm also old school: the whole suing culture thing has never sat right with me. I really didn't want to spend my days hanging on for handouts. I just wanted to get well and work; it's what I've always done. What good would it do me anyway? I still didn't have a current diagnosis and, before entering into this mess, I'd been handed that medical disclaimer to sign. It seemed that, in the event of something going wrong, the doctor's back was totally covered. But *mine?* Meh, not so much.

Back home I watched from my bedroom window as spring turned to summer. I could see that weeds had taken my once pristine garden hostage, which seemed to mirror what was happening in my ailing body. Downstairs I overheard my youngest ask, *"Hey Mom, why, is our grass so long?"* The world through a kid's eyes; you have to love them. The *only* thing she had known in her short life was that Dad's immaculate garden had *always* been kept on-point. Maybe she thought the grass fairy came and did it, who knows?

I had now been seriously ill in bed, alternating between shivering and sweating, for six *long* months. More doctors' appointments ensued and yet a solution remained as elusive as ever. Such bright doctors trying to unravel a complicated problem without, it seemed, a thread of *common sense* between them.

Naively, I was still convinced that I was about to shake this off any day. But my symptoms continued to ebb and flow with annoying repetition. The only thing to change was the unkempt view from my window. Order and pride quickly fled and already the fall season was upon us. Fall had long been my favorite. This year, watching maple leaves fall to the ground was a little harder to do because it signaled the end of *another* missed season and winter was now approaching.

When it snows in the northern mountains of New Hampshire there is no telling when it will stop; that year the snow came early. I needed to be outside plowing the driveway but, through no fault of my own, this was no longer an option.

As I watched the snow quicken, a local contractor pulled into the drive with a rusty yellow plow attached to the front of his truck. Holding his collar to the wind he quickly made his way to the back door. Apparently he had heard of my plight and offered to plow the drive in exchange for hot coffee. With every spare penny being counted this was certainly one less thing to worry about.

As things continued to go from bad to worse, the thought of Christmas coming filled me with dread. This was the first time I'd been unable to provide for my family and it was proving difficult to accept. A new question began to churn in my brain like a toxic worm—*What use am I if I can't even provide for my own family at Christmas?*

Leaving behind only silent footprints in the snow, someone stepped in and donated a large bag of Christmas presents along with the simple note that read "Merry Christmas." While this anonymous of act of kindness was appreciated, it was also deeply humbling. I was now finding a new awkwardness in accepting that which I had not worked for. The brick wall I was hitting took hold of my ridiculous male pride and began to shred it.

With a streak of stubborn independence still running through me, I *always* felt more at ease struggling than accepting offers of help.

I'd been standing on my own two feet from a very early age and now my claims that I'd never needed help from anyone became irrelevant background noise. Life was teaching me some pretty harsh lessons, and it became clear that my need for self-reliance had perhaps been mistaken for constant defiance. With illness still hitting me hard, I really wasn't in a position to argue.

As the rest of the festive world continued to turn with selfish repetition, the strain on my beautiful wife's face was becoming plain to see. Worry had replaced optimism and her once raven black hair now displayed streaks of pure grey. This wasn't an easy time for *either* of us and, at times, it showed more than we would have liked. The next morning, seeing her brown leather suitcase packed on the neatly made-up bed, made me wonder if things could get any worse.

I wasn't going to beg her to stay, for begging is not my prideful business; but I guess turning to say goodbye was simply too much emotion for one day. It was obvious we still cared about each other the way only families can.

Still visibly upset from an earlier argument, she wiped away a fresh tear and put the suitcase away. No matter what life was throwing at us, we were still inseparable best friends and, from this point forward, no matter how distressing this illness became, it was clear we were in this together.

As Christmas 2011 ended, it also brought with it a naïve glimmer of hope. A new year was looming and we both longed to put the current heinous one behind us. What we didn't know was that things were about to take a dramatic turn for the worse.

Chapter 3

DEATH BY A 1000 PAPER CUTS

January 2012 brought with it our sixth wedding anniversary. The past year hadn't been easy and the new one didn't appear to be getting any easier. We celebrated the day by visiting a neurologist from a neighboring hospital. Who says romance is dead?

The test being carried out today was to check the nerves in my legs. This was accomplished by sending an electric pulse down the nerve via a needle. With each turn of the dial, a pulse shot down my leg, causing it to twitch involuntarily. Something about seeing this bizarre reflex set my wife off; evidently she has a warped sense of humor and eventually needed to excuse herself from the room.

Now alone with the sadist in the white coat, I found myself nervously lying on the neurologist's bed in my underpants waiting for the next jolt. The neurologist gently put his hand on my shoulder and encouraged me to *just-relax.* This led me to believe at least one of us in the protocol was failing to grasp the fullness of the situation. Generally speaking, whenever a man carrying a clipboard electrocutes you, just *relaxing* doesn't come easy.

We cannot solve our problems with the same
thinking we used when we created them.
– Albert Einstein

Polite conversation soon turned to my home town. Apparently he knew of my primary doctor quite well and spoke of her fondly. Fifteen minutes later he declared that I could stop "relaxing" as the nerves in my leg had apparently passed the test. He then handed me a bill for $530 and sent me on my way. *Sheesh, thanks, doc.*
However helpful this irrelevant information may have been to the neurologist, it really wasn't that helpful to us. Maybe it was my growing frustration with the medical profession but, some days it felt as if the whole diagnostic progress had closed ranks for fear of being sued. That

left me in the unenviable position of trying to convey the message that I was a worker, *not* a shirker, and my only goal was to get myself back to work.

I'm actually a real person, so it began to seriously bother me that I was being viewed by some people as just another malingering sick guy shuffling from appointment to appointment. At my core I was still somebody's son, husband, brother, and dad. It registered that I had now been *seriously* ill for almost a year. For someone who rarely got sick this was proving a hard to accept.

Adding to the problem, the doctor who had inadvertently set me on this path was still unable to provide answers. While I waited, my previously robust immune system began acting like a fragile candle in the wind. *I'd never had an allergy before in my life!* Now suddenly watery eyes, sneezing, and itching all became a daily annoyance. My immune system had obviously been spooked, but nobody seemed willing to connect the dots.

Over the coming months, things quickly continued downhill. If I could get out of bed at all, it was often on my hands and knees. Using a metal walker for the first time made me realize how far my previously robust health had fallen. With so much going wrong in my body, I wondered whether (and how) anyone could possibly fix it.

Adding to my endless list of problems, I now found myself needing to use the bathroom every five minutes making rest impossible.

I really needed this symptom like a hole in the head. Being kept awake around the clock with frequent urination soon began to wear me down. The sheer stress of being forced to scramble urgently to the toilet all night long meant that any time I briefly fell asleep my teeth would constantly grind together.

While the whole town slept, I was awakened again and again by the urgent need to visit the bathroom. In the moments I fell asleep in between, my jaw began clamping down so hard that I'd seriously have to

36

put my fingers in my mouth just to try to ease the tension. It wasn't long before I had a cracked tooth and needed to see a dentist.

Back in the U.K. I had a great dentist. Simon was one of those people who just got on with the job without any drama. Our agreement had always been this: he fixed what needed fixing. I paid his bill and left. No fuss, no problem. But this was rural America and, just when I needed it the least, I had the misfortune to come across a dentist whose specialty was incompetence. Somehow he managed to turn a cracked tooth into a pulsating abscess. And, not content with that, the tooth he filled didn't fit right. *I know, right? Can I catch just one break?*

For a while, when you really don't have a choice, you learn to adapt. Rather than go back to the dentist, I took some sandpaper and began sanding down my own tooth. As crazy as it sounds, it worked. Sadly, I was having less luck with the urgent trips to the bathroom.

My latest coping strategy was to sleep a few minutes at a time. Sometimes I did this with my forehead on the toilet roll holder. At some point I went back to the doctor and begged for a solution. She ordered a series of urine tests. Go figure – *they all came back normal.*

With some degree of desperation, I went home and did my best to cope. Every night the same pattern repeated: normal people went to bed while I shuffled painfully from bedroom to bathroom, bathroom to bedroom using a walker. The longer I went without a full night's sleep; the harder life became. When you live on the fringe for long enough, it's isn't long before hopelessness overtakes you. Then it's only a matter of time before *something* has to give.

When I was a kid, my dad once took me to visit an underground cave. Deep inside, Dad stopped and turned his flashlight to a constant drip above our heads. Then he shone the light on the floor and showed me a small hole in the stone.

At the time this meant little to me other than I got to put my whole finger in a cool hole, but to Dad it was an opportunity to illustrate that even a small but constant drip could wear away even something as solid as stone.

As a tsunami of symptoms now raged, I was beginning to understand *exactly* how that stone must have felt. For now, lack of sleep, along with my newly pulsating tooth abscess, conspired against my every positive thought. Each night I'd walk the darkest corridors of my mind and this was rapidly becoming a regular and unsustainable occurrence.

As I sat helplessly counting what seemed like an insurmountable list of ailments, it surely felt like the beginning of a slow death from a thousand paper cuts.

As a previously active person, I was horrified at the thought of losing what was left of my independence. It's a little unnerving when you live with good health for most of your life and then suddenly your legs become strangely tight for more than a year. It was incomprehensible to think of one day being trapped in a wheelchair, but by that time it was no longer a question of if, but rather when.

SICK-NOTE

It was around this time that the doctor, whose advice I had first taken on that fateful day at 10:30 am on February 16th 2011, sent a letter to my house. It started by stating that she was leaving to take up another job in a different practice. At some point she used the phrase, "It is with a heavy heart that I am leaving."

It crossed my mind that holding onto furniture as I walked across a room was good reason for a heavy heart. Watching my wife struggle to pay for groceries was good reason for a heavy heart. Hearing concern stretch across the Atlantic in my mum's voice was reason for a heavy heart. But skipping town for a better paid fucking job? *No, that* was *not* good reason for a heavy heart. And, given my situation, maybe even a tad insensitive!

Make no mistake – I was now being slammed hard against a brick wall of ill health. Around the clock I faced debilitating fatigue, tightness in my muscles, weak arms, irritability, weak legs, confusion, painful eyes, heart palpitations, hot sweats, cold sweats, new food sensitivities, twitching muscles, new seasonal allergies, jaw clenching, and sleep deprivation with ongoing horrific nightmares – all matched by an equally worrisome fresh crop of fatty lipomas that had suddenly begun to spring up. Oh, and let's not forget that pulsating tooth abscess. And just for good measure, excessively frequent trips to the bathroom.

I'm guessing that last paragraph took you less than a minute to read so to help you better understand this next part, try this: when you go to bed tonight, set your alarm to go off at midnight. When it does, hit the snooze button every 10 minutes for the next six weeks. If, at any point, you sleep through the alarm, start the whole process over again to ensure that you get no more than ten minutes sleep per night for the next month or so.

Okay, I really don't want you to go through that. *Allow me save you the trouble.*

It really isn't very long before this routine, which had become my existence for months and months, became *overwhelming*. Sooner or later even the most persistent people will hit a breaking point.

UNSUSTAINABLE

I'll be the first to admit, in this life I've made my fair share of mistakes, none of which I'm particularly proud of. As a troubled teen I often ran with the wrong crowd. I got married at 19 and there are no prizes for guessing how that worked out. But for the past 10+ years as my environment changed, so did my values.

So while I don't ever pretend to be perfect, I'd like to point out that during my entire second attempt at marriage, I'd remained faithful and honest to my wife. This has always been the glue that holds us together as a family. Like most people, we have our ups and downs, but she had skillfully and successfully turned me into a dedicated family man and *that* is now the quality that defines me, which is why this next part isn't quite so easy to write.

It's very easy to judge someone from the sidelines, but the day our *every* thought becomes tainted by illness, the feeling of letting everyone down quickly becomes relentless. Sooner or later the stress of prolonged fatigue will come to an *unsustainable* breaking point. I know what you are thinking because I thought it too: if this is no longer sustainable then how can it be stopped?

As problems go, this one caused me *considerable* anguish. As the night air cooled, it eventually gained a mathematical probability. Determined to spare someone the inconvenience of cleaning up my mess, I found myself outside, kneeling before God with an open heart and a loaded gun; a sure sign that a previously robust man was now on the edge.

Trembling like a pathetic wet dog, the fear of the unknown finally gave way to a sweaty but insistent right hand. As if it even mattered, I glanced at my watch and, at 4:22 a.m., I lost all hope. Without further distraction a cold metallic snap went off next to the right side of my head – which then echoed away endlessly into the blackness of the night.

The deafening silence that followed was interrupted by a pounding heart fueled by a steady supply of fresh adrenaline. If nothing else was going right for me then at least math appeared to be on my side. Eventually, my two bleary eyes dared to open, which gave me the presence of mind to accept that I still belonged to this world, albeit as a dead man walking. I have to tell you that, when you reach this point, the only question to cross your deeply tormented mind is this: *why am I being forced to endure this nightmare?* Either way, enduring it seemed like the better choice. And in that moment, that's what I was determined to do.

By then, the doctor who had inadvertently lit the fuse to my health problems had moved on with her heavy heart to a better paying job. So I met with several new "specialists" to review my medical records. Two of them were really nice and one was actually quite arrogant. Not one completely understood the complexity of what was happening to me.

Symptoms were screaming out to be heard but nobody was listening. Suppressing symptoms is what doctors do best so I was offered drugs to pacify me. But I wasn't looking for easy painkillers to mask over symptoms; I wanted a *solution*. To me, at least, this type of thinking is no different from a fireman climbing into a burning house only to cut the wire to the smoke detector. The twisted logic of *no alarm = no problem*, tends to work best when it's not your house that's burning.

During each and every visit to the doctors, my wife stood firmly by my side and, with great dignity, we thanked each doctor for their time. She would then help me up out of my seat and through the door. The day my wife took the initiative and brought home a used wheelchair from a charity shop was one of the lowest moments of my life. Even now, as I write this several years later, that day still makes me choke up.

I remember being annoyed that she had even brought it to the house. Stubbornness told me I didn't need it, but the truth was that I'd probably needed it some time ago. I was afraid that if my wife saw me sitting in it she might begin to see only the chair. It also crossed my mind that once I sat down I might never get up again. To be clear, I hadn't lost the use of my legs, it had just reached the point where using them was too slow and too painful.

Reluctantly I handed over my walker and took my first seat in this damned ugly looking metal contraption. I felt humiliated, as if I had given up. Turning my face to hide the frustration, I was determined *not* to let even the smallest tear roll down my face, but they did anyway. Admitting defeat wasn't something I took lightly but by now my self-worth had begun to drip out from under me.

It's not until you sit in a wheelchair that you begin to see the world from a very difficult perspective - literally. It might not look it, but getting a wheelchair to move is cumbersome and hard work on the arms, especially when you don't feel well to begin with. It's also not easy to feel like a man when you are frequently having conversations with everyone else's navel.

Sometimes it's all just too much. I might have complained about the chair a wee bit much because a week later my mother in-law drove 223 miles from Massachusetts to deliver an electric wheelchair direct to my door. Like her, it had a few miles on it, but I'm guessing it still must have cost her a small fortune.

Having power wheels enabled me to get outside with a certain level of mobility. A few hours later, that battery and I were both exhausted and my new toy was placed temporarily on hold for recharging.

And there I was, slouched deep in an electric wheelchair and needing a moment to be alone. I was now *fully* aware that, when the medical profession screws up, lasting solutions are elusive. The irony is, on that February 16th 2011, the procedure I got myself roped into was described as being both *safe and effective* with zero mention of a downside.

Mainstream medicine, with all its money and power, had failed me. I was now just another little guy slipping through the medical cracks without a diagnosis or cure. Even science with its pristine reputation for accuracy was sulking in the corner, still wondering if Pluto was a planet or not.

Hanging on for someone else to figure out my health problems had been the plan for two long years and for too long. The problem was now becoming bigger than both of us. Unless we did something, *anything*, to fight from our corner, my cause would soon be lost.

NEW DOCTORS

Meeting with new doctors can be frustrating in the best of times. There are times when that new doctor can be a little more human than we like, especially when faced with a problem (that's you) that won't go away or doesn't fit into any typical example or pattern.

If we *aren't* careful the onus of blame can conveniently be shifted onto the patient. This ensures that, at the end of each shift, messy problems fit into neat little boxes. *Do you see what's going on here?*

When a doctor doesn't have the time, experience, or persistence to figure out your complex health problem, sooner or later conceit takes precedence over their desire to understand, as well as over their understanding. The doctor is basically saying "Hey, I don't actually

42

understand your complicated symptoms but I'm paid to be smart, so it can't possibly be me. So, for now, let's say that you are the problem!"

This repulsively flawed logic only serves to protect the ego of an ignorant person who lacks facts. The sheer arrogance of any doctor to make this distasteful suggestion was sure to be the last.

I wasn't to blame! I had done everything asked of me. Back in 2011, I was blissfully minding my own business. It *hadn't* been my brilliant idea to provoke my immune system into a total meltdown.

I'd since turned up for every appointment and sat quietly and respectfully while being prodded and poked. I'd be damned if I was now going to allow someone to add insult to my injury. I hadn't bought this on myself in any way shape or form. *Enough of this horseshit. I was done!*

Whatever it took, **whatever** I had to sacrifice, **whatever** I had to learn, I was determined to do it or drop dead trying. My dad used to say, *"A determined man will always find a way; a lesser man will find an excuse."* I was done having my destiny be controlled by the ignorance of others. I certainly wasn't going to sit back and subject myself to more of this nonsense. Now I was ready to roll up my sleeves and fight my own corner and boy did I have a point to make!

> *Survival was my only hope, success my only revenge.*
> – Patricia Cornwell.

When the human spirit hits the right motivational spot it has an uncanny ability to triumph over adversity. History books are full of people whose inner determination refuses to be told something can't be done. Remember those two bicycle repairmen who once asked the question, "If a bird can fly, why can't man?" Aviation, as we know it today, came as a direct result of the Wright brothers' persistence. But I wasn't looking to fly; I only needed to walk.

For sure, the road ahead of me looked uncertain but I held one distinct advantage over every expert that had thus far failed me. That advantage was my *unbending persistence*. When doctors went home at night I was no longer a priority. Rather than sit around waiting I was going to make *myself* my own top priority.

I'm a firm believer that *all problems* have solutions and I was now being challenged to find mine for myself. Let's take stock of what I had going for me, (a) I had a point to prove, (b) I'm persistent, (c) I was still of this world and (d) I had a family to feed. *For most people that will do it.* I was still being kept awake around the clock and by now I had gotten used to it, so I began using that time productively. Every night while my family and the town slept, I began the slow and laborious process of trying to figure out what had gone so terribly wrong with my health.

I can assure you that learning highly complex medical problems from the ground up, while dealing with an ongoing illness, financial hardship, sleep deprivation, and the demands of a family, was no easy task, but today I walk unaided and sleep through the night. My mind is at peace and I have energy to be able to work on demand. Yes, a few stubborn quirks remain but 95% of my original symptoms are now *under my control*. Given the severity of my earlier condition, I regard this as a remarkable success. *Here's how I did it.*

Chapter 4

CRACKPOTS AND CATS

When faced with a long list of complicated problems, knowing where to begin becomes key. Sadly, this pivotal piece of information eluded me and several years of failure followed. But giving up wasn't something I do readily or particularly well.

My wife has often referred to me as being the most persistent man she has ever met; to me each defeat became a new learning experience. This gave me a *defining* and favorable edge over most of my doctors who – I was quick to notice – all went home at 5 p.m. My persistence had no such limitation.

The fact that I had already survived through so much gave me renewed resolve. If I had to work until I dropped to find my answers, then so be it. *Clearly there was only going to be one eventual outcome; how long it would take to get there was a different matter.*

I also knew my *own* body better than anyone else, and I'm guessing you know yours too. When our health becomes adversely affected 24 hours a day it gives us ample opportunity to get to know our symptoms. If anything, it helps to have a little more skin in the game.

Maybe you can't see it yet, but if you are enduring a difficult time at your *own* brick-wall, I urge you not to give up. If I can have dragged myself out of the hellhole I was in, then there is **hope**. And all the tools I've picked up along the way are right here in this book.

There is always a formula for getting from point A to point B. Here's mine: don't be too quick to dismiss the internet as a valueless entity full of crackpots and cats. Every single day people learn new skills simply by tapping into this free global communication network. Everything from how to build a boat to how to bake a cake is there in the public domain.

*If you can read, you can learn everything that anyone ever learned,
but you've got to want it.* – Ricky Gervais

A realization hit me that schools and doctors were no longer the *ultimate*
gatekeepers of all knowledge. At my fingertips I suddenly had access to a
colossal library holding endless amounts of medical information.

So far, every logical thought that my own doctors applied had hit a glass
ceiling, but computers work best by exchanging and connecting *unlimited*
free information, so there isn't any glass ceiling to hit and there is no five
o'clock quitting time, either.

I soon found *vast* amounts of knowledge and experiences shared by
academics, physicians, and professors right there on my desktop – for
free. For anyone with a burning desire to learn, Dr. Google is a tool of
infinite possibilities. The biggest problem I faced wasn't a lack of
information *but how to sort through it all and filter out what wasn't useful
or valid!*

Day after day I read just about any medical article I could get my hands
on. I read until my eyes hurt and then I'd switch to listening to audio clips.
I'd often fall asleep with my headset still on. Happily for you, this book will
spare you many years of the trial and error I put myself through.

For anyone with a persistent nature, having access to information and
sources 24/7, and being able to view them indefinitely becomes an
incredibly helpful tool. If I misunderstood any part of a subject, I could
simply go back and find a video lecture on it and then play the same loop
over and over and over and over until something eventually clicked.

Then I discovered TedTalks.com, which gave me a way to tap into some of
the brightest minds from around the world. At night I'd watch hours of
medical YouTube clips. Every time, I'd come away having learned
something new but, with so much information to wade through, I was
frequently left with more questions than answers.

For sure I had an absolute mountain to climb; I was facing the same problem that smarter people had failed to identify but, with no alternatives to fall back on, what choice did I have but to keep learning? Rather than let it consume me, I devised a plan to **refine** my search. I figured if someone held a PhD, obviously they had to have a certain level of credibility. *This was my new benchmark and these were the minds I would seek first.*

I became completely submerged in the task ahead of me, losing all track of time. Birthdays came and went, as did the 4th of July, Christmas, and the Super Bowl. Days, nights, weekends and cookouts all passed me by as I sucked information from anybody that had it.

Several years passed and people around me noticed that my social skills were becoming increasingly awkward. I was no longer able to hold a conversation without its somehow relating back to the topic of healing. Everything else became a distraction. Finding the answer wasn't just something I needed to do; *it had become an insatiable passion.*

You need a lot of passion for what you're doing because it's so hard.
Without passion, any rational person would give up."
– Steve Jobs.

My appetite for medical knowledge knew no bounds. I'd read while sitting in the bathtub and I'd read on every car ride as my wife drove along, talking to herself. I'd even wake in the middle of the night and begin reading. It's funny how we dislike being taught and yet, when something is important to us, we have an unquenchable thirst to learn.

Finding answers was on my mind the first thing in the morning, the last thing at night, and just about every moment in between. It wasn't uncommon for me to be fact-checking long before my wife woke up and long after she had gone to bed. Yet, despite all these efforts, so much of my own puzzle remained elusive.

THE COLLECTIVE POOL

With no one paying for my *web-ucation* my *only* goal was to press on and find something that worked. In a bid to find the missing pieces, I began to question *everything* by cross-referencing what I had already learned. In doing so, a rich vein of fresh thinking opened up that, until then, hadn't even been on my radar.

I began finding larger clumps of the puzzle from the most unusual places. There were other people who were also suffering and keen to share *their* experiences. And many were farther along the path and willing to share what they had learned. Health forums are full of regular people just like you and me. Some are there enjoying being able to give back to the collective pool, others are there searching for answers.

Health forums are *not* to be used as a standalone tool but rather as a way of tapping into people with similar problems, and then *splicing* two sets of information together. On the one hand I was becoming well read from PhDs with great expertise, and on the other hand I now had access to people with valuable *firsthand* experience. Piece by piece I was beginning to get a grasp of the scope of the problem.

The task ahead remained both tantalizing and daunting, but for the first time I felt there was light at the end of a hideously dark tunnel. I began putting the small things I had learned into practice and this allowed me to take one tiny micro step forward at a time. As with so many other persistent people before me, my progress was often sidelined by a spectacular, but short-lived, failure. But as time went on, my thousands of hours of intense research began to pay off. Whereas I had for so long felt frustrated by my lack of progress, now my quest no longer felt hopeless, and the smallest victories empowered me.

As I applied the techniques I was learning, I began to enjoy a slow but steady improvement in my overall symptoms. I was now moving around on a cane and doing so with a huge smile on my face because I was having success where my doctors had not.

So how does a layperson find his or her way out of a medical maze when fully trained doctors remain clueless? That same word keeps coming back: **persistence.** Had this trait not been instilled in me from a very early age I wouldn't be writing this. My dad had always admired this characteristic more than any other. He often said things like, *"People are free to mock the man that tries, but they should never underestimate him."*
Today, as I write with enthusiasm, I have seen a 95% improvement in my original symptoms and this has been accomplished without taking *any* medications. Zero. Am I totally free of all symptoms? No, but the majority of my symptoms are reduced to the point where they no longer control me: *I control them.*

I am extremely thankful for my hard-fought gains and hope this book will save you the kind of frustration I had to go through. In 2011, had I known what I know now, *the devastating decline in my health could have been averted altogether* or at least my recovery would have happened much sooner.

This process has left me with tremendous compassion for anyone who is frustrated by illness, and a strong sense of obligation to share what I have learned. Up until this point writing about my past hasn't been easy but, with the stage now set, my writing shackles can finally come off!

My challenge now is to take these fundamental concepts and convey them with genuine empathy *without* their sounding like mundane, medical mantra. Over the course of the coming chapters I'll set out to explain the many things I did to improve my health.
This is what excites me.

I see this as my *bonus* life. If it had to end tomorrow, I would accept that, but today I am obligated to share the things I have learned in the hope that they will one day help you too.

Come, we have much work to do.

Chapter 5

YOU DON'T HAVE AN ILLNESS, YOU HAVE A LABEL

In its most basic form, every *living* thing on this planet is made up of cells, from plants to animals, from trees to humans, wherever there is life there are cells. Just as a house is made of thousands of bricks, trillions of tiny cells make up your eyes, lungs, brain, fingers, nose, toes, and just about every other bit of yourself you can think of. Nerves, blood, muscle, tissue, and even bones are all completely composed of cells.

When looked at under a microscope, you and I are little more than a mass of cells tightly wrapped in a living *breathing* layer of skin. Essentially, cells are the building blocks of *all* life and the smallest living unit that can replicate independently.

What's the relevance of knowing that we are fundamentally made up of trillions of microscopic cells? *Think about it ...* if we are to accurately manage what ails us, our first goal must be to break down what is complex into something *manageable*. Looking at a problem in its most basic form (the cell) allows us to quickly develop a fresh perspective of what an illness really means to us.

Lord knows illness can be complicated enough, and to some, what you are about to read may seem like an *over* simplification, but try to keep in mind this is just the base on which we will soon build as each chapter unfolds.

> *If you can't explain it simply,*
> *you don't understand it well enough.*
> – Albert Einstein.

As you read this paragraph, your old worn out cells are being replaced. This turnover forms an essential cycle of life. We can think of this process as similar to deleting unwanted photos from our cell phone; once that space is freed up, the overall system works better. Keep reading, there is a point to all of this that is about to become clear.

To make way for healthy new cells the body makes a judgment call to either keep, kill, or recycle damaged cells. When cells are recycled, the body eats them, a process known as autophagy which stems from the Greek word, "self-devouring."

When a cell is deemed damaged beyond repair it's encouraged to commit suicide, a process often referred to as apoptosis. Under *normal* circumstances cells do this in a tightly regulated fashion. When old cells "forget" to commit suicide, problems begin.

If we assume that a healthy organ is made up of mostly healthy cells, we can also assume an *un*healthy organ must have a quantity of *un*healthy cells. What we are doing here is breaking the problem down to its most basic form. Illness is reflected in the structure of our cells and this is true for just about any illness from A to Z.

Cancer is the most *obvious* example of an overzealous set of cells malfunctioning beyond the body's ability to regulate them. A diagnosis of cancer can be alarming enough, but if we look a little closer at the problem, the bigger issue is *always* being played out at the cellular level. The term *cellular* is simply a word relating to the cells. **The more health issues you have, the more relevant simplification becomes.**

Let's look at it another way: a basic four-digit PIN is all we need to provide financial peace of mind. Our money remains securely locked in the ATM because the number of possible number combinations that would have to be tried to hack into it is just too great. *Now imagine trying to unlock a health problem that could have any one or several of hundreds of possible causes!*

Worse, is the strong likelihood that the causes of illness may overlap, making the total number of possible causes truly daunting. This overlapping of symptoms makes the diagnostic process all the more difficult to navigate. This was something I was forced to deal with during my own recovery.

By breaking down the problem to the cellular level, we can see it from a totally different perspective. In every organ of the body we either have a collection of healthy cells or not so healthy cells. When it is the latter, we call it illness.

It could be argued that in the case of something like glaucoma, cells are *not* the root cause of the problem. Intraocular pressure on the optic nerve, which goes on to damage to the eye, is the problem. But while it is true that fluid pressure is responsible for causing the optic nerve to degenerate, cells always remain the basic structure of a healthy optic nerve. We could *endlessly* debate such diagnostic variables and in the process remain *firmly* rooted in disease. **The bottom line is this, in its most basic form the body is tied to its cells, and so too is illness.** The importance of this will become clearer as we move forward.

I know what you are thinking because I thought it too: *even if illness is nothing more than a set of wacky malfunctioning cells, how does this help me?* First let's replace the **how** question with a **why** *question.* When we ask the **why** question we are forced to dig below the surface for answers.

WHY?

Asking WHY our cells have turned sickly on us is a smart question to ask and the answer is relatively straightforward. For a cell to form or rebuild it requires key nutrients. It rarely bodes well for a cell to be made up of toxic elements.
When new cells build, they take from whatever nutrients the body has at its disposal. A nutrient can be thought of as any substance that provides nourishment essential for the maintenance of life and growth. *The quality of these new cells greatly depends on the quality of the raw materials fueling the body.* Think of a carpenter trying to build beautiful furniture with rotten wood.

Quality nutrients are needed to build quality cells. These nutrients come to us in the foods we eat; this is the fuel the body runs on, whether it is junk food or *super* food. Here we see the birth pangs of problem cells. A *lack* of key nutrients flowing *into* the cell will affect the cell's overall quality and optimal integrity.

TOXIC

With quality nutrients, cell walls remain permeable, allowing the exchange of oxygen carrying nutrients to come in, and the free flow of toxins out. Anything of a toxic nature adversely obstructs this rebuilding process.

When any part of our body becomes ill, either something is missing in our healthy cells or it has been replaced by something toxic. In short we are trying to build a house with substandard bricks and rotten wood.

I'm using the word "toxic" here in its broadest possible sense. Indiscriminately, it could be used to describe any pathogen or foreign matter that has the potential to penetrate your cells and make you ill, be it a virus, fungus, bacteria, pesticide, drug, heavy metal, chemical, liquid, gas fumes, contaminated food etc.

The list of *potential* (known) toxic substances is impossibly long. We will, of course, be looking at many of these toxins in more detail *along with effective ways to remove them from the body.* For the sake of simplicity, we can also think of the word toxic as *any* substance poisonous to the body.

The body (that's you) is aptly designed to filter out such toxic substances and it does so in a highly efficient fashion. Problems arise when more toxins than the body is capable of removing flood *into* the body. Unfortunately, humans, in our pursuit of progress, have become highly destructive creatures, gleefully contaminating the world we live in and, along with it, ourselves.

Sadly, it has become impossible to avoid dangerous levels of toxicity, *hence, awareness becomes all the more important!* As a rule of thumb, if you have a pulse then you have some degree of toxic exposure. To take this a step further, we could say that anything you come in contact with that's manmade almost certainly has a toxic element to it.

The body relies heavily on the functioning of the liver, kidneys, lungs, and skin to filter out these harmful toxins. In fact, *our entire health hinges on the ability of these organs to cope.* Once these vital organs begin working overtime, it's easy for the whole system to become overrun. A tipping point usually occurs when the prolonged demand remains too great for the body.

> *It doesn't matter what your doctor calls it,*
> *it ALWAYS involves toxicity.* – Dr. Sherry Rogers

Imagine a bucket of water catching water drips from a ceiling, only this bucket has a small hole in its side. As each new drip lands in the bucket another oozes out from that hole in the side. As long as the drips coming in match the drips going out, the bucket doesn't fill up. One drop in, one drop out maintains a steady level.

In this analogy, think of the drips coming into the bucket as your daily exposure to toxins, and the hole on the side of the bucket as your detoxification organs working to keep the bucket from filling up.

If the drip coming from the ceiling begins to speed up and outpace the rate at which water leaks out through the hole, the water level in the bucket will rise. When the water level reaches the rim of the bucket is when we find ourselves at the edge of illness, or at the "tipping point." And when the water spills over the sides of the bucket, it's a sign that your body can no longer cope with the demand being put on it. Life is good when we prevent toxins from building up to the point where they overtake our detoxification capabilities.

The good news is that by the end of this book you will have a clear plan for how to reduce your exposure to toxicity *and* how to get clean nutrients into your cells. Once the cells get fired up, *good things happen!*

Common sense suggests that our first goal must be to reduce the number of *new* toxins coming into the body. *At least until the gravity of the situation is assessed.* There is no point in bringing nourishment to a toxic cell. That would be like putting a fresh bandage on an open cut before washing all the dirt off your finger.

If repetition is the mother of all learning, let's remember that new cells are constantly replacing old, worn out cells. These new cells are made from the raw materials that *we* provide from the things we ingest, whether those are carrots, cucumbers, or fizzy colas. A cell with a toxic element to it is not a healthy cell and illness ensues.

LABELS

Having any illness can make it seem as if our world is coming to an end. Going into a hospital can be a daunting experience, and trying to make sense of it all can drive a person to despair. As a patient, you will typically deal with an organization well versed in terminology unfamiliar to you. Enduring any long term medical problem *with* a firm diagnosis can be terribly frustrating. Not having a diagnosis is even worse.

Once we become ill, the first thing a physician wants to do is give the illness a name. A diagnosis is simply a descriptive term relating to a *specific* part of the body – that's all. No matter what ails you, I'd like to suggest that you really *don't* have an illness, **what you do have is a label,** which has been *handed* to you in relation to something that's going awry at the cellular level.

A complicated diagnosis can leave a patient feeling helpless. A synchronous diaphragmatic flutter for example certainly has a serious ring to it, but most of us know it as a hiccup. And that transient lingual papillitis? That's nothing more than a bump on the tongue. *I know right? Who talks this way?*

This type of terminology can soon become overwhelming, especially if you aren't feeling well to begin with. The next time a doctor provides you with a complicated diagnosis you could try saying to yourself, *"Nope, what I have now is a label."*

Looking at a diagnosis this way helps to *charm* the mystery out of complex medical terms. Osteoporosis, as I'm sure many will already know, is the label given to reflect the condition of certain bones, but again keep in mind that even bone is made up of cells. We could just as accurately say that something is going wrong with the cells that make up the bones.

By taking the complex and breaking it down into workable parts we begin to unravel a tangled web of symptoms. An autoimmune condition affecting the cartilage of the joints carries an arthritis label, but once again we know that *all* cartilage is made of cells. A cancer found in the blood carries the leukemia label, but *again* blood is made up of cells.

Each and every part of the body has its own label, but regardless of the label being applied, *something untoward is happening at the cellular level.*

The suggestion that cells play such a pivotal role in our health might be a different way of thinking to the current mainstream understanding of illness, but that tide may be turning. In 2016, the Nobel Prize for medicine was awarded to Yoshinori Ohsumi of Japan for his work on none other than **cells.**

Ohsumi's discoveries are directly related to the importance of how cells recycle their content, how they break down proteins and non-essential components for energy and destroy invading organisms. I guess another way of saying it is that cells are working out whether to keep, kill, or recycle themselves.

As each new chapter unfolds we will first look to *reducing* the amount of new toxins coming in, and then find ways to remove older toxins that may have built up in the body over time. Getting the *toxins out and allowing the nutrients to flood in is the* essence of reclaiming good health.

TED

To help you get the most of this book I've assembled a collection of influential but *short* video clips that can be found at the end of certain chapters. Think of this book as interactive.

The first video clip is an important one and can be found in today's homework assignment. It's a TEDx Talk given by a British doctor who makes a bold claim that he can make diseases disappear. That's quite a remarkable claim, but in this short video he actually proves it! *You will find many of the principles in this inspirational video mirrored throughout this book.*

What did we learn from this chapter?

A diagnosis is nothing more than a label and it shouldn't define who we are. Complicated problems remain complicated unless we break them down into *manageable* parts.

Daily contact with a known variety of heavy metals, chemicals, viruses, fungi, bacteria, and pesticides is not only a given in today's world, it is commonplace. A smart first step in the right direction is to first *reduce* the amount of daily toxins we absorb in order to help lift the overall burden from the body.

Having a tipping point can at times also be a positive thing. Illness has a unique way of focusing us on habits we need to change and motivating us to do so. Once we become *sick of being sick* we become more open to new ideas.

Cells can be found throughout our whole body, *what you feed them is up to you!*

Homework: I'd like to invite you to watch a short TED Talk by Dr. Rangan Chatterjee. If this is a paperback version, a simple Google search will take you there. For my online homies, simply click on the link below.

"How to make diseases disappear?" by Dr. Rangan Chatterjee.

Chapter 6

BEHOLD, HOUSEHOLD TOXINS

In all forms of illness something close to you is either making you sick or keeping you sick. The purpose of this chapter is to help you find out what that is. We do this by eliminating as many potential problems as possible. Once we have this important step out of the way we can begin moving forward at speed.

Before setting out to tackle a problem we must first have a basic understanding of **what** the problem is and **where** it comes from.

Keep in mind that toxins coming into our cells can be insidious; they drip, drip, drip all around us in such a subtle way that all too often we are simply not aware of them. Maybe you are reacting to something in your home, the food you eat, or even those medications or supplements you take.

This is a process of elimination, so let's start with the most obvious first.

If you are currently taking any kind of medications stop what you are doing (even reading this!) and immediately check the insert to see if your symptoms match any of the known side effects. This is an important step, which is why it's placed so early in this chapter. Know that *any* medication can cause a reaction. (This is a topic we will explore in more detail later.) If you hit a match, bingo! Talk to your doctor to replace or reduce the dose.

Now that *that's* out of the way, we have a lot of ground to cover so let's push through together. Before we know it, we could begin to see some tangible progress being made. So here we go.
You would think every product that finds its way to the supermarket shelf would be rigorously checked for toxic ingredients. Unfortunately, you would be wrong. Many household items do indeed have a deadly toxic element to them. I hate to be the one to break it to you, but we live in a fallen world; expecting any corporation to police its own income stream is at best a naïve and at worst outright foolish. Any substance that has a

toxic element to it has the *potential* to build up in the body. Sometimes this build-up happens quickly; sometimes it will happen over time. Until we make ourselves more aware of these toxic products they will continue slipping past us with ease.

Without a basic understanding of our toxic exposure, the pieces of the puzzle will *always* remain elusive. Imagine a healthy, colorful goldfish swimming around in a glass bowl full of pristine clear water. In an ideal world, this is how our environment should feel.

Now picture the same goldfish trapped in a plastic bowl full of unfiltered, dirty water and forced to use its delicate gills to breathe in the murky water. This is representative of the world we have made for ourselves, but instead of gills we humans **use our skin to breathe**.

You may not have thought about it before, but your skin is alive and intelligent; it's also the body's *largest* organ. This protective layer is so vitally important that it's considered to be the body's third kidney! As one of the body's main detoxification organs, it needs your help. Here's why.

Skin is super absorbent. Whatever we put onto the skin goes *into* the skin which in turn gets dumped into the bloodstream. Oils, cosmetics, bug sprays, creams, perfumes, deodorants, and underarm antiperspirants can be particularly problematic, *especially if you aren't well to begin with.* No one forces us to use them, yet as sure as night follows day we continue to add them to our toxic burden, drip, drip, drip. If our goal is to stay away from illness then we should begin by making the life of our living, breathing skin easier.

Still not convinced?

Okay, try this. Every day for the next week try spraying perfume or bug spray on a delicate living houseplant and watch as the leaves begin to curl up and die. Our skin is absorbent in the exact same way.

To add to the problem, we then restrict the body's ability to regulate itself by wrapping it in layers of manmade fibers. Go ahead; take a look to see if

60

the shirt you are wearing right now has the potential to stifle the *largest* most sophisticated organ in your body. Below are some common fibers that are known to affect the skin:

Polyester is made from synthetic polymers that come from esters of dihydric alcohol and terpthalic acid. If you are trying to let your skin breathe, polyester is perhaps one of the worst fabrics you can wear.

Teflon is increasingly being added to clothing because it makes it wrinkle-free. Most clothing labeled "no-iron" contains carcinogenic PFCs, but don't take my word for it. Even the U.S. Environmental Protection Agency (EPA) recently announced that PFCs are cancer-causing compounds.

Acrylic fabrics are polycrylonitriles which, according to the EPA, have known carcinogenic qualities.

Rayon is treated with chemicals like caustic soda, ammonia, acetone, and sulphuric acid – all are believed to survive regular washing.

Nylon is made from petroleum and is often given a *permanent* chemical finish that can be harmful to delicate skin. Many stain resistant and wrinkle-free fabrics are treated with perfluorinated chemicals (PFCs), like Teflon.

Throughout this book the idea is to first bring awareness and then offer a viable solution, so what's the alternative to manmade fibers?

Long before these manmade materials came along we all used natural fibers like cotton, hemp, or wool. These products remain easy to find and make a good replacement. Natural fibers allow the body to cool *without* leaching toxic chemicals onto the skin.

*Tip - Whenever you catch yourself reading what Kim Kardashian is wearing you might want to spend an equal amount of time googling what **you** are wearing... just sayin'.*

Keep in mind that we also spend a third of our life in bed so be sure to use cotton bed sheets rather than polyester. Will doing this one thing change your health? Perhaps not, however, the rest of this chapter is loaded with other small changes and when they are tightly grouped together, yes, collectively they *do* have the potential to compound and become quite significant, especially if you aren't feeling well to begin with.

I might as well get this out in the open: the rest of this book requires some degree of effort on your part. Think of this effort as the currency of wellness. As we now move forward it might be helpful to grab a pen and paper to make side notes. The good news is that each of the following recommendations in this chapter is easy to implement. In most cases finding a solution is relatively inexpensive, the much bigger problem is remaining blissfully *unaware*. Once we have these bad boys checked off our list we will begin looking into a wide range of interesting topics. For now, let's stick with a few basics and work our way up.

A good place to find toxins in any home is the kitchen. Anti-bacterial hand soap sounds good in theory *but it should be the very first thing you throw out*. Antibacterial soaps contain agents such as triclosan and triclocarban. The dangers of these two agents are many and well documented. They are *proven* endocrine disrupters and should have been banned years ago as they *are now* doing in the U.S. Replace your antibacterial soap with a regular bar of soap like the one Grandma used to use, but even then check the ingredients. The least toxic brands are usually found in your local health food store.

WATER QUALITY

Water is water right? *Wrong*. The quality of your drinking water can vary dramatically. Whatever else you have to save on, **don't** allow the water you drink be a compromise. The human body (*that's you again*) is made up of approximately 65% water, even more in infants. *That's a pretty big deal,* especially if you are relying on someone else to do this step for you such as a municipal company.

If we know that water flows through more than half of the human body, then the quality of the water coming into your home is pretty important, right? Soft drinks and beer don't count as water, *but hey – nice try.*

Bottled water is an improvement over soda for sure, but it really isn't the *best* solution. You need *quality* water **and so do your cells.** Plastic bottles can leach Bisphenol-A (BPA) into the water you drink. BPA is a synthetic estrogen that can mess up your hormones and has even been linked to some cancers. It takes energy to make plastic, usually in the form of oil. At some point, when there is no clean water left to drink we will be forced to understand we can't drink oil. *But I digress (often).*

Despite the picture of a pristine mountain river on the label of the water bottle, some water brands are simply filtered water, which begs the question: why not cut out the middleman and invest in a good quality water filter for your house? If your house **doesn't** have a water filter, then your kidneys become that filter! *I know, right? Kidneys are delicate organs and we should be protective of them.*

Not all water filters are the same; some will filter out more contaminants than others, just as some cost more than others. Depending on your situation an element of diligence will serve you well when choosing a new water filter. But ANY filter is better than no filter!

There are lots of filters on the market and you need to find one that fits your budget *today* rather than waiting until tomorrow or next week. You can always upgrade later. Berkey manufactures a range of decent clean water filtration systems, they are quality built, simple in design, and *effective* at what they do.

Being on the *quality* end of the spectrum these filters aren't the cheapest on the market but, over time, the cost of buying a good filter is offset by not having to buy plastic water bottles. I'm not endorsing any product here and you can buy whatever product you like so long as it works for you.

There are lots of types of water filters out there, but you tend to get what you pay for. Reverse osmosis filters have become popular because they remove a whole range of impurities. While there are benefits to this kind of system, be aware that this type of filter typically employs a series of filters so you may need to restructure and re-mineralize the water. You can sometimes do this by adding minerals back into the water and allowing a jug of filtered water to sit in the fridge overnight. Sometimes this can be done *automatically* during the filtration process. We will talk more about water later. A Google search will yield lots of information about how to replace minerals that have been filtered out.

Whichever filter system you choose, be sure to look at it objectively. If a filter is doing its job correctly then it's going to need replacing at some point, be sure to stay on top of this by writing the date of installation directly on the filter.

Yes, this all takes effort but clean water is critical to your and your family's the health. Come on now, this is important, let's **not** pretend you didn't hear me. Think of it this way, most people have a hobby that takes an equal amount of time, effort, and a certain amount of money. Regardless of your situation there is always a solution, it really depends on how you prioritize things.

If you want to kick this up a notch, you should test the quality of the water coming into your house. This is easy to do, and compared to having an illness, it's relatively inexpensive. Simply Google a water specialist firm in your area. They will come out to your home, take a sample, and do the water test for you. If a problem is found (*and it usually is*) a filter is the answer. To stay on top of things, do this annually.

Tip – If you go with the Berkey water filter you can periodically test it by putting red food dye in the water. If the red dye bleeds through into the filtered water, you know the filters need replacing. Berkey filters allow minerals to pass into the filtered water; red dye doesn't have any minerals so in theory none of that dye should come through to the water you drink.

Once you have your water checked off the list, the single biggest potential problem now lurking in your house is hidden mold. And I'm not talking about the black stuff around the bathtub. What I'm referring to is a much bigger issue and potentially far more dangerous.

Mold that is obscured from view can unleash untold devastation because it's not always obvious. In this situation, **testing is essential**. When we are exposed to hidden molds symptoms can range from brain fog to chronic fatigue and just about everything in between. Some people may even express anger or suffer from stubborn weight gain.

The idea here is to become your own detective. Start by asking yourself whether any health issues correspond with a recent house move. It pays to be vigilant, so water damage should be cleaned up quickly. But what lurks beneath carpets and behind sheetrock often goes unseen. If you are unsure, ask your neighbors if your street has flooded in the past.

Unless hidden mold is on your radar, it can make connecting these health dots a real challenge and even more serious health issues can be overlooked by your doctor who, as a rule, is perhaps not even considering toxic mold as a factor.

Mold can build up anywhere there is the slightest moisture. Moisture could be coming from an *unseen* leaking pipe in the ceiling, wall, or under the floorboards. Be on the lookout for any tell-tale signs such as brown water marks on ceilings.

Keep an open mind and be aware that some people are far more sensitive to mold than others. Some toxic molds can absolutely affect people mentally as well as physically. The good news is once you pinpoint a mold problem, life gets a whole lot easier

To help you do this, there is currently a test called an ERMI mold test. It's an objective, standardized DNA based method of testing that will identify and quantify molds. At the time of writing, the test costs around $290. *I know, right? But again, think in terms of lost work hours, doctor's appointments, medications, and even failed relationships.*

ALTERNATIVES

As we continue to shine the spotlight on toxins around the house, try to look at this process in a positive light. There is a very good chance that something in this chapter is stressing your system and once we remove it, health improves. Until we find that stressor, the smartest thing we can do is begin stacking the odds in your favor. We'll do this by removing as many **known** toxic items from your environment as possible. To help you do this, keep reading.

Take a look below your kitchen sink. There you will find some of the deadliest of all household poisons. Many of these products contain carcinogenic ingredients. Carcinogenic simply means the substance or product has the potential to cause cancer. Keep this in mind when you're wiping down countertops with these harsh chemicals – the last place we need carcinogens is where we place our food!

Look, I get it, we obviously need to clean our houses, but a less toxic option would be to use 3% hydrogen peroxide. You can buy this from any pharmacy. It's inexpensive and does a stellar job at killing bacteria, especially on countertops.

Three percent hydrogen peroxide comes already diluted in the bottle; it's the same stuff that's sometimes used to spray directly on cuts and scrapes to clean them. Three percent hydrogen peroxide is quite a mild strength, it's NOT going to burn holes in your clothes, that would be a different strength altogether. I sometimes use greater strengths to increase the oxygen in my cells, but that's a whole 'other story for another time.

For now, let's stick with household toxins found in the kitchen. Wooden cutting boards are said to trap 200x more toxic bacteria than your toilet seat. (Eew, now that's nasty.) When you use hydrogen peroxide on cutting boards, any bacteria left there will actually turn white and fizz. It also works pretty well if you get any meat/blood spills on the kitchen counter, when you hear the 3% hydrogen peroxide fizz, it kinda lets you know that it's doing the job.

The cleaning power of these natural alternatives can outperform toxic chemicals *for less money!* It makes no sense to keeping buying toxic poisons that are known to damage your cells.

You can use 3% hydrogen peroxide wherever you would a carcinogenic chemical and it's generally much safer around food than any of the usual household cleaners found in the store. You can gargle with hydrogen peroxide ... how many other things under your sink would you do that with?

The skin is super absorbent, anytime you hear the word toxic try to also hear the word *insidious* – all of those harsh toxic chemicals have the potential to build up over time like the drip, drip, drip in the bucket.

The aim of this chapter is to provoke you into looking at toxic possibilities, any one of which could suddenly lead to your very own eureka moment!

Rather than use a harsh toilet cleaner, alcohol can be just as effective at killing bacteria. Simply turn a regular bottle of (cheap) vodka into a spray by pouring the vodka into a plastic spray bottle. Hey-presto, you now have an effective cleaner *without* any carcinogenic ingredients and nobody thinks you are an alcoholic.

We like to think of air pollution as being an *outdoor* problem, but every time we let rip with that odor neutralizer or air freshener we release a dangerous concoction of chemicals. It is well documented that these chemicals hang around in the air and irritate the lining of the lungs. If your house smells for any reason, simply open up a couple of windows, *it's free!*

Spray disinfectants and bug sprays sound good in theory but again both are known to irritate the delicate linings of the respiratory system. Lungs are important, we need them to work optimally as they form a vital part of the detoxification system, which helps to *remove* toxins. It really doesn't help to keep breathing in harsh chemicals.

When it comes to cleaning glass, vinegar and newspaper cleans best, and without toxic side effects. You can use regular baking powder with a squirt of lemon to clean just about everything else!

If you are looking to improve the overall air quality in your home/office/bedroom, then plants are an inexpensive way of doing it. NASA has done detailed scientific research in this area bringing ample credibility to the topic.

Tip-
If you don't have a green thumb, ask the sales assistant before you buy. Some plants are robust, others are picky. Getting this right in advance makes life just that little bit easier.

COOKING

Staying in the kitchen, here are a few more things to check off your list. Be especially aware of any nonstick pans. Teflon is polytetrafluoroethylene (or PTFE for short), as it heats up it releases toxic gasses that have been linked to organ failure, reproductive damage, cancer, and other harmful health effects. *I know, right? Who makes this stuff?*

Also begin thinking about the oils you cook with. When cooking with the *wrong* oil at high temperature, free radicals are formed. As a rule of thumb, if your frying pan is producing smoke while you cook, you are producing free radicals.

Free radicals are highly reactive uncharged molecules. Free radicals cause damage by adversely altering lipids, proteins, and even DNA, all contributing to a preventable cascade of diseases. In plain English, a free radical is very much like a drunk at a party, unless he quickly finds his partner (aka an antioxidant) he will roam from room to room kicking tables over. Once damage occurs everyone wants to know who invited the jerk to the party.

Technically speaking, your body produces a *small* amount of its own free radicals. As with most things, the problem only occurs when things get out of balance. If you have more free radicals than your body can effectively deal with, the imbalance manifests in numerous ways. Antioxidants are important because they help neutralize free radicals.

Prevention will always outperform cure so you might be better off cooking with something like avocado oil, clarified butter (ghee), or coconut oil. Generally speaking, these oils are much healthier for cooking because they are more resistant to heating. Oils to **avoid** at all costs are corn, canola, soybean, safflower, and sunflower. These oils have *unstable* fats, which not only make an abundance of free radicals they destroy the nutritional properties of your food.

POTS, PANS, AND DISHES

Aluminum saucepans were once quite popular; however, we now know that trace amounts of aluminum can leach into the food as the pan heats up. *When the amount of aluminum consumed exceeds the body's capacity to excrete it, illness follows.* An added concern is that recent research has found high accumulations of aluminum in the brains of Alzheimer's patients. A good quality set of stainless steel pots and pans is a much better option.

Lead is a known neurotoxin and dangerous heavy metal. Even in small amounts, lead causes a wide range of serious health problems. While we have all heard of the dangers of lead paint, few of us make the same connection with the dishes in our kitchen cupboard.

Brightly colored dishes may look pretty but are often covered in a glaze containing low levels of lead. If buying cheap dishes has the potential to make you ill, then any savings you enjoy are counterproductive. Simple quality dishes may serve you better.

As a side note, lead is also found in many cosmetics which when applied directly to the skin can be absorbed into the bloodstream.

Tip-
Apple pectin can be a helpful ally in chelation of lead. At the correct dose it can help pull lead out of the body. Heavy metals are an interesting topic that's covered in more detail later.

BATHROOM

I cannot tell you *why* manufacturers think it's okay to put harmful ingredients in our bathroom products, but what I *am* telling you here is that they most certainly do! Let's not forget, Johnson & Johnson was recently forced to pay out millions of dollars for failing to disclose the alleged cancer link to its baby powder!

> *Treat the earth well:*
> *it was not given to you by your parents,*
> *it was loaned to you by your children.*
> – Ancient American Indian Proverb

All this is not meant to feel like 101 ways to make your life more difficult, we're simply looking at ways to **reduce** your toxic burden.

Most people start their day by brushing their teeth, taking a shower, and then rolling on some kind of underarm deodorant. Let's take a closer look at these daily occurrences.

When it comes to oral hygiene, it's hard to get away from fluoride. There is already so much controversy surrounding fluoride that I'm going to sidestep it all and leave you with this single thought …

To function optimally your thyroid needs iodine. There's nothing too controversial about that statement until you realize that both iodine and fluoride appear on the same periodic table as halogens.

This basically means that *both* fluoride and iodine are chemically similar; that's a pretty big deal if you happen to be a thyroid.

The thyroid is a small butterfly shaped organ located in the base of your neck, but don't be fooled by its size. The thyroid performs a *precise* set of functions, one of which is to slowly release hormones that control the way your body uses energy. Some believe that fluoride has the ability to block iodine absorption.

Once the thyroid is compromised the *whole* body suffers. A daily and constant hit of fluoride may have the potential to cause fatigue, increased sensitivity to cold, heat, dry skin, and facial puffiness. These are some of the *many* symptoms of a poorly functioning thyroid.

Changing our hygiene and dental habits is as easy as changing our brand, most health food stores carry alternatives and playing it safe is perhaps the better option.

If enough of us make the switch, then perhaps corporations will begin to sit up and take notice. When it all seems too much, I like to think of it this way: we get to vote three times a day with the food we eat and maybe once a week with the toiletries we buy. Business follows money, period.

Regular store bought shower gels and some soaps have toxic ingredients that can range from aluminum to parabens. In 2004, British cancer researcher Philippa Darbre PhD found parabens present in malignant breast tumors. Parabens are well known to mimic/disrupt estrogen in the body and are found in many cosmetics. If our goal is to find *lasting* solutions, the first step must be to **limit** anything with a toxic element.

Grab your shower gel, deodorant, makeup, and anything else that comes into contact with your skin. Look at the label of ingredients; a quick Google search should shock you to the core.

Toxic ingredients are in our shampoos, soaps, deodorants, and shower gels to name but a few. You may choose to ignore this information, but starting today it becomes difficult to say you didn't know about it.

Sadly, toxic chemicals are a relentless, integral part of our modern day existence (*some call this progress*) yet the ongoing damage to our world is profound. We *can* all do our bit to stop these toxic invaders from seeping into our homes by switching to greener brands.

Remember, ANYTHING that goes onto the skin goes *into* the skin and is then absorbed into the bloodstream. Oils, cosmetics, creams, perfumes, bug deterrents, deodorants, and underarm antiperspirants are particularly toxic to the skin.

LEAD

It has to be acknowledge that government agencies have done a remarkably good job at alerting people to the dangers of lead paint, even to the point of handing out large fines to any contractor attempting to remove it without the correct safety equipment.

The dangers of lead paint are real and far reaching, and full credit where it's due — bravo to the environmental agency.

But if it's the goal of the government to steer us away from danger, why stop at lead? Why isn't the same level of attention being directed to other household toxic products such as the mercury found in light bulbs?

Many of these bulbs were pushed on the public as a way to save energy, they are now declared so toxic that some local dumps won't take them. Check to see how many of those curly shaped light bulbs you have in your home *and FFS be especially careful not to break one!*
We have become so entwined with these toxic products that it's no longer possible to completely avoid them all, but we can certainly try to minimize our personal exposure to them.

OFF-GASSING

Like any good detective, we are searching for clues in every corner of the house and always keeping an open mind. It's worth noting that new furniture, rugs, and plastics ALL have the potential to "off-gas" with dangerous chemicals. Off-gassing (also known as outgassing) refers to the release of airborne particulates or chemicals. This is something to be aware of in a small bedroom, especially for those with young children.

Fire retardants can be particularly problematic. These can be found in a mattress, pillows, and even your favorite armchair. As pillows are next to our face for long periods, try to replace them with the least toxic option. Again knowing the root cause of something can be halfway to finding the solution. You could also check for apps that help you uncover toxins in everyday household products. *I know they are out there.*

CARBON MONOXIDE

Let's not forget our old friend carbon monoxide which can come to us at home (*or* at work) through a faulty furnace. Carbon monoxide is sometimes referred to as the *silent* killer and yet detectors are incredibly easy to install and, compared to death, offer good value for the money.

RADON

If your downturn in health coincided with a move to a new house then hidden mold and a change in water quality are certainly suspects to check for. The other sleeping giant would be radon. Radon is a colorless, odorless, radioactive gas formed by the radioactive decay of the small amounts of uranium that occur naturally in all rocks and soils. Radon can lead to serious lung damage and is another known carcinogen.

If radon is found to be present in your house, the solution can be as simple as venting the air out from your basement or installing a plastic membrane under the concrete. Again, the much bigger problem is being *unaware* of it. The possibility that radon could potentially be seeping up from your basement floor is real. The good news is that testing is relatively easy and inexpensive.

EMFs

Okay, last one. EMF stands for Electromagnetic Field which is a field of energy created by electrically charged objects. The most common sources for high electromagnetic fields include proximity to power lines, transformers, appliances, flaws in a building's internal wiring system, and stray currents on utility pipes – sadly, it doesn't end there. Utility companies are now installing "smart" meters across the US which add to the frequency burden. So it seems our exposure to EMFs is going up by the day, especially as we demand better phone coverage and more Wi-Fi signals.

Wi-Fi and cellular phones have become an omnipresent part of our lives and I fear the allure of technology is too great for me to overcome in this paragraph. I did once hear someone say, "If trees gave off a Wi-Fi signal we would all be out planting them; too bad they only produce the oxygen we breathe."

This sounds about right to me, hence the reason I have not owned a cell phone for the past fifteen years – although my wife seems to think it's because I have no friends to call. In truth, I just prefer to use email as a way to communicate.

When using a laptop, it's important to restrict direct contact between you and it. Ideally keep your laptop on a desk, if that's not an option, then at the very least place a buffer (like a thick book or cushion) underneath it. There is now increasing evidence to suggests that laptops, when used incorrectly have the potential to cause fertility problems. To help limit your exposure special EMF protective mats can be purchased online. These types of mats fit neatly under the laptop to shield you from harmful radiation, they can also prove useful for children's hand held devices.

EMF testing for the home is available in most areas and seeing your personal level of exposure on a meter gauge is a sobering experience. Half the battle is won if you know exactly where your highest EMF reading is coming from. Electric blankets can also be particularly problematic and should *always* be turned off at night.

To help defuse some of those electromagnetic fields one solution is to install a "grounding mat" in your home. Grounding mats can again be purchased online or you can make your own. They are pretty simple and inexpensive to make; this option is covered in more detail later.

Are there more household toxins out there? Yup, lots, but with so much ground to cover the aim of this chapter was never intended to be an all-encompassing list of possible household toxins, but rather a tool to highlight areas of concern.

On the upside, for those of us who are surrounded by neighbors, Wi-Fi routers can be a perfect opportunity to mess with people. Simply name *your* Wi-Fi network something like, "Mobile Police Surveillance" or "Shut Your Damned Dog Up" or, my personal favorite, "Tell-my-Wi-Fi-I-Love-Her." Or if you are feeling particularly fresh, "Tell-**Your**-Wi-Fi I love her". Lol.

What did we learn from this chapter?

To be able to identify potential problems we must first know what they are. It's essential to do whatever is within your power to reduce the flow of toxins coming into your home. We can absolutely influence the companies that make toxic products to change their ways by buying from their green competitors.

If you have recently moved to a different house, be aware of whether the onset of any of your symptoms corresponded with the move. Any house that suffered a flood in the past will have a higher susceptibility to mold and this type of mold isn't always visible to the naked eye.

Any water filter is better than no filter. Without clean water all things die, sometimes this can happen *slowly*. Have your water tested.

Homework: Install a water filter and then begin to remove any toxic cleaning substances from your house. If you have the financial means, immediately test for mold, radon, and carbon monoxide.

If you *don't* have the funds, do one test at a time as funds become available. If you are unsure, Google each of these terms for more information.

Chapter 7

BUILD A PERSONAL TIMELINE

So far we have exposed a range of household toxins that have the potential to adversely affect our health. What say we now switch gears and begin to shine the spotlight on *you*?

Today it's not uncommon for your doctor to take a blood sample. But when we rely on blood tests alone, it's like putting all our detection eggs in one basket. And by doing so, we run the risk of doing a great disservice to the patient (yup, that's you again).

Before handing over our health to a computer, every informed patient should know that regardless of what the printout says, *symptoms should always trump bloodwork numbers.* Even some seasoned health care providers have this simple logic a little twisted. With an infinite number of variables, health by the numbers can be a novel concept. Let's take a look.

In a perfect world, diagnostic bloodwork is an incredibly useful tool, *no question about it.* However, this process isn't always perfect and even slight fluctuations in our personal biometrics can produce unsatisfactory results. If for some reason your lab results have sent you on a fruitless mission, it can help to go back to basics. This was how old school medicine was practiced long before all those computer printouts came along.

If conventional bloodwork testing has worked for you in the past, then more power to you, but for many, the sheer complexity of our uniqueness can be difficult to capture by lab work alone. It's worth noting that not all complaints are *immediately* picked up in the bloodwork. Sometimes test results are misinterpreted or the results might simply fail to be in the optimal range at the time of the test.

Are you getting this? I'm saying some biomarkers have been shown to fluctuate at different times of day. Some test results have the potential to show one reading in the morning and a completely different reading later in the day. Again, I'm not dismissing the value of bloodwork; I'm simply offering a different perspective when results are stagnant, inconclusive, or confusing.

To give you a feel for this chapter, let's use an example of a patient with a kidney issue. When all is not well in the kidney department, the body is going to start sending out clues in the hope you will pick up on them. When we learn to listen, we may begin to notice changes in the amount of urine being produced, or perhaps a swelling of the legs, ankles, and feet, which can happen when the kidneys fail to eliminate water waste. These are just a few tell-tale clues. When it comes to the kidneys, there are many others.

The skin is often referred to as the third kidney and with good reason. When the kidneys become overtaxed, the skin is used as an added filter. Here we might see changes such as an annoying itchy skin rash. Other signs might include puffy eyes, unexplained shortness of breath, excessive drowsiness or fatigue, persistent nausea, confusion, or pain or pressure in your chest. The point is this: once we learn to pay attention, these clues are everywhere.

If your health problem has remained without a solution for any length of time then clearly what you have tried hasn't been working. But when we start to connect the dots we become more in tune with our body.

Being in tune with our body also has other benefits. Not everyone has the means to run a full-panel test. Running endless bloodwork tests is far from cheap. For that reason, some insurance companies simply won't cover certain tests. For many of us this can result in having to pay out of pocket for these types of services. My European homies obviously have no such worry as they have a mostly free health care system. Being the crazy socialists that they are, they also have free police and free fire stations. But I digress.

Maybe you have money to spend on medical testing, maybe you don't. For those of us with limited funds there can be *other* ways to achieve the same goal. When the fancy elevator back to wellness appears to be broken, there's always the old reliable set of stairs.

Personally, I haven't had a blood test done for more than five years, although I suspect that when I feel like crap my biomarkers are off and when I feel good I know I'm moving in the right direction. *I know, right, it's a rebellious concept. Hear me out.*

As soon as we learn to pay *close* attention to our own symptoms (clues) we become a better informed patient. To guide us, some simple detection techniques can be particularly effective.

The body is constantly sending out symptoms as clues in an attempt to get you to pick up on them. All too often, though, we rush to *mask* over these important clues with painkillers. Let's not forget that the convenience of being relatively pain free is a *short-term* solution and *no* drug is totally free of side effects. Being on the lookout for clues can reveal a problem is coming our way long before it's picked up in our bloodwork.

When a long term health problem remains undiagnosed for any length of time, it's entirely possible and predictable that your stubborn illness has its roots in *several* different places. To help us better see the clues, here are a few self-testing tricks that I've picked up along the way. Some of them may seem a little strange at first but trust me on this because they all work. This information can be applied to *any* health issue, small or large. Generally speaking, *we are looking for patterns* as opposed to a single event.

SIX MEN

To help us find those elusive answers you are once again being steered into the role of detective. Let's jump straight in as we hunt for clues in the form of **your** symptoms. Here's an example of how this might work in practice.

When trying to figure out a difficult to understand illness, it's helpful to employ Rudyard Kipling's six honest serving men. (*They taught me everything I know.*) Their names are **What** and **Why** and **When** and **How** and **Where** and **Who!**

All things have a starting point; some illnesses are easy to trace because they have an undisputable starting point. Let's use an example of someone being involved in an unfortunate skiing accident who suffers a broken leg. In this example, the correlation between time and event is pretty clear. The cause of the injury is an accident and the clue trail starts and ends on the ski slope.

But not every illness is quite so cut and dry. Let's now imagine someone swinging an axe when suddenly a tendon in the wrist snaps. This time around the sequence of events is not as straightforward as it was in the skiing accident. How so?

Think about it – tendons are pretty tough, they are designed to work hard. It's not normal for them to give way that easily. If it were, the human race would already be extinct.

The trick here is *not* to accept that shit just happens, there is *always* a reason. Maybe in this instance we need to look a little closer at the history of the patient, after all a snapped tendon isn't something that happens every day. And in fact, this patient has probably chopped wood in the past without snapping a tendon.

We know that tendons are usually pretty robust and under normal circumstances they are capable of handling normal daily workloads that can include things like swinging an axe. As with most medical mysteries, *there has to be a reason.*

Prior to the tendon snapping, let's first ask **what** is different. Perhaps when we look to earlier events it may reveal an interesting pattern. Who knows, *maybe* in the months leading up to the tendon snapping an infection was present. These days, an infection will often lead us down the antibiotic road. Given that in this example we have a snapped tendon perhaps it would be prudent to check whether any of those possibly prescribed antibiotics have any known side effects that might include weakened tendons.

Bingo! In this example we could suspect a frequently prescribed antibiotic by the name of Cipro. Research this drug and you will quickly find that one of its known side effects is snapped tendons. *I know, right? Ouch – why would they?*

As with so many side effects from pharmaceutical drugs there can sometimes be a total disconnect in time (i.e. the tendon snapped several months after the person took Cipro) and *unless we are looking* for this piece of vital information it can easily be overlooked by both you and your doctor. Obviously there could be other reasons for the degeneration of tendon tissue and here Cipro is being used purely to make a point. But given its dangerous track record, it remains a strong suspect. Without analyzing previous details, this puzzle would have remained unsolved. Whenever we look *backward* in time at our symptoms (clues) a specific sequence of events usually unfolds. To help you find these patterns we need to build a simple framework. When we are looking for answers *nobody* knows your story better than you do. You live with yourself every day. Everywhere you go, there you are, looking back at yourself. This makes you both an expert witness *and* the perfect detective.

Sometimes we are quick to hand this responsibility over to others, if that has helped you in the past then more power to you. I am a *firm* believer in doing whatever works. However, for some of us it didn't quite work out that way. We found ourselves trapped in a repetitive cycle of going to doctors but never quite finding a *lasting* solution.

Again all things have a starting point, and unless we find ourselves standing directly below a coconut tree, illness rarely falls out of the sky. If we hope to find an end to what ails us we must have a plan to better understand **when, where, and how** it all began.

In the old days, a physician would carefully listen to a patient's symptoms (clues) and then ask a series of probing questions in an effort to uncover the root cause of the illness or complaint. This is how *good* medicine was practiced. Today much greater emphasis is put on running your blood through a computer. Once that happens, your sample results are given a number and that number is checked against a list of other numbers. If matching two pieces of dry ink somehow fixes your problem, great, if not, you may find yourself back on the merry-go-round of chronic illness. I actually lost count of the number of blood tests I managed to pass while feeling deathly ill. *I know, right? What's up with that?*

A prime example of a test that has become pretty hard to fail is the standard thyroid test. Despite a catalogue of *physical* symptoms to the contrary, the thyroid-stimulating hormone (TSH) test usually concludes that everything is fine. Passing a TSH test when you aren't feeling well serves as little comfort, and in the real world it rarely provides a complete picture.

Typically, most doctors don't run a *full* thyroid blood panel nor do they spend sufficient time investigating the patient's more obvious physical symptoms. The TSH test can be the equivalent of a plumber coming out on a cold day to fix a broken heating system and only checking the thermostat. The analogy of a broken heating system is an apt comparison to an underperforming thyroid as both can leave you shivering in the cold or becoming overheated when it's warm.

The nature of TSH testing fails to look at the overall picture. Looking at the thyroid in isolation fails to take into account that the liver also plays an important role in converting the main thyroid hormone T4 into T3.

Too often, focusing on a set of limited variables yields limited results. On the other hand, asking well-targeted questions allows the exploration of the most likely cause. Hold onto your hat as we now embark on an exercise in medical inquiry that will allow us to explore the most likely cause of your illness when everything else has failed. Before we set off on this path, it's worth noting that whatever health problem you may have, it usually has more than one component to it. The good news is that this book is crammed to the absolute brim with suggestions to help you find your answers.

For this exercise you will want to grab a pen and a blank sheet of paper. If at some point in the past your doctor hasn't listened to you (or failed to fully understand your symptoms) *then this is your time.*
Okay, you are going to take your plain sheet of paper and list ALL your symptoms. Start the list with the symptom that is giving you the *biggest* problem and then work your way down the list to include lesser complaints. *Stay with me on this, it's a very simple but highly effective way of making sense of your medical maze.*

If your symptoms are vague, or you really aren't too sure, try starting from the top of your head and moving down your body to the tips of your toes. As you journey down through your body, list any and every medical problem that you've experienced or that concerns you. Give this task some careful consideration as even minor things can later become important clues. If you aren't sure, that's okay, simply choose three health problems you wish you didn't have and write those down.

It would be unusual for any illness to have just one symptom; there is usually a pattern. However, don't get too freaked out if your list seems too short or too long. Everything in the body is connected. What ails you in one part of the body will logically throw up symptoms in another part. If you want to put this theory to the test, try dropping a hammer on your big toe and see if your eyes water. *Whoa, just kidding!*

Okay, once your list is complete, check that all your symptoms are in order of priority, starting with whatever bothers you the most. What you should now have is a piece of paper with a list of all your symptoms starting with the biggest problem at the top and the absolute smallest problem at the bottom. *Got it? Okay, good.*

Once you have *that* paper filled out, put it to one side and pull out a second blank sheet of paper. Only this time we are going to do something a little different. Turn the sheet of paper sideways (landscape orientation) and at the top write the word **Timeline.**

*Tip - If you have a lot of symptoms you could potentially run out of space. To solve this problem simply add more pages to your **Timeline** sheet with adhesive tape.*

As you look at your new **Timeline** sheet of paper you need to write today's date on the far right hand side. Over on the far left side write the date when you last felt well. *Done? Perfect. Now bring back your list of symptoms from the first sheet of paper.*

The idea is to now transfer those symptoms onto the **Timeline** sheet in some kind of *chronological* order. It doesn't have to be perfect, at this stage we are just trying to get a sense of **what** when wrong and **when**.

Some illnesses may have a long history to them. If this is you, *hang in there* and, as mentioned, simply add more paper to your timeline sheet to stretch it out. *If* at any time your **Timeline** sheet begins to look like a biblical scroll, you might want to stop what you are doing and seek out a little divine intervention.

For the rest of us, what we should now have in front of us is a sheet of paper turned on its side (so it's 11 inches across the top, or longer if you've had to tape sheets together) with the current date on the far right hand side and a start date (when you last felt well) on the far left. The space in between those dates will have *approximate* dates of when each of your symptoms first appeared.

All we are attempting to do here is *match* up your list of symptoms with approximate originating **dates**. Doing this on paper allows you to see patterns that you might otherwise miss. Yup, this all takes a little effort on your part, but keep moving forward. The cost to you is *low* and the rewards are high. It might just be the reason why no one else has figured out your annoying health problem.

I accept that this might take a little time to finish and that's okay too. Sometimes sleeping on it will help you fill any missing blanks. Asking your healthcare provider for a copy of your medical records can also be helpful. If you don't have access to your records *progress is always better than perfection,* just do the best you can with what information you have available.

Once you have your timeline sheet complete, take a while to look at it from different perspectives. Maybe ask a friend to look over it with you. Examine your timeline for patterns; a group of small insignificant dates (or symptoms) grouped together can suddenly start to have a significant meaning. Once clues start to surface, look hard at the dates surrounding those issues.

From a set of seemingly *obscure* clues an awful lot can be discovered. Some people like to do Sudoku puzzles. I find these types of health problems far more interesting and here's one simple example that mirrors many others.

For arguments sake, let's say you have managed to get all the way down to your big toe before you've found the first symptom (clue). Here in the joint of that big toe you notice a sharp pain, maybe on a scale of one to ten you note the pain as being right up there at an eight. *Perfect, let's run with that as our first solid clue.*

An educated guess would suggest you have case of gout. So far so good, but how does this information help you? Well, most of the time you'd take yourself and your big toe along to the doctor's office. Here's how this works in practice: you tell the doctor you keep getting an excruciating pain in your big toe. He or she sticks a needle in your toe to take a fluid sample. This sample goes off to the lab and your doctor later confirms you have Hyperuricemia (gout to the rest of us). A follow-up appointment is made to discuss your treatment options. You leave with a pocket full of pills that later go on to tax your liver, kidneys, *and* wallet. *If only there were another way before getting to this point.*

Please don't get me wrong, if this were a more serious condition, your best option would always be to go directly to your primary doctor. But all too often we take up the good doctor's time with benign, non-life threatening ailments without pausing to consider the *least invasive options first.* Instead, we find ourselves in a self-perpetuating loop of taking pharmaceutical drugs and never finding a lasting solution. These types of drugs are great at alleviating pain but they are rarely aimed at addressing the root cause. To get off *this* particular merry-go-round we only need to ask ourselves a few probing questions.

Ready?

Okay, this time what say we try something different with our gouty big toe? Rather than paying for the good doctor's time (and draining our own valuable resources) let's begin by asking the all empowering **why** question. When we ask "why" we start to develop a whole new picture.

Unless the toe has recently incurred some kind of trauma (*duh*) it's really *not* a normal thing for your big toe to be in such pain. If gout is the usual culprit for that pain, then *why* is that? That's a smart question to ask and with a little detective work we'll find the answer is a build-up of uric acid. But why stop there? Clearly it's *not* a normal thing for the body to suddenly start pumping out excessive amounts of uric acid in the joint of the big toe, so *why* now? By continuing to press the *why* button we move a little closer to finding a *lasting* solution.
According to old wisdom, excessive uric acid may be related to the things you eat. For example, it could be due to an over consumption of red meats or, as newer thinking suggests, even the fructose in fruits can be the culprit. Either way, having this *new* information provides us with a whole different approach.

In this version of gouty events it could be worth trying to reduce your daily intake of acid forming meats as a good starting point. If that doesn't work, then try taking all fruit out of the diet for thirty days. Some gout sufferers swear by drinking 12oz of water along with the juice of one freshly squeezed lemon. Either path could lead to success rather simply popping more pills.

Exhausting the least invasive option first (in this case a change in diet) may even bring faster results. If all else fails, you still have the doctor's appointment to fall back on.

This is just one short example to demonstrate the **why** question, and we could have used a hundred other examples. The point being made is this: even a single big toe can reveal a wealth of information. Think what else we could discover when you begin to look at the body as a whole!

UNTURNED STONES

Good police detectives leave no stones unturned. They often find evidence in unexpected places. If you want to be active in your own recovery treat it as if it were a crime scene. When filling out your timeline sheet, make a note of any recent medications, surgeries and/or medical procedures. Your body is *dying* to give you these clues!

Whenever you find yourself sitting in a doctor's office listening to a damning diagnosis don't become a tourist visiting your own health, be sure to ask questions. Before you sign up to become an unpaid guinea pig, ask *why* do you suddenly have illness X-Y-or Z? If your doctor can't answer the *why* question, then how on earth will he or she begin to treat it?

A spike in symptoms may overlap with a hospital or even a holiday visit. *Always* be on the lookout for patterns, and be aware that some of the side effects of medications can have lingering effects which can mean you miss the connection between the cause and the effect. Remember the snapped tendon story. If you aren't sure, a simple *process of elimination* can be helpful.

Like any good detective, we need to pay particular attention to *anything* that's manmade or an unnatural occurrence in the body. When listing medications, don't forget to add things (if applicable) like the "humble" birth control pill. That alone has the potential to upset a woman's estrogen levels. Given that the theme of this chapter is all about empowering yourself to find your answers, I'm going to resist the temptation to go off on an estrogen tangent. Needless to say, the potential of the birth control pill to *adversely* affect a woman's body chemistry is great, and screwed up estrogen levels can manifest in more ways than this chapter has the time to discuss. If this is you, know that the side effects of taking oral birth control will absolutely warrant doing a little of your own investigative research.

When looking at your symptoms, be guided by your intuition. *Your intuition is probably the most underused tool you have at your disposal.* Deep down you know when something isn't right. It's well documented that specially trained dogs have the ability to sniff out cancer. I often wonder is it the cancer they can smell, or are they simply able to *sense* when something is wrong? Or could it even be that they are picking up on their human subject's sense that something isn't right?
I guess we don't know what we don't know. Perhaps these dogs have never been conditioned to believe their *instinctive* senses are wrong. As far as the dogs know, their intuition is working just fine.

Taking a step back and looking at events on your *own* timeline can reveal more than you might think. Try to keep an open mind when looking for patterns. Some people will react to vitamins; others have been known to react to certain medical procedures. Both will have the same thing in common ... a start date!

Be sure to add any recent dental visits to your timeline. It's often said that health *starts* in the mouth *but so too can illness.* An abscessed tooth can be a drain on the entire immune system and even the adrenal glands.

Every single action you take from root canals to white fillings can have a detrimental effect on your health. Once cut off from the immune system, root canals can become miniature hotels for infection.

Those white composite fillings often contain BPA (Bisphenol A) and "silver" fillings contain trace amounts of mercury, a known neurotoxin. If this is news to you, don't panic, all these subjects will be covered in more detail later.

As we continue moving forward, let me again urge you to take your time and try not to feel overwhelmed. Your answer is in here somewhere. Yes, there is lots to think about, but let's keep it in perspective. Each time we become aware of one of these stressors we have an opportunity to fix it, and in doing so the overall burden to the body will be lessened.

FREAKY CLUES

Once you learn to look a little closer, you will notice clues are littered all around us 24/7. Some of these clues will become more obvious than others and once you reach this point it can become difficult to switch off your clue antenna. Here's an example of that.

I once went into a hardware store and needed a little help finding a drill. A sales assistant led the way and we spent a few minutes chatting about the drill I was interested in buying. He was a nice enough fellow and as I thanked him for his time I felt that I should probably warn him about his high blood pressure because left unchecked it can have *deadly* consequences.

He hadn't mentioned it during our short conversation so when I asked him how his high blood pressure was doing, he was actually quite surprised that I knew it had only recently gone up. He went on to say that he had only left the doctor's office *that* morning and had left with a diagnosis of hypertension (high blood pressure).

He knew he hadn't seen me at his doctor's office and by now he was very curious to know how I had somehow picked up on it. Looking for clues had become such an ingrained habit for me that I saw the answer right there in his fingernails as he pointed to the item I was buying. When a person has high blood pressure the half-moon shape at the base of the fingernails becomes quite prominent, with the exception of the little finger which doesn't have a half moon at all. Surprised, he admitted he had never even noticed his fingernails before, *nor had his doctor.*

Had he known what to look for *earlier* maybe he could have seen the warning signs coming. He was very grateful he now had a tool (literally at his fingertips) to monitor his blood pressure at times when he couldn't get to his BP machine. He asked if there was anything *he* could do to help his condition. I mentioned that (as well as working with his doctor) he could try getting more *natural* potassium in his diet from foods like avocados instead of eating more bananas, which are high in sugar. Sweet potatoes have natural potassium in the skin, and wild caught salmon is also helpful as is drinking hibiscus tea. Sometimes these simple changes can be more helpful than popping pills.

The fingernails *alone* can tell us about *far more* than just high blood pressure. Go ahead, take a look at the shape, color, and texture of your fingernails and then check them against a friend's, you will quickly notice that *your* fingernails are totally unique to you. Watch closely and you will see that your fingernails change and they *always* tell a story.

TIMING

Timing is everything in this life, sometimes we have to be aware that some people *want* to hear these insights, and some people don't. My wife is an accomplished knitter and I recently met with some of her friends at a small social gathering. During introductions, I shook hands with a middle aged lady and noticed she had dry skin. I also noticed she was the only person wearing a sweater in a room full of people wearing T-shirts. A quick glance at her eyebrows revealed that the *outer* third of her eyebrow had completely thinned out indicating a possible thyroid problem as the reason for her dry skin.

As I watched her crunch on her second cup of ice within fifteen minutes, I wondered if the root of this lady's thyroid problem was anemia – people often crave ice when they are low in iron. As I now sat silently observing this lady from the other side of the room my wife came over and discreetly reminded me of the agreement we had made *before* leaving the house. Her side had gone something like this: "These are my knitting friends, try not to freak any of them out." My point? Clues are all around us, and they are helpful, but sometimes discretion is wise.

If you felt this chapter got a little too weird too quick, then you might want to hold onto your hat because I've saved the best (or weirdest) for last. So *here goes nothing* ... each and every day your body delivers new clues for you to observe. Once you learn to read *these* signals you are well on your way to self-discovery.... so here's the scoop – on poop.

POOP

If we eat healthy every day we can expect to expel a stool every day. Good digestion always starts in the mouth, so be sure to chew your food rather than rush it. To help you remember, think of it this way: the better you chew, the better the poo. The size, shape, color, and texture of stool tell a very interesting story.

Diet, certain medications, and even vitamins can all change the color of stool, but a "normal" stool should be somewhere on the brown spectrum, which indicates the liver is excreting enough bile. *I know, right? What's bile?*

Think of bile as similar in function to dishwasher detergent which helps clean excess oil and grease from the dishes. In its most basic form, bile acts the same way.

A stool with lots of holes drilled into it could be a sign of a parasitic infection; this can be quite common and something that will rob your body of vital nutrients. A normal stool shouldn't stink up the bathroom, and if it has you hanging your head out the bathroom window then it could be a sign of malabsorption.

Is it me, or would it be weirder if I left out *talking about these important clues?*

Either way, the good news is that much of this is diet related. Diet is inextricably tied to *good* health and it's a subject we will obviously cover in more detail. They say a picture is worth a thousand words. With that in mind, you can access a free medical chart called THE BRISTOL STOOL

CHART via a simple Google search. The Bristol Stool Chart is better able to show clearly in pictures what I am attempting to describe in words.

PEE

The color of your urine also holds invaluable information or clues. Again, medications, vitamins and diet can change it, but in most cases healthy looking pee should be the color of straw. If it happens to be clear on a *regular* basis, then it's possibly passing through your kidneys a little too quickly and could be a warning sign of trouble in that direction.

If your pee is dark, it could be a sign you are dehydrated. If it's dark orange *and* you are passing pale stools it could be a sign of a malfunctioning liver, if this is you, pay close attention to the whites of your eyes which may also begin to show a yellow tint. The liver and kidneys are organs to help us rid the body of toxins and it's important to have them working optimally.

If pee is cloudy or murky it could be a sign of kidney stones forming, but you won't have to second guess when stones are ready to expel as the pain to the kidney will be excruciating. Kidney stones can sometimes be related to problems with the *parathyroid*. Although the parathyroid and thyroid are both located in the same area of the body, they perform totally different jobs. The primary job of the parathyroid is to regulate the body's calcium levels. *But I digress.*

If pee is cloudy, murky, and foul smelling it could be a sign that you have a UTI (urinary tract infection). If diabetes is suspected the kidneys will do their best to get rid of excess glucose and the pee may smell sweet. If you really want to put this to the test, you *could* try tasting the urine rather than doing the finger prick test. *Whoa!* Hang on, I didn't say you had to drink it, I said *taste* it.

I know to some this may all seem a little gross, but the aim of this book isn't to tickle your ears with things that are pleasant to hear, it's to help you stay well or get well. Once you get over the mental hang-up of checking your pee and poop for clues, it can be used as highly effective diagnostic tool.

This is *your* fight; if progress with your health has been stagnant then let's not get too comfortable blindly following the instructions of doctors and hoping for the best. Use these tools to become an active player in your own recovery.

Finally, before people start jumping all over me on this, might I point out that whenever Bear Grylls drinks his own pee on national television he's applauded for sharing an acceptable survival technique and quickly becomes the darling of the day. I'm simply saying don't be afraid to use these tips *which can also aid in your own survival.*

What did we learn from this chapter?

Symptoms are important clues that should be investigated rather than suppressed. If you are stuck on that merry-go-round of illness it's absolutely okay to play a bigger role in your own recovery. Remember, *nobody* knows your situation better than you do.

Homework: create your own Timeline of symptoms and look at it objectively.
Recommended Reading: *Never Be Sick Again: Health is a Choice, Learn How to Choose It,* by Raymond Francis. M.Sc. This was one of the first health related books I read; it was also one of the most helpful.

Chapter 8

HOW DID WE GET HERE?

Rest assured, solutions are coming, but to get the most out of this book it pays to have an open mind. Fortunately, there is a simple thirty-second technique to help you do this. Whenever you hear an idea that's different from your own, try to resist the initial temptation to rush in and pour cold water on it. Instead, *challenge* yourself to listen to new information with an *open mind* for a minimum of thirty seconds.

This doesn't mean we'll have to agree with opposing opinions, it will simply demonstrate a willingness to be less rigid in our thinking. If we can learn to suspend our inclination to disregard those whose views differ from ours – at least until we've heard them out – our minds will become a fertile breeding ground for new ideas. If you can do this, even in short bursts, you will have gained something valuable in the process: a more flexible mindset as well as a better understanding of the other person's point of view. Moving forward this becomes a very valuable tool that will ensure your mind has the freedom to breathe.

Once we let go of our rigid thinking *we are in control* of our thoughts as opposed to our thoughts being in control of us. In this life there are no shortages of opportunities to practice this technique, even as we move through this chapter.

Ready?

Recently, my wife and I visited my elderly aunt who is in a nursing home. While we were there it became clear that my aunt had no clue who I was, or even where *she* was. This once dignified woman was now trapped inside a sickly body and relying on a range of medical services to prevent her from sitting in cold, damp underwear. As a result of crippling illness, she had been confined to a bed for quite some time, unable to walk or talk.

As I looked around the nursing home it became clear that my aunt's situation was being replicated all around us. Withered bodies were being spoon fed in front of television sets airing mind-numbing shows. Seeing people like this weighed heavy on my soul.

On the opposite end of that spectrum meet 102-year-old Edie Simms of Missouri. Edie should be an inspiration to us all. In her long life she had many experiences, but getting arrested was not one of them – but it was on her bucket list.

For her 102nd birthday, Edie called the local police department and asked to be taken into custody. Not content simply to be ushered into the back of a waiting squad car, Edie put her hands in the air and asked to be handcuffed! (You can see a clip of this on YouTube.)

When you hear this lady talk it's obvious that her outlook on life is what keeps her going. She spends much of her time helping the "younger" residents at the senior home where she lives. Helping others has been Edie's formula for living a productive life, and her simple advice is backed by actual scientific studies showing that at the neurobiological level our brain lights up whenever we give social support to others. Although after 102 years, I suspect Edie probably already knows this.

On the flip side of Edie's story sits senile dementia. Unfortunately, sharp minds like Edie's are now few and far between. Alzheimer's Disease International estimates that in 2015 46.8 million people worldwide were living with dementia. This number is expected to double every 20 years, reaching 74.7 million in 2030 and 131 million in 2050.

While there are lots of theories for this anticipated increase, it's important to recognize that health problems aren't confined to the older generation and statistically speaking, a child born in the U.S. today has a lower life expectancy than those in the generation before.

The presumption by some is that our ancestors have given us bad genes. Personally, I take issue with this argument *more than any other* because it suggests we are powerless to control our destiny. This type of thinking instills a victim mindset which is not only *unhelpful,* it's deeply flawed. In my humble opinion, debunking the bad genes theory is essential for recovery.

Spend enough time sitting in your doctor's office, and sooner or later you will hear that your suffering is genetic. In case you missed the subtle message here, this little gem hints that *you* are somehow to blame for your illness and there isn't anything much anyone can do about it. This way of thinking obviously presents a bigger problem to you than it does to the doctor treating you.

The common suggestion is that we are all predisposed to illness through our genes. But this misconception doesn't take into account that, historically speaking, our ancestors' genes *had* to be pretty robust for the human race to survive this long. Nor does it take into account the toxic world we have made for ourselves and that we now live in. Today, much of our highly processed diet comes loaded with toxic additives and excess sugars.

The "bad" genes hypothesis also tends to gloss over a vast array of toxic *environmental* factors. If you grew up in cramped squalor and suffered from head lice, then so did your siblings. If you grew up in a home full of mold and damp, there is a pretty good chance you developed some chest problems and so did your siblings. If you grew up in a house next to a toxic waste dump, then so did your siblings. If cancer shows up disproportionately high in these family units, does anyone ever stop to ask **why?**

Think about it, if your mom ate junk food for breakfast, lunch, and dinner then as a kid so did you. When *both* become diabetic does anyone stop to ask if this predisposition came as a direct result of bad genes or as a result of a bad diet?

The short answer to that question is *always* going to be no, in part because doctors receive so little training in the field of nutrition. *Now* we start to see a very different picture and one that challenges the concept that your cause is lost to bad genes.

When we apply a little flexible thinking, these connections begin to look a lot less like genetics and more like common sense.

Perhaps all those medical pundits are referring to our *early* ancestors? Well, let's have a look, shall we?

Today we owe our freedom to those brave souls who gave up their lives fighting in the First World War. It's well documented that during that war more good men were lost to poor sanitation than to enemy bullets. Wait a second … *what*? It's an indisputable historical fact that a lack of basic hygiene caused more deaths than flying bullets.

It's a tragically sad statistic I know, but it's important to understand that between 1914 and 1918, lack of basic hygiene killed more men than rapid machine gun fire did!

Think about it, during that time a plumber's wrench had the potential to save more lives the surgeon's scalpel!

If only those helpless men stuck in the trenches had been given more access to hot water and soap, fewer deaths would have resulted. Today we know that bacteria are easily disrupted from spreading from person to person with effective hand washing, hence the reason we have all become overly obsessed with doing it.

THE PLAGUE OF LONDON

As we continue to move back through human history let's consider the dark chapter in our history when plague swept across Europe. Cramped living conditions and poor sanitation has always played a role in spreading disease around the world. It's *rarely* taken into account, however, that during that period, hot showers and basic hygiene standards hadn't yet been invented. On the flip side, we could just as easily argue that improved sanitation has helped to **reduce** the spread of communicable disease.

Some historians believe that jumping fleas were behind the spread of the London plague, others believe that as populations grew, so did the growing problem of human waste which was often left to accumulate on the ground.

It's often been said that you could smell London long before you saw it. Can you imagine living in a city full of backed-up human waste?

Back then, primitive sanitation disposal meant emptying a filthy bucket of waste *directly* into the street, which meant the general population walked over raw sewage. This happened day in and day out, year after year. No toilet paper and not a bar of soap anywhere. *I know, right? Rather than look objectively at the evidence let's blame the plague on fleas.*

The Black Death wasn't a case of bad genes. It was most likely caused by poor sanitation. Despite the practice of leaving piles of open raw sewage in public places populations in cities continued to explode as did disease.

NO SHIT

Before we poke a finger at our ancestors' genes, let us remind ourselves that poor waste management and disease go hand in hand. Quite remarkably, right up to the late nineteenth century, indoor toilets were still considered a luxury! It really wasn't that long ago that "soil-men" were still being employed in towns and cities across the U.S. and Europe to remove human waste from our homes and businesses.

This was done typically at night and by hand by a four-man team consisting of a hole man, a rope man, and two tub men. The hole man crawled into the cesspool and filled the buckets. The rope man hauled up the buckets full of human waste and passed them to the two tub men who put them on the truck. These poor unfortunate souls carried these buckets of slopping waste all night long – now that's what you call a shitty job. As for the spills? They were often left in the yard where young children played during the day.

In pre-sewer America, imagine seeing an open sewage cart being pushed along Fifth Avenue with human excrement dripping over the sides. On a hot summer's day, it's often said that the stench would hang in the air making people gag as they scurried away.

When we look back at disease, let's not be in a rush to discount the obvious advantages of a modern flush toilet. Again, if we put our flexible thinking goggles on, ask who's really saving more lives here, doctors or plumbers?

So where does this all fit in?

It's easy to take our *current* standard of sanitation for granted but who knows, had the same standard been applied earlier in history then maybe the plague of London (along with many other diseases) could have been eradicated much sooner. Either way, nineteenth century sanitation continued to improve and your ancestors' genes not only went on *to survive,* they positively thrived. *Hoorah, for indoor plumbing and hot showers!*

Today we face a new threat from pesticides, pollution, parabens, plastics, and other petroleum-based products, *and that's just the letter P!* To blame our toxic world on our ancestors' genes is not just incorrect, it's actually a little insulting to them.

No?

Okay, let's try this.

Regardless of your ethnicity, your ancestors' *robust* roots are heavily carried in your DNA. If we again pull back the curtain of time 2000+ years we find an army of Roman soldiers who thought nothing of marching 25+ miles a day while wearing a hefty 65 pounds of body armor.

That's actually the equivalent of a bag of concrete! If your early ancestors' genes were so predisposed to weakness, how did the Romans manage this?

From the intense heat of North Africa to the cold and damp of Northern England, these determined Roman foot soldiers had no choice but to walk to the battlefield. No cough drops from the pharmacy, no last bus home. And after days or weeks of marching, these formidable warriors had a ferocious fight to the death to look forward to.

Imagine if earlier this morning you and I had been told to march twenty-five miles down the road while carrying a sixty-five-pound bag of concrete, only to find ourselves at the end of this delightful trek panting on a battlefield and standing toe-to-toe with a fully kitted-out Roman soldier. How do you think we would fair?

I think we are about to get our toxic butts kicked.

THOSE STUFFY VICTORIANS

Perhaps the blame for all our modern illnesses lies with those stuffy, oh-so-proper Victorians. Looking back to the Victorian era and based on the things they built, it's easy to see how our ancestors' minds worked.

From the early 1800s, the *meticulous* Victorian architects worked diligently to capture a stunning look that has yet to be rivaled. Across Europe you can still find these magnificent tall buildings standing to perfection, a true testament to all the craftsmen involved in building them.

By comparison, **our** modern architectural legacy too often includes quick-build metal boxes. And while this type of structure may be suitable for industrial units, it has a distinct emphasis on cheapness rather than quality. When we compare Victorian building standards to these soulless metal boxes, it becomes difficult to argue that building standards have improved. Clearly our ancestors got a lot of things right and maybe we shouldn't be in a rush to leave them buried in the past.

Compare the trim body shape of those Victorian figures to the high obesity rates today. They obviously got something right, right? According to bbc.co.uk/science the incidence of obesity is set to *treble* in the UK alone. You can rest assured, whatever is going is wrong here hasn't got a whole lot to do with your great grandparents' genes. Nope, seems to me they handed us some pretty good genes.

ME MATE DAVE

Earlier this week I visited an old school friend who was busy renovating a Victorian style house. He mentioned how difficult it had been to find workers who could replicate the same meticulous Victorian standard. To make his point he showed me a recently fitted door and complained that it was as crooked as the builder who fitted it.

It begs the question, how far has our current standard fallen, if the generation we once considered to be the "unwashed masses" is still to this day outperforming its offspring in so many ways.

As we talked, me mate Dave was busy assembling a flat pack set of IKEA drawers. I decided to leave when it became painfully obvious that the included two-page instruction pamphlet had gotten the better of a fully grown man. It also left me pondering, what was it those Victorians got right in construction a hundred years ago that we seem to be missing today?
Surely with all our modern day advancements we should be thriving far beyond anything imagined 100 years ago. Maybe in our rush for progress we forgot to bring along our common sense. Our insatiable desire for modern convenience often creates toxic by-products that have become an all too common part of our lives. *But it doesn't have to be this way.*

What if we somehow managed to tap into that strong work ethic that our Victorian ancestors had and spliced it with the best of our clean technology today? Maybe if we enthusiastically embraced our ancestral genes rather than blame them for our modern diseases we could begin to create a better world for ourselves. Whatever is going wrong with our health, it's a little too convenient to blame it all on our ancestors.

Moving forward, let's challenge ourselves to look at problems differently. Maybe if we took the same diligent care of our bodies as we do our houses, our careers, and our cars one day we could look forward to getting arrested on our 102nd birthday like Edie Simms.

Think of it this way, this shell we call our body is the home of our spirit; if we don't take care of our body – where are we to live?

What did we learn from this chapter?

When we look at historical diseases and their role in human history and their effect on the human race, it's worth remembering that squalid living conditions and a lack of personal hygiene have *always* played a pivotal role in disease. These are well-documented historical facts.

To accomplish what they did, your early ancestors must have been a pretty hearty bunch. By comparison, we now seem hell bent on making ourselves extinct.

Given the current statistics for dementia it seems quite questionable that, as we've been told, we've "never had it so good," and that living longer as we do isn't all that great if the case for longevity includes being spoon fed in front of a continuously droning TV set. Maybe our early ancestors' genes were stronger than people would have us believe.

So let us now look for solutions.

Chapter 9

THE CORNERSTONE OF HEALTH

Throughout this book I've tried to use simple comparisons to help make a point. Continuing in that vein, let's say that the human body is similar to a motor vehicle because they both rely on a set of systems to function properly. The car has a transmission system, an electrical system, and a braking system. It would be difficult to argue that any one system is more important than the others. We wouldn't want to be rolling down a hill without a braking system, nor would we want to be going up a hill without a transmission system. In short, all the systems are relevant.

The human body has eleven systems. Okay, let's zip through these: the skeletal system has 206 bones and can be thought of as the frame of a car. To help those bones move around we use the muscular system. We also have the respiratory system, the immune system, the reproductive system, the endocrine system, and the excretory system which includes filtration into the urinary system, yada, yada, yada.

Obviously we need blood pumping around the body and this is done via the circulatory system. We also have the integumentary system. If you aren't sure what that last one looks like, simply take a look in the mirror; it's everything you see on the outside like your skin, nails, hair, etc.

We also have a nervous system (my personal favorite). This bad boy is the *only* system that comes into direct contact with all the other systems. It links them all together much like the electrical wiring in your car and is similarly controlled by a complex onboard computer, which we humans call the brain. However, instead of using electric wires to carry the signals, the nervous system uses nerves to convey all information to and from the brain.

All these systems play an important role in our health and it would be foolish to think that any one system doesn't somehow affect the others.

GOOD NEWS

If you were counting (I know your type!), you have noticed that so far I've only named ten systems. That's because I've saved the best for last. This last system is so important it deserves its very own section. Any idea which system it is?

Here's a clue, *unlike* the many others systems *you* get to choose how well this one works, that's good news for anyone looking to have greater influence over their health. This last system provides fuel for the body and is called your digestive system, and every single day of your life you can choose to *enhance* this system or continue to damage it.

Based on my own lived experience and six years of meticulous research, I suspect that more illness begins here, in your *digestive* system, than anywhere else.

Why?

Think about it, the digestive system is home to a whopping 75+% of our immune system. If that hasn't just knocked you off your seat, let's try saying it another way.... *Death begins in the colon. I know, right? Bummer.*

Oh, but the fun doesn't stop there. Gut bacteria manufacture the majority of the brain's supply of serotonin. *Wait a second, are you catching this?* The digestive system is heavily affecting other systems! Serotonin is a chemical that's widely regarded by some researchers as being responsible for maintaining positive mood balance. Perhaps this is why the digestive system is often referred to as the body's *second* brain, and yet we think of depression and anxiety as something that affects only the mind.

BAD NEWS

Statistically speaking, so many chronic health problems have their roots firmly planted in the gut. These are by no means limited to hormonal problems, diabetes, chronic fatigue, inflammation, fibromyalgia, eczema, rosacea, anxiety, depression, Crohn's disease, IBS, celiac disease, and some pretty serious autoimmune diseases such as hashimoto's thyroiditis and rheumatoid arthritis to name but a few. To be clear, problems aren't confined to bloating or gas. Hell no, those are just basic clues to tell us we are doing something wrong, the overall issue is much bigger.

But the job of the gut or gastrointestinal tract (GI tract for short) isn't to cause illness, it's to digest food and absorb nutrients. To save any confusion, let's define what the GI tract is. In its most basic form the GI tract is responsible for digesting foods, absorbing nutrients, and expelling waste. *That's its job.* It starts at point A (the mouth) and ends at point B (the anus). What happens in between largely depends on the choices *you* make. *This is your job.*

Like the skin, which we talked about earlier, the GI tract is *alive* and intelligent; perhaps this is why we have "gut-feelings" about certain things, it's certainly not some dumbass design that has suddenly decided to malfunction. *I know what you are thinking because I thought it too ... if the GI tract is behind so much potential illness what's going wrong here?*

DO THIS

Humor me, for the next 24 hours what I'd like you to do is write down EVERYTHING you swallow, be it solid, fluid, vitamin, or pharmaceutical, etc. If you need to, carry a small pocket-sized notebook around so you don't miss anything. The next morning let's take a hard look at what you wrote. Something on that list is a problem; I just know it is. The aim of this section is to help you find out *what*.

Your digestive system is smart *but it's not magical.* If you put garbage in, garbage comes out. The digestive system can only work with the raw materials you give it. Make no mistake, everything we put into the digestive system is a choice, nobody is forcing us to buy processed/junk food.

Whatever it is you are feeding yourself *that* is the fuel your body runs on – whether its carrots, cucumbers, or crack. This in turn is fed to your cells. *Oh look, we've just come full circle, remember toxins out, nutrients in?*

Indian medicine and Chinese medicine are known to date back *thousands* of years and to this day they continue to stand the test of time. Both Indian and Chinese medicine regard the digestive system to be the cornerstone of all health. By comparison, western medicine with all its *modern* sophistication, offers little in the form of nutritional training to either its nurses or junior doctors. *Wait a second, are you catching this?*

The health of the digestive system is reliant on the foods we choose to swallow, yet science- based medicine doesn't value nutrition enough to train its doctors extensively in this field.

HOSPITAL FOOD

This lack of nutritional training creates an obvious disservice to the patients they treat. To take this a step further, we could argue that hospitals should be the one place where food is the absolute best money can buy. Sadly, it's usually exactly the opposite. *I know right? WTF? (Where's the food?)*

Given the explosion in both Type 2 diabetes and obesity, we would expect that doctors be given *more* nutritional training, not less. To be fair, I've yet to meet a doctor without a bright mind. These dedicated men and women are gifted in so many ways and yet results are often stifled by adopting a flawed approach to nutrition. Let's not forget, this isn't a new concept, 430 years B.C. Hippocrates was wandering around and saying outrageous things like:

ALL disease begins in the gut.

Personally, I believe most doctors *are* smart enough to figure this out for themselves, but for them to veer away from a path they have been trained to follow would almost certainly attract substantial criticism from their peers with their rigid thinking.

During my illness I was sometimes hooked up to some pretty fancy machines costing hundreds of thousands of dollars and yet the whole time no one ever thought to look me in the eye and say, *"Hey, quick question for you sir, what type of fuel are you running your body on?"* For all they knew I could have been stuffing my face twelve times a day with Twinkies... *just sayin'.*

THE BIG SQUEEZE

These days we ride our digestive systems pretty hard and to be fair it's doing *exactly* what we ask of it. Everything we swallow is pulled apart and squeezed in an attempt to extract all the juice and nutrients, these nutrients then run along the sides of the intestine wall where millions of tiny finger-like projections called villi are waiting to absorb them. Once all key nutrients have been extracted, any leftovers are sent out as waste.

Keep in mind that villi are *extremely* sensitive. This is good news if you have just eaten a *clean* apple, and not so great if you have just eaten chocolate flavored bacon chips washed down with a diet coke. I'm sure many of you already knew this, but don't worry if you didn't because I'm going to continue walking you through the whole process.

Astonishingly enough, the standard food pyramid is heavily influenced by the corporations who stand to benefit from the foods they recommend. With illness now spiraling out of control, it's difficult not to question the wisdom of their nutritional advice.

The whole GI tract is an incredibly delicate organ. If we feed it foods it likes, life is good; if we feed it foods that are laced with antibiotics, harmful additives, excessive sugars, pesticides, and growth hormones our reward is health problems. *I did mention that the digestive system is the cornerstone of all health, right?*

There is an unmistakable correlation between how we treat the GI tract and how it reacts. Treat it well and it will serve you well. **You can't put bad things in and expect good things to come out.** Almost two and a half thousand years later, Hippocrates is back again. He said it this way: "The bodily process of digestion and absorption is one of the most important to our health." Today this statement appears truer than ever and

Hippocrates is still considered to be one of the most outstanding figures in the history of medicine.

As we learned earlier, symptoms present themselves as the body's way of trying to get our attention. Constipation, bloating, acid reflux, gas, and stomach pain are all signs that the GI tract is no longer tolerating our poor food choices. I hate to be the one to tell you, but your gut doesn't like all those grains you keep forcing it to deal with.

Grains are found in things like bread, cereal, and pasta but they also sneak into lots of other products. Before this book ends you will know how to spot them.

Grains are the seed of the crop, and nature designed these seeds to survive if something came along and ate them. Maybe that is the reason grains can be so problematic for certain people. Hello gluten types. Although, this can be a much wider issue than just gluten and here's why. Often when people go gluten free they exchange one grain for a different one. Unfortunately, that doesn't always work out too well. It would be like quitting one brand of cigarettes and exchanging it for another.

Let's flush this one out early, it's not just gluten that's causing the problem, *all* grains can be harsh on the digestive system.

Grains also have a twisted cousin and it goes by the name of corn. Corn is similar to grain in that it was designed by nature to be a part of the plant's reproductive system. For that reason, corn is notoriously difficult to digest. I'm sure you've noticed that when corn comes out the other end it often looks just like it did going in. Corn is the seed of the crop, and because it's so cheap to produce it is often used in food as a filler. Adding to the problem, 90% of all corn is now genetically modified. But even organic corn can be harsh on the digestive system.

Let's look at this as a positive. You aren't even a quarter way through this book and already we have identified two of the biggest players for causing digestive issues. Grains and corn.

What you choose to do with this information is up to you. Obviously eliminating these products from your diet today would be a huge first step in the right direction. Rather than letting this information overwhelm you, you can begin to incorporate the simple step of reducing grains even as more nutritional news continues to pour from the spout.

What did we learn from this chapter?

If you are plagued by any multi-faceted health problem of *"unknown"* origin, always look first to the gut. Learn to respect your digestive system; it plays a *huge* role in making or breaking your health. Death *begins* in the colon.

Think of food as fuel for the body and then take responsibility for the way you eat rather than handing the responsibility over to the supermarket. Unless you are aware of the devious tactics supermarkets adopt they will *always* get you to buy more of what you don't need.

Homework: make a comprehensive list of anything that passes your lips over the next 24 hours and then begin to analyze those items as if they are clues left at a crime scene. And look at them with this question in mind: is this nourishment or junk?

Chapter 10

IT TAKES GUTS TO LEAK

Certain foods can be harsh on the gut, no question about it. Over time, the delicate lining of the gut can become irritated and inflamed. Once this happens, it's been suggested that the lining becomes permeable, allowing food particles to ooze through and enter the bloodstream. *Let's explore this theory.*

From the time we swallow it, to the time it leaves the body, food is intended to remain **inside the digestive system.** For it to stray outside the digestive system and enter the bloodstream is both unusual and unnatural. In fact, some might say this is almost as unnatural as the way we now grow our food. *Ah, but I digress.*

It's fair to say that most sections of the food chain are now routinely sprayed with some pretty heavy duty pesticides. This has become an everyday farming practice and nobody seems to mind. However, many of these pesticides contain EDCs (endocrine disrupting chemicals) which work to kill pests by disrupting their central nervous systems. Some of the newer insecticides also work by disrupting the guts of insects. *Hmm, I see.*

In recent times, food has undergone some pretty radical changes. "Modifying" our food sounds good in theory, but I've yet to hear anyone say with confidence how this will affect us long term. Throw into the mix literally thousands of food additives and preservatives and maybe we shouldn't be all that surprised when people experience digestive issues. All this brings us back to the theory of a leaky gut and perhaps we should start with a visual understanding.

In your mind's eye imagine holding a bicycle inner tube, then take a pair of scissors and cut it so that it becomes a single straight line. Next place the inner tube on the floor. As you look down at it, imagine it is your digestive system. The design is similar. Both are hollow tubes with an opening at the top (the mouth) and an exit at the bottom (your butt).

Now imagine putting a banana into the top of that inner tube and slowly squeezing it all the way down until it arrives out at the bottom end. Once again, this is very similar to how your digestive system works. Food has gone into a tube at the top and then *squeezed* all the way down until it came out at the bottom as waste.

When we try to do the same thing with certain grains or seeds you can bet they are ultra-harsh on the inside of the tube. To make this point, let us now imagine taking those same scissors, only this time make several microscopic nicks anywhere you like along the inner-tube. If we again attempt to push a through a banana (or any other type of food you can think of) you will notice that small food particles squeeze through some of those nicks. *Hold this image. Got it?*

Hopefully this mental image is able to demonstrate the "theory" behind the syndrome commonly referred to as leaky gut. Once tiny food particles begin oozing out, they cause a much wider problem. Instead of finding their way to the bathroom with the rest of the food gang you've eaten and digested, these tiny particles find their way into the bloodstream. *That's not good, right?*

Not if you happen to be a protein by the name of gluten. The immune system is *not* expecting to see a piece of your bacon sandwich floating around in your bloodstream. As far as the immune system is concerned, all bacon sandwiches are (and should be) safely trapped **inside** the inner tube (your digestive tract). When the immune system spots the bacon sandwich in the bloodstream, it gets a little freaked out and sends the whole system into red alert. Those proteins found in gluten are treated as foreign invaders. *Boomshakalaka, say hello to your new food sensitivities.*

In certain people, the gluten found in wheat, barley, and rye has the potential to cause a wide range of reactions ranging from a feeling of general fatigue to mental confusion *and just about everything in between.* It also pays to keep in mind that although oats don't contain gluten, they certainly can become cross-contaminated with gluten during processing. The good news is you can get *certified* gluten free oats, but it pays to be sure of the source. The bad news is some people are still going to react to even gluten free oats.

INFLAMMATION

Given that the standard western diet is heavily reliant on grains, unwarranted attacks can become frequent and systemic inflammation is your reward. As we move through these chapters you will learn that inflammation plays a *pivotal* role in illness.

A small amount of localized inflammation can be thought of as a well-guarded campfire with a practical benefit. However, inflammation left to linger can soon become a rampant forest fire. The connection between illness and this type of out of control inflammation is well documented.

It seems that doctors are better equipped (or more apt) to hand out pills than they are dietary advice, and the theory of a permeable gut lining doesn't always sit well with them. But doctors *do* agree that gluten has the potential to cause damage to the intestinal lining, and when those intestines become inflamed it can be harder for the body to absorb nutrients.

Yet merely mention the notion of a leaky gut in your physician's office and you can expect to be met with an uncomfortably long stare. Keep in mind that the pharmaceutical industry is like no other. It generates higher profit margins than the oil industry! Big pharma has no interest in your nutritional needs.

Many of us have been conditioned to think the answer to our health problems lies in swallowing more pills, but trying to medicate our way out of a poor diet is just poor judgment.

With so many diseases labeled "unknown," maybe the leaky gut theory should be given a little more merit or, *at the very least,* explored to the fullest.

If you were paying close attention you may have noticed that the keyword I keep using to describe all these events is "theory" so you might now be asking **why** this is still a *theory*? Well, clinical trials cost millions of dollars and this "theory" simply isn't sexy enough to pay for those clinical trials. Put simply, there's no money to be made from telling you to change your diet.

LEST WE FORGET

The remarkable story of doctor Ignaz Semmelweis began in 1846 when he took his first medical position as an appointed assistant in a maternity ward at Vienna General Hospital. Shortly after doing so he noticed that some wards had a disproportionately higher infant mortality rate than others.

Ward 1 gained a particularly bad reputation, so much so that many local women preferred to give birth in the street and, statistically speaking, their chances of survival actually improved! Young doctor Semmelweis was told by his seniors that the reason for these higher deaths was a "poisonous gas" that often came into the ward. But doctor Semmelweis was quick to notice something else.

Ward 1 was directly next to the mortuary and it was a common practice for doctors to perform autopsies in the morning and then work in Ward No 1 in the afternoon.

Back then hygiene wasn't properly understood and a scalpel used in an autopsy was often later used to cut an umbilical cord. Even basic hand washing wasn't in place until Dr. Semmelweis introduced it as standard protocol.

But here's the rub.

Despite the obvious improvements that included an immediate reduction in deaths, the views held by Dr. Semmelweis were not part of the general medical beliefs at the time and were met with hostility. He was not only attacked by senior medical figures; he was actually dismissed from his position. *I know, right? Keep reading, it gets even worse.*

Ward No 1 doctors went back to their old ways and fatality rates immediately returned to their level pre-1847. Dr. Semmelweis was so incensed by such ignorance that he wrote open letters to his main critics calling them "ignorant murderers." It takes courage to challenge such embedded beliefs, and for the next 20 years Dr. Semmelweis desperately tried to warn people that germs from a dead body needed to be washed off a doctor's hands before attempting to deliver a baby!

Unfortunately, the status quo had just about enough of doctor Dr. Semmelweis and his germ theory and in 1865 he was tricked into visiting a mental asylum. When he tried to leave, Dr. Semmelweis was forcibly restrained and put in a straitjacket. His injuries were such that they became infected and two weeks later he died. Dr. Semmelweis was buried in Vienna and very few people attended his funeral. Today his theory is saving lives. Who knows? Perhaps in time we will look back and find that the leaky gut theory has merit equal to the germ theory.

> *Those who do not learn history are doomed to repeat it.*
> – George Santayana

I appreciate that some readers may already have quite a comprehensive understanding of these concepts while others may be hearing these things for the very first time. In either case my goal is to always leave you with an abundance of relevant information presented in a way that's easy to absorb.

If you must, continue to fight the idea that the digestive system is the cornerstone of all health, but sooner or later something is going to click. When it does, this renewed understanding will serve you well.

IT'S NOT YOUR FAULT

You might not hear this all that often, but the poor food choices you make are not entirely your fault. You *should* be able to go into the supermarket and pick out anything on the shelf to nourish the body. But somewhere along the line everything got twisted and today we are more likely to find foods high in calories and low in nutritional content than the reverse.

It's not easy to find a product on the supermarket shelf that doesn't have some kind of harmful additives, colorings, preservatives, artificial flavors, or high fructose corn syrup, etc. This begs the question, *what's up with food?* As a rule of thumb, if you can't pronounce the words on the label, chances are the tiny villi in your intestines aren't going to like it.

I was once at my local food store and noticed an elderly lady in the parking lot struggling to load a heavy grocery bag into her car. It took me but a second to help lift the bag into her trunk and she was duly thankful. As she drove away waving, it made me wonder if she understood the meaning of the words on the labels of the foods I'd glimpsed in her bag, words like acesulfame-K, Aspartame, and monosodium glutamate.

Perhaps the onus shouldn't be on the shopper to have to read the fine print on every label. With so many potentially toxic food additives, it can be a full time job just keeping up with them.

The hard way is to read every label; the easy way is not to buy food *with* labels. *I know, pretty radical right? Hold onto your hat, more is coming.*

You may view your local supermarket as a convenience, but remember it's a business, and as such it is there to make money. If the supermarket is creating meaningful jobs and making it easy for you to gather food, that's great. But someone needs to ask, if food is playing a role in illness why can't we just go back to having simple ingredients that are less harmful to our body? That kind of food and those ingredients can still be sold in supermarkets for our convenience.

If you aren't sure *what* to buy or *where* to buy it, no need to panic – this book is here to help. The good news is that if you choose to eat three times a day then you also get to vote with your feet three times a day, a topic we will be coming back to in more detail. The bad news is it's actually easier to buy crack cocaine on the street than it is to buy locally raised organic chicken. *I know, right? What's up with that?*

BE KIND TO YOUR SMALL INTESTINE

For sure the digestive system is super important but the problem isn't confined to what we put inside our belly, it's also what we **do** to our belly that can affect our health. For this exercise we need a small cloth tape measure similar to the type found in a sewing kit. *Got one? ... Great.*

Today more than ever we spend a disproportionate amount of our time sitting down; we do it in our cars, at our desks, at the movies, even while we eat. Hell, you are probably doing it right now! While **sitting down,** grab that cloth tape measure and run it around your waist and make a note of the number. Now stand up and do the same thing. What you have are two very different numbers, *am I right?*

Now take off your pants (trousers to the rest of us) and measure the inside of the waistband. *Forget what the label says,* just measure it and then write *that* number down. Finally do the same thing with your underwear while in the *"unstretched"* position.

Now compare all four sets of numbers, suddenly it becomes clear that our clothes have the uncanny potential to restrict the free movement of our small intestine for maybe *sixteen* hours a day! If you suffer from bloating this whole restrictive process will be magnified tenfold, especially when you are sitting. Throw in a few leather belts and buckles and we really compound the problem.

The goal here is to try to avoid *unnecessary* discomfort to the small intestine. Keep in mind that the accurate sizing of our clothes depends largely on who made them. It can be a costly mistake to simply grab "your" size and go. Always take the time to try new clothes on *in a sitting position* and make sure you aren't shooting yourself in the foot by restricting the very cornerstone of your health. Also be aware that our body shapes can change from season to season, it's not uncommon to gain a few pounds in the winter.

Your digestive system needs you to wear clothes that are *comfortable*. If you happen to be a total fashionista and currently wearing ultra-skinny jeans, then I realize this news is probably falling on deaf ears. Try to keep in mind that hospital gowns come in limited colors and generally speaking are less flattering than jeans. Organ compression can lead to serious digestive problems down the road. I'd really like to prevent that from happening to you. *Now go burn those skinny jeans.*

As we move through this book together I'll continue recommending key people for you to check out on YouTube, this ensures **all** gaps are plugged.

This time around I'd like to suggest that you take a look at the leaky gut through the eyes of Dr. Darren Schmidt. I love this guy; his videos are always clear and highly informative yet simple enough not to be a distraction.

Over the years I've literally watched thousands of hours of medical clips to gather all this information for you. I find Dr. Schmidt's style refreshingly different, which helps keep my interest in the game. You can find him in today's homework assignment below.

What did we learn from this chapter?

Once gluten becomes a problem, switching to gluten free products is unlikely to be helpful. To help you turn this corner, it may be more helpful to go *totally* grain free.
Remember that many of the great medical discoveries were first mocked and even vilified by the medical establishment. For the sake of your digestive system, consider buying whole foods that come without labels. Try to wear comfortable clothes.

Homework: check out Dr. Darren Schmidt talking about leaky gut on YouTube. His videos are always a breath of fresh air.
For e-book users here's the direct link.
https://www.youtube.com/watch?v=j1T5LLfk6L8

Chapter 11

ALKALIZE TO ENERGIZE

While we are all uniquely different, we all share this one thing in common – our blood needs to be slightly alkaline for us to stay healthy. Every single day we owe our lives to a delicate balancing act between the two states of alkalinity and acidity. *So what does that mean?*

The pH range is quite small and to help us measure the state between acidity and alkalinity we use numbers ranging from zero to fourteen. The lower the number, the more acidic, the higher the number, the more alkaline. For example, battery acid would be around 0 and household ammonia around 12. The number 7 is represented as being unbiased or neutral – neither acidic nor alkaline.

The body strives to keep our blood pH tightly regulated at approximately 7.35 to 7.45 (slightly alkaline) and it generally does an excellent job. However, there isn't a huge margin of error and even *slight* differences can have *serious* health implications.

When blood has excessive acidity it goes by the name of acidosis. Acidosis can lead to numerous health conditions and even death. The American Association for Clinical Chemistry (AACC) categorizes acidosis as lower than 7.35, which really isn't too far away from 7.45.

We don't want to be too acidic or too alkaline. When the pH of the blood becomes *too* alkaline it is referred to as alkalosis. Alkalosis occurs **above** 7.45, again bringing with it a whole host of health problems. We could conclude that blood pH has a narrow range of 7.35 to 7.45 and stepping outside of those parameters brings big trouble. Try to remember these sets of numbers, before this chapter ends I'm going to ask you about them.

So by now you are probably thinking, if this whole pH thing is so important, what the heck keeps it in balance? That's a really great question and I like the way you are starting to think. It's sometimes said that knowledge is having all the right answers, but *intelligence* is asking the right questions.

The pH of the body is kept *within* this range in part by the kidneys and lungs. When the body becomes too acidic, the kidneys help restore balance by using common electrolytes – sodium, potassium, magnesium, calcium, plus chloride, phosphates, and sulfates – to buffer acidity. Put simply, this buffering system helps keep you alive.

Here's the rub: if the body is kept in an acidic state for any length of time, minerals used to buffer that acidity may become depleted. The body doesn't want you to die from an excess of acidity and will do *whatever* it takes to keep the blood pH from slipping below 7.35. *Can you see the problem yet?*

When the body runs short of available minerals, it takes drastic action by stealing minerals from the bones, cells, organs, and tissues. This isn't an ideal situation and can be thought of as the body pulling the emergency brake just to keep you alive.

Minerals are critical to our overall health not just to buffer acidity but also to keep the cells functioning properly. Cells devoid of minerals cannot dispose of waste or even oxygenate optimally. As mentioned earlier, you and I are nothing but cells from head to toe. **Now** *do you see the importance of this?*

A lack of minerals will *hinder* the absorption of vitamins and allow toxins and pathogens to accumulate in the body. Ultimately this will lead to a suppressed immune system. All of this stems from a body striving to keep itself from becoming too acidic. So what would make the body too acidic?

STRESS

There are several factors and one of these can be stress. But as we all know, stress is an omnipresent part of life that we can never fully get away from. The best we can do is manage it. *I know, right? That's much easier said than done.*

We all get stressed from time to time but the good news is that by the end of this book you will have an effective strategy for reducing stress. If you find yourself doing a job you hate or, even worse, working **two** jobs just to surround yourself with bigger and better things, then it might be worth re-evaluating what's really important to you – more stuff, or more health? When stress gets to the point where it's making you ill, then clearly you have the right to choose another path. Sometimes owning less can lead to more health.

I once made this same point to an elderly Scotsman who happened to be a retired accountant. As I watched him work himself into the ground I joked with him there are no pockets in a shroud and for sure he couldn't take any of his money with him. He looked me squarely in the eye and said, "Son, if I can't take it with me then I'm not going." He's dead now so I guess I was right and he was wrong.

While so much of stress can be self-inflicted, it can also come from the people with whom we surround ourselves. Maybe you have a toxic friend in your life that's adding to your stress – some people are just wired that way. You can't change them, but you *can* change your exposure to them. And I suspect deep down you already know this.

Given the importance of this topic, you may find it desirable to periodically monitor your pH. This can easily be done at home. For this test you will need a set of relatively inexpensive pH testing strips, often sold in your local health food store. The kit is inexpensive and comes with litmus paper that you will pee on. Simply match the sample test strip with the various color shades found on the box.

There is a right way to do this and a wrong way.

The wrong way is to pee on them as soon as you get them home or, God forbid, try to pee on them while standing in line at the store (generally speaking never a good idea). My point is that rushing to do the test will *always* give you a false reading, so it's a waste of both the litmus strips and your time.

The *right way* is to wait and pee on them first thing in the morning after you've had a minimum of six hours of sleep. This will give you an accurate reading.

For some, dealing with stress and drinking (bad) coffee go hand in hand, so now we have two things contributing to our acidity. Shall we go for three? How about alcohol, smoking, irregular eating patterns, or lack of exercise? All these things are known to be acid forming. If you **are** a coffee drinker, don't panic, there is an easy way around this problem. Keep reading.

Diet can also play a part, although not in a way that most seem to understand. The body is designed to buffer out all acidic food, but each time the buffering system is called into action it depletes vital minerals from somewhere else in the body. Great if you have an abundance of buffering minerals at your disposal, not so great if you are trying to supplement your way out of a bad diet that's mineral deficient. *Are we there yet?*
If you were paying close attention earlier, you noticed that I said the *kidneys and lungs* help keep pH balanced, hence the reason exercise is important because it gets the lungs working. I'm sure many of you already understand the benefits of regular exercise, but if the idea makes you cringe, then I bring good news because the following doesn't require you to join a gym or buy a new pair of running shoes. *Check this out.*

Here's an exercise that isn't dependent on the weather and you can even do this while listening to music or watching your favorite television show; your cells really don't care, they just like to move. To do this you will need one of those small inexpensive yoga-type trampolines. And all you do is bounce on it real gentle and stop whenever you like. The idea isn't to put you off doing this, the idea is to encourage you to do whatever feels comfortable and then stop. *Why?*

Cells like don't like to be stagnant and they react well to movement. Imagine a balloon half filled with water. Now in your mind's eye walk with that balloon held out in front of you. As you move, so does the water in the balloon. This is how the energy in your cells reacts to movement.

124

Using a mini trampoline indoors means you can do this in the privacy of your home any time and you don't have to worry about people pointing at you in the gym. Now that you have this information I know you are smart enough to work out a simple bouncing program for yourself without me nagging you.

Compared to jogging on the sidewalk, this form of fun exercise cuts down on that harsh repetitive impact to the knees and you never again have to worry about stray dogs trying to bite you as you jog along the street.

If gentle bouncing isn't your thing, then I'd like to invite you to walk in any direction for 30 seconds and come right back again. Excellent, you have just exercised for a whole minute, what say tomorrow we shoot for 2 minutes? The point is this, committing to an intense exercise program can be enough to talk some people out of doing it entirely. Better to do a little at a time rather than none at all.

If you really are a couch potato, then this next tip is just for you. Whenever you go to the store make a habit of parking your car in the far corner of the parking lot. Yup, I'm talking about the corner *farthest* away from the store. *Why?*

For some folks this might be the only walk they get today, and walking helps to get the lungs working which in turn helps to contribute to the overall balancing of pH. If you are disabled by illness, then try to move whatever you can to get your blood pumping. It's important to do the best you can, *not the least you can.*

Unfortunately, the standard American diet (SAD – aptly enough) is a little tilted toward acidity. Fast food, fried food, soda, and sugar are all acid-forming. These foods are the exact opposite of what we need to eat to be healthy. Take a look at the list below and see which of these things you consume on a regular basis. And this is by no means a complete list, but you can use it as a rule of thumb.

- meats are acidic
- vegetables are alkaline

- cola is acidic
- water is alkaline
- processed foods are acidic
- whole foods are alkaline
- cheese is acidic
- goat's milk is alkaline
- lemons are acidic *outside* the body
- lemons become alkalizing *inside* the body

As you've probably noticed, some rules tend to have exceptions, and today the exception is lemons. When a lemon is sitting on your kitchen counter, it is acidic (pH below 7) but once you eat that lemon and it is fully metabolized, it becomes alkalizing (pH above 7)

Rather than inundate you with a long list of foods that are highly acidic, try to keep in mind we are simply looking to keep our body in *balance.* Fortunately, at this point you don't have to overthink this concept because everything you are reading is now beginning to pull you in this direction *automatically.*

If at any point this all gets to be too much, try to remember this simple rule of thumb. At every meal cover at least half your plate with dark leafy vegetables; doing this will help keep those excessive portion sizes under control. Greens also help detoxify, and they help alkalize. Good fats are pretty important too, and this is something you can look forward to learning about later in the book.

TEST FAIL

Now, let's see who's been paying attention. If I asked you for the pH of the body I'm sure you would quickly recall the numbers 7.35 and 7.45, and you would be wrong. The pH of the *blood* is 7.35 and 7.45 but the body has a stomach, and boy is the stomach highly acidic – with good reason.

On the pH scale, the acid in the stomach is quite low, somewhere between 1 and 3 which can easily dissolve metal! *I know what you're thinking because I thought it too: if the acid in my stomach can dissolve metal, why doesn't it eat right through the lining of my stomach?* That's another great question and the short answer is that the stomach has a mucous membrane and a wall of cells that are constantly replaced; as one layer burns through, another steps in to replace it.

We seem to find ourselves once again looking at the importance of the digestive system. It really is the beginning and end, the alpha and omega, the *cornerstone* of all health. The acid in our stomach needs to be able to turn whatever we eat into a liquid mush for better absorption. This is the reason for ultra-*strong* stomach acid, also known as hydrochloric acid, or HCL.

Again, allow me to repeat that good digestion starts in the mouth and properly chewing food aids the whole process. Once swallowed, food travels down a long tube called the esophagus. At the end of that tube is a small muscular valve that opens up just enough to allow the food you just chewed to drop into a bath of stomach acid. See diagram below.

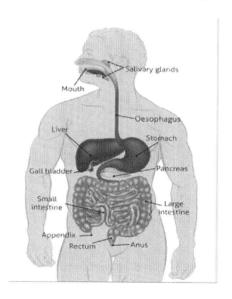

The stomach has been working this way since the beginning of time and you kinda have to marvel at the design. Once the food has been turned into liquid it is ready to move onto the next stage. *Oh, but wait, there's a problem. Can you see it?*

Food drops down the shoot into a bath of acid – splash! Food turns into soup; soup then oozes out a little at a time into the small intestine, so far so good, right?. *Meh, not so fast...what if the stomach acid has become weak through illness, neglect, abuse, or simply through time?* **The whole process of digestion hinges on this pivotal stage.** If the acid isn't strong enough, a whole chain reaction of negative events can begin to unfold. Not least, nutrients will struggle to be fully absorbed. Remember, we need the nutrients to power and rebuild our cells.

Bloating, belching, flatulence, indigestion, diarrhea, and constipation are all clues that something isn't quite right with the stomach and, in certain circumstances, a person with weak stomach acid may also suffer from heartburn. *Wait a second, did you catch that?*

But isn't heartburn treated by the million-dollar antacid industry? *If only it were that simple.* If this is you, my question is this: how has years of taking antacids been working for you? Has it fixed the problem or does it just keep coming back, again and again and again?

Some believe that antacids can add to the problem by making *already* low stomach acid even lower. The stomach then strives to balance itself while all the while you continue trying to *override* it with alkaline pills. Now you are caught in a constant dance with yourself. Sometimes, we need to get out of the way and let the body do the job it was designed to do.

Obviously if you are taking a *prescription* antacid that is something you need to work out with your doctor to ensure this approach is right for you. While you are there, it might be worth getting tested for H-pylori which is a type of bacteria ALSO known to *reduce* stomach acid ... *just sayin'.*

A lack of stomach acid is believed by some to be the culprit that allows the valve at the end of the esophagus to open back up. Known as the lower esophageal sphincter (LES), this valve is a muscle that contracts much the same way the anus does. It forms an import seal to keep the acid from slipping back up into the esophagus where it can cause damage and heartburn. Some schools of thought suggest that the LES valve has some sensitivity to the acid in the stomach, and when the stomach acid is too low it may be fooled into opening back up. Hence, antacids aren't really helping the problem.

According to the late, great Mr. Einstein, the definition of insanity is doing the same thing over and over and expecting a different outcome. If taking antacids hasn't fixed the problem, it *may* be worth trying a different approach. *Increasing* stomach acid rather than decreasing it is easy enough to do and before we end this chapter I'll share with you the best way to do it.

For now, the problem is much bigger than heartburn. Weak stomach acid has a domino effect effect throughout the remaining stages of digestion. The slushy soup is now a semifluid mass of partly digested food with the fancy name of chyme or chymus. It's then expelled by the stomach into the duodenum. (See previous diagram.)

Without wanting to confuse you with lots of fancy names let's just work with the primary rule of physics and say that all shit rolls downhill, and in this case, it passes a whole bunch of important sensory checkpoints on the way down. These checkpoints scrutinize the quality of the chyme, which for now we'll just call slushy soup.

In theory, if the quality of the stomach acid is good, so is the quality of the slushy soup. If not, then it's a case of too bad, so sad, because when it comes to shit there is no going backwards.

Once our slushy soup enters the small intestine, enzymes are eagerly waiting to break things down even more. This can present a problem if the hydrochloric acid in the stomach hasn't done its job properly.

The three main enzymes the body uses to aid in digestion are amylase, protease, and lipase, but many other specialized enzymes also help in the process. Cells that line the intestines also make enzymes called maltase, sucrase, and lactase, and each is able to convert a specific type of sugar into glucose. We need these enzymes to help us absorb our nutrients. **Do we need to know all these terms as a lay person?** Probably not, but I know it disturbs some people when I use terms like slushy soup. But I digress …

Two more enzymes by the names of renin and gelatinase then come into play. Renin acts on proteins in milk, converting them into smaller molecules called peptides. These are then fully digested by pepsin.

Gelatinase digests gelatin and collagen – two large proteins in meat – into moderately-sized compounds whose digestion is then completed by pepsin, trypsin, and chymotrypsin, producing amino acids. *I know, right? Who thinks like this?*

If weak stomach acid allows partially undigested food to move through the digestive system, the whole delicate balance is disrupted. A domino effect occurs as the liver, gallbladder, and pancreas also pick up on the lack of acidity in the slushy soup and react accordingly. *If weak acid in the stomach isn't doing its job optimally, it's a safe bet that neither is anything else.*

Rather than trying to bolt the stable door after the horse has fled, it might be prudent to pay particular attention to *increasing* stomach acid. Stomach acid also plays an important role in protecting us from bacteria that may be on ingested food.

In some people, it's thought that chemotherapy can reduce stomach acid. If this is you, you may notice a sudden increase in acid reflux and this chapter becomes all the more relevant.

To recap: We need strong stomach acid to help us break down our foods, especially proteins. Strong stomach acid also helps kill off any harmful bacteria that may come in with food. Weak stomach acid on the other hand can cause a whole host of health problems.

Before we get into this next part, let me once again stress that the following information should serve only as a guide to help you in your own research. It cannot and should not be substituted for medical advice.

Okay, here's one way I test to see if my stomach acid is running low.

1 First thing in the morning, mix 1/4 teaspoon of baking soda in 4-6 ounces of room temp water.
2 Drink the baking soda on an empty stomach.
3 Time how long it takes before you belch.
4 If you have not belched within five minutes, stop timing.

In theory, if your stomach is producing adequate amounts of stomach acid you'll likely belch within two to three minutes. Early and repeated belching may be due to *excessive* stomach acid (but don't confuse these burps with small little burps from swallowing air while drinking the solution). **Any belching after 3 minutes indicates a low acid level.**

Because we are all uniquely different, timeframes may vary a little. This test is only a basic indicator and you might want to do more testing to determine the level of your stomach acid with your doctor. This test is a guide and *not* to be considered accurate enough to rule out low stomach acid. To rule out low stomach acid you will need to also try what's called the Heidelberg test or Betaine HCL challenge test.

If stomach acid is found to be too low, there are lots of ways to increase it. One is to use a supplement called Betaine HCL, which is best taken with protein.

Another is to take a tablespoon of apple cider vinegar (ACV) 10 mins before each meal to help increase stomach acid. Simply mix the ACV in 8 oz. of room temp water and drink (*for health, not taste*).

Ayurvedic (Indian) medicine suggests that you can raise your stomach acid by mixing one freshly squeezed lemon, 4 oz. of water, approximately three knuckles of chopped raw ginger, and a half teaspoon of sea salt. Leave this mixture to pickle for a few days and then take a teaspoon of the mixture before meals. It's an acquired taste, but I actually got used to it and then my body craved it. Keep in mind that Ayurvedic medicine is more than 3000 years old and it's still going strong. As ALWAYS, however, check with your doctor *first* and then, as with anything new, start with a small test dose and go slow.

If you take only one thing away from this chapter then let it be the value of your stomach acid. Putting our health back together is a process. And slowly, piece by piece, we are now bringing pieces of the puzzle into view.

What did we learn from this chapter?

We need the *body* to be slightly alkaline but the *stomach* needs to be quite acidic to help digest food. Stomach acid is super important to good health.

The body strives to keep our blood pH tightly regulated and it generally does an excellent job of doing so. If your body's pH is not balanced, you *cannot* effectively assimilate vitamins, minerals, and food supplements. You can test your pH with litmus strips by doing it *the right way* (so no peeing in the aisle of the health food store).

Getting gentle exercise helps regulate pH because it gets the lungs working. Committing to a short but regular exercise every day is a 100% improvement over doing nothing.

Homework: to help you better understand this concept take a look at a short YouTube video entitled *"You thought you understood acid/alkaline diet... until you saw this!"* By Peter Glidden

E-book readers simply click this link YouTube clip by Dr. Peter Glidden,

Chapter 12

FARMER FRED

As a society, it seems we have become accustomed to having large portions of the population in a state of ill health. Today, we don't bat an eyelid when we see someone speeding down the road in an electric wheelchair while breathing on a portable oxygen tank.

Growing up in the 70s, things were a little different. I went to a rather large inner city school but I cannot recall a single kid who took medication or who had allergies. *I know, right? What changed?*

In any given school year, you could count the number of sickly kids on one hand – even though we know schools are notoriously full of germs. And the truth is, some of those kids were suspected of faking it just to get out of gym class. If our current epidemic of health problems were mirrored in any segment of the animal kingdom, it would be quite shocking.

Imagine driving through the rolling English countryside on a sunny day and coming upon a large sign with the warning: KEEP OUT, 1 in 2 COWS WILL SOON BECOME SERIOUSLY ILL!

Maybe we should look at the problem from *that* perspective. In the following scenario, humans are played by cows and you can think of the vet as our well-meaning doctor.

COWS

Farmer Fred wakes early one spring morning and sets off to feed his cows. He notices something odd and picks up his pace. On closer inspection, his cows look lifeless, tired, and show little interest in their food. The farmer eagerly rattles their food bucket in a bid to grab their attention "Don't you want your feed today?" he asks. A pool of large, vacant eyes stares back at him. Adding a spackle of enthusiasm to his voice he offers it a second time. "Come on girls, it's your favorite, soy and corn." *(I know, right? Cows used to eat grass.)*

The next morning Fred telephones the vet to explain that his cows just don't seem themselves. "They probably have CFS," says the vet.

Fred's silence prompts the vet to continue.

"I'll come take a look this afternoon."

Fred's cows are obviously an important commodity to him; they are his livelihood. As he anxiously waits for the vet to arrive, his mind becomes preoccupied with tracing back his steps. He knows for sure his cows weren't ill yesterday, and logically he's thinking something must have changed. *But what?*

Before he has time to identify the problem, the vet arrives and Fred loses his train of thought. The vet examines the whole herd and confirms that Fred's cows do indeed have a form of CFS (Cow Fatigue Syndrome).

"Is it serious?" Fred asks.

"Totally," says the vet.

Fred presses for more details, "What causes it?"

"Not sure," the vet replies.

"Well, then how do you fix it?"

"No clue."

The vet opens his brown leather medical bag and begins to inject each of the cows. By the end of the day, Fred has a huge bill to pay and illness continues to sweep through his herd.

For the cows, feeling ill becomes their new "normal," and by the end of summer Fred has again noticed something very odd. A third of his cows have become grossly obese.

Fred's wife asks, "Did you think to maybe change their feed?"

Fred reminds her that *he* is the head farmer and she is *not* a vet.

Again the vet is called out and this time he declares an outbreak of cow diabetes. "Not much we can do Fred, diabetes rates are climbing."

Before long, because of complications of advanced diabetes, some of the cows have had limbs amputated and nobody wants to eat steak for dinner.

As the autumn winds begin to blow, Fred again finds himself pressing his vet for answers. This time his concern is that after drinking town water from the outside tap some of his cows are shivering with cold.

"Hmm, looks like a real nasty case of hypothyroidism," says the vet. Neither of the men think to check the water and the vet leaves with the words, "See you soon, Fred," hanging ominously in the air.

As winter rolls around, Fred's situation goes from bad to worse. Sadly, some of his cows are now dying. Without flinching, the vet delivers another blow. "Fred, I hate to tell you, but your herd has cow cancer and eventually it will affect one out of every two cows."
The vet proceeds to cut, burn, and poison all the cancerous areas, the same way his father did it, and his father before him. As he leaves the farm, the vet thanks the farmer for his payment and tips his hat to bid the farmer good day.

A month later Fred telephones to confirm that the vet's math was indeed correct and 50% of his herd has now been wiped out. Sensing Fred's disappointment the, the vet quietly utters the words, "I'm so sorry for your loss," and hangs up the phone.

Shortly before retiring to bed, Fred breaks the devastating news to his wife. "In all my years of farming I've never managed such a toxic herd." This time his wife remains silent and allows Fred's incompetence to run free. Perhaps she has been conditioned not to question.

Winter arrives, there is snow on the ground, and Fred diligently closes his books for the year. Despite heavy losses, Fred takes some comfort when he notes that his grain bill for the year was much lower than usual. Fred's wife, who is looking over his shoulder, notes that although the grain bill was lower because they had fewer cows to feed, their vet bill was dramatically higher for the year. Once again she quietly accepts that it's not her responsibility and leaves it to the "experts" to figure out.

As winter turns to spring, Fred shrugs off his losses and adopts a positive, upbeat attitude. It's spring, the season for new life and new beginnings! But Fred's optimism is short-lived as each new calf is born. Both he and his wife know that their weakened herd is *not* sustainable. Eventually everything they have worked so hard for will be lost.

Fortunately, Fred and his sickly cows are fictitious. And when we hear this story, it sounds absurd. But if we analyze the numbers from this imagined story, they are **not too far from our own!**

We humans are now experiencing alarming rates of chronic fatigue, obesity, diabetes, autoimmune diseases, and cancer. A hundred years ago, cancer was likely to affect three people out of every hundred. Today it is estimated that cancer will affect one out of every two men and one in three women (Cancer.org).

Yup, cancer is now wiping out *large* sections of the human population. Despite the astonishing amounts of money being spent every day, we are actually no closer to a cure than we were a hundred years ago. *Wait a second – did you catch that? Can that be right?*

Over the last twelve months, just think how far technology has come. That phone in your pocket isn't just a phone, it's a camera, a personal computer, even a live streaming video recorder! Forty years ago it would have been a struggle to fit a calculator in your pocket! Hold that thought for a second and then ask how far we have come with cancer.

A little over a hundred years ago, aviation wasn't much more than a man flapping around with paper wings, and yet today we can jet across continents in just a few hours. In **every** other field, technology has moved efficiently forward at breakneck speed, yet when it comes to advancements in cancer treatment, we are still using the same questionable techniques of cutting, burning, and poisoning cancer and science-based medicine is actually no closer to a cure than it was when the Wright brothers were doing their thing.

The twisted irony is that anyone who claims to have found an inexpensive and *natural* cure for cancer can expect to be scoffed at and persecuted, ensuring stagnant, but highly profitable progress for pharmaceutical companies for generations to come. According to the American Society of Clinical Oncology (ASCO) newly approved cancer drugs can average as much as $10,000 a month, with some therapies topping $30,000 a month! *Wait a second, are you absorbing these astronomical figures?*

Sadly, waving cash at cancer offers little comfort to those whom it visits, and the cut, burn, and poison technique looks set to continue for another hundred years. No matter how much money is thrown at the problem, it appears that a solution isn't destined to come from within.

> *It is difficult to get a man to understand something,*
> *when his salary depends on his not understanding it.*
> – Upton Sinclair

For now, let's stick with the cow comparison. According to the CDC's own website, it is estimated that by 2050 diabetes will affect one in four of us. Some sources believe we are *already* past this point. The damaging effects of diabetes to business alone are huge. Just in the U.S., the economy takes an approximate annual hit of $245 billion through medical costs and loss of wages. The *human* cost of amputation is *incalculable*.

A worrisome uptrend in autoimmune conditions has become an omnipresent part of our bold new world. Everything from food allergies to ALS has its roots deeply embedded in the immune system, but the immune system is far from dumb, so what are we doing to make the immune system so confused that it turns against us and attacks us?

In our story, a third of Fred's cows were labeled obese. According to National Institute of Diabetes and Digestive and Kidney Diseases (NIDDK), this is also true of a third of U.S. adults.

We could continue with these startling numbers all day long but the point has already been made. **The moral of Fred's story is clear: if we do not want to become like his cows, then we must stop acting like sheep.** Learn to question *every* diagnosis and look at your situation subjectively. Had Fred *paused* and looked at his situation a little more closely and carefully, maybe a *better* solution would have presented itself.

What did we learn from this chapter?

Capitalism is alive and well in the pharmaceutical industry.

Chapter 13

THE MAGIC PILL

We all know Illness is inconvenient, and with bills to pay we sometimes make choices out of sheer panic. *No work, no pay, must fix* – I totally get it. The short term solution is to keep swallowing anything that promises relief; whether pharmaceutical or even a supplement. While the rationale for swallowing handfuls of quick-fix-pills is understandable, it can easily become unpredictable. *Why?*

There can be a lot more to the process than first meets the eye. Choosing the right pill isn't particularly easy, nor is it a straightforward proposition.

Regardless of the promises made on the label of that bottle of supplements, swallowing handfuls of pills could be adding to your health problem. Depending on our level of understanding, supplements can be either a Godsend or a curse. Here's where that madness begins.

The body strives to be in balance and it works hard to do so. In our rush to get well, *any* supplement can have an overwhelming effect on the body. During illness, the liver and kidneys may already be pulling double shifts. These are the main filtering organs and they must process everything you swallow. *Let's try looking at it this way, okay?*

In your mind's eye, imagine a delicate set of scales with a white feather on one tray and a small pill placed on the other tray. If the two balance each other out, then this is your body in a state of equilibrium. This harmonious adjustment can be the difference between feeling well and feeling ill. Today more than ever, it's much easier to disrupt this fine balancing act than it is to keep it.

The job of the liver and kidneys is to keep you alive by means of filtering and detoxifying. *Your* job is to stop making this process harder.

Swallowing a pill to overcome illness is a bold move; if it's working for you stick with it. But you should know that once the liver and kidneys become overtaxed, symptoms can manifest in a whole bunch of different ways.

While the body does its best to keep these different elements in perfect balance, it's possible to become our own worst enemy. Common sense and moderation appears to have fallen out of fashion and been replaced by a new concept that is completely detached from reason.
Besides being constantly bombarded with toxins, we add to our body's burdens by asking it to deal with mega doses of unnatural compounds. In *theory*, EVERY supplement sounds good, but if we took *every* supplement that *sounded* good in theory, **we would soon need a suitcase to carry them all around in.** And remember, what might work for one person doesn't necessarily work for another.

TIPPING POINT

All things being equal, the liver and kidneys do a great job of filtering out what is harmful, but in illness there comes a *tipping* point when these overtaxed organs become sluggish. As the body struggles to cope, those amazing results you were promised on the bottle will soon feel like a big fib.

When the liver and kidneys are no longer filtering optimally, indiscriminately swallowing pills has the potential to advance the situation from sluggish to damaged. The situation then becomes far more fragile and new sensitivities to medications or supplements can begin to develop and even small doses can leave you feeling as if your health is a candle in the wind, about to be extinguished with the next gust.

We are all desperate to find that magic pill. *I get it*. But it's easy to be blinded by all the benefits to health that products X, Y, and Z offer. It may be prudent to balance out the euphoric enthusiasm that often accompanies a product's literature by spending an *equal* amount of time researching the same product for its known side effects.

So first, I'd like to draw attention to the possibility that *any* new supplement can send you into a tailspin and then give you some strategies to help you stay on the right path. The aim of this chapter isn't to discourage or confuse you; it's simply to make you aware of a *vastly* underreported subject that very few people in the field are keen to talk about.

I accept that this chapter isn't going to sit well with some health coaches and – depending on what products are being sold – it's either going to piss you off *or* be the most interesting thing you read today. I might be swimming against the popular tide here, but it beats drowning in numbers. *Shall we jump in?*

It's often said that the only difference between table salt and poison is the dose. My point is this: *too much of anything is a bad thing.* Popping pills without fully understanding this premise is foolhardy and doing it in mega doses *can be downright dangerous.* Don't make the mistake of writing a check to your body that your body cannot cash.

MAGIC PILL

We live in a fast-paced world with the widely held belief that more is more, and taking supplements in mega doses is surely a good thing, *right?* If only it were that easy. You may have diligently done your homework and read review after review before pressing that buy-now button, but keep in mind one person's food can easily become another person's poison.

That glowing review Mrs. Jones wrote relating to product X, Y or Z isn't going to automatically isolate you from the adverse reaction Mr. Smith had. Look, we all desperately want to swallow a magic pill that will end all our health problems, but alas, that's not the way it works in practice.

So what's the solution?

Know that the body deserves to be in balance, so **work with it not against it.** Using *selective* supplements that work synergistically in small groups can bring much better results. However, without a firm foundation of understanding it will rarely translate into a successful outcome.

A good rule of thumb is this: if you aren't 100% sure of why you taking a supplement don't buy it. Whatever it is you decide to buy, make yourself accountable by writing yourself a note listing three reasons why you think supplement X, Y, or Z is going to work, and three reasons why it may not. Now we are thinking *logically* with our heads as opposed to acting out of fear, wishful thinking, or blind panic. *Been there, done that, no thank you very much.*

MULTI

There is a misconception held by many that all vitamins, supplements, and herbal formulas are good for you. In good faith we take that **multivitamin** in the hope that we are covering all the bases. While there is some merit to this way of thinking, it's not without problems.

Many multi vitamins are synthetic; they are low quality imposters of the real thing. Often large retail stores will import supplements from abroad where quality controls can easily be sidestepped. It's widely reported that inferior supplements can arrive in your medicine cabinet laced with toxic dyes. Some are even cut with talc!

These types of synthetic vitamins are cheaper to make so they make more money for the company selling them. Buying these types of products based on price will always take you on a fruitless mission. *Make no mistake, over time cheap synthetic vitamins will hurt you.* They simply *cannot* be absorbed properly and will pull the whole body out of balance.

Okay, so what else do we need to know?

Vitamins fit into two groups: fat soluble or water soluble. These groups determine how vitamins are dissolved and stored in your body. Fat-soluble vitamins reside in the body's fatty tissue and liver and are used *as needed* by the body. By contrast, water-soluble vitamins dissolve in water and are generally *not* stored in your body. It's worth remembering that *both* have the potential to cause toxicities when taken in excess.

If you are a total newbie, try turning to your local health food store for advice. Generally speaking, small independent mom and pop type stores tend to sell *better quality* supplements than the big box stores, but again moderation will often serve you better than excess.

Quality is not the only thing to worry about. How about *quantity?* This measurement is often a preference set by manufacturers themselves. Your health guru may tell you that you need vitamin X-Y-Z *and he or she may or may not be right.* But common sense should dictate that *anything* new that you introduce into your body should always be taken in the smallest dose first to see how you react. The term to remember is *start small and go slow.*

For anyone looking for that elusive quick-fix pill, I'm aware and accept that the following sentence is about to make me about as popular as a piranha in a hotel swimming pool, but here goes nothing: **supplements cannot act as substitute for a poor diet.**

PLAY SMART

If a true nutritional deficiency exists, perhaps a much smarter way is to "selectively" steer towards *specific* (high quality) supplements. To make this point think of a rifle with a high powered telescope on the top. Now compare that rifle to the bluntness and accuracy of a shotgun. If the two weapons were laid side by side and the goal was to hit a bullseye, might the smarter choice be accuracy?

Smaller more accurate groups of selected minerals and vitamins often work better than a broad based multivitamin which could be thought of as a shotgun approach. Many of these smaller groups tend to work together synergistically. This term simply means various components are working together to produce an enhanced result. Now that we have all that cleared up, problem solved right? *Meh, not so fast.*

Even if the stars aligned perfectly, you got the *exact* brand, the *right* quantity, and you even managed to accurately diagnose your own deficiency, the problem doesn't automatically end there. **Vitamin supplementation fails to work optimally in a body that is lacking in trace minerals**. This is important to know because all too often the emphasis is put on vitamins, but without sufficient *minerals* vitamins are worthless. It's *minerals* that make up the lion's share of the nutrients your body needs.

To some degree, the body can adapt to minor deficiencies – much like a car with a rear tail light out. The car still runs even with the broken light. Some deficiencies left to fester can become life threatening; the heart, for example, is one organ that needs a ready supply of potassium and magnesium!

The good news is that given the correct raw materials the body can begin to repair itself – no, seriously, the body does it all the time. In order to do so, the body (that's you) requires approximately 90 essential nutrients that include 60 essential minerals, 12 Amino Acids, 16 vitamins, and 3-4 essential fatty acids. Yes, there are more but these are considered "essential" for the simple reason that the body cannot produce them and they must therefore be consumed.

Don't worry if this seems like a lot to take in, this whole process becomes easier to understand as we move through each chapter.

KEEP IT SIMPLE

In a perfect world that highly touted supplement you just ordered online would come to you at the speed of light with a fully refundable money back guarantee that, once taken, your health will immediately spring back. *Alas,* the world we live in is far from perfect; sometimes we are derailed by our own lack of understanding and sometimes people *make claims online that are downright deceitful!* Anything man can put in a box and sell has the potential to go wrong (or be an outright lie).

For this reason, *when trying anything new it just makes more sense to keep it simple*. Think back to our earlier example of your four digit banking PIN. If you take four new supplements and something works for you, great! But how do you know which one worked?

On the flip side, if you feel *worse* after taking them, how will you know which supplement caused the problem? The ideal solution for people with an easily overloaded system is to *start small and go slow*.

SELF TEST

The promise of benefit is always seductive; if we find ourselves stuck in a desperate cycle of popping pills it can become a challenging habit to break. The only sure way to prove to ourselves that we have *not* become dependent on popping-pills is to try this easy self-test. Ready?

Refrain from taking ANY supplements at all for seven straight days. I know people who absolutely **cannot** do this and still refuse to admit they have a problem. I also know people who *have* done this and have seen great improvement as their bodies come back into balance on their own. If you have to, put all your supplements in a cardboard box and have someone save them for a week or so. It's just a week!

Think of it this way, what if today you suddenly found yourself marooned on a beautiful desert island **without** *any* of your supplements (or medications), the only protein available had to be wild caught each day, the only vegetables had to be freshly picked from the land, and the *only* drink was pure water or fresh coconut milk – how do you think your health would be a month from now? *I know, right? It makes my head hurt too.*

If you do find yourself stuck in a pill popping loop, then the next step is to get yourself a week-to-week day planner. Write down the kind of the supplement you take, and then in brackets write down the time and the reason you take it. If you can't list the reason then why are you taking it?

This simple tip helps (a) serve as a record, (b) plot progress and, (c) keep you accountable. The latter can be quite revealing when you look back over the week. Make this process as simple as you can so it doesn't feel like a chore to do it.

Here's an example of how to keep a simple record for someone with a system that's already out of balance or easily over loaded.
Tuesday 22nd November

8am L-glutamine powder x 1 half teaspoon (gut repair)

1pm Milk Thistle x 1 (liver detox)

3pm AHCC x 2 (immune system)

7pm Topical DMSO (knee pain)

10pm CBD oil (sleep)

Am I saying these are the supplements you need to take? Nope, never did say that, *this is just an example.* But notice how the times are spaced out. This (a) helps us highlight what is working and what is not, (b) prevents us from overloading the liver and, (c) makes it easier to maintain a state of equilibrium. Once health improves, the amounts can increase, but for now the last thing we need to do is add to the burden of a body that's already struggling to cope.

Yes, there are some supplements that work well together synergistically and we will be looking at those in closer detail, but for the moment we are attempting to tackle a much bigger issue which is keeping the body in balance. Also, if you took everything on this list at 8am in a mega dose how would you work out which supplement is working and which supplement gave you a bad reaction?

Remember, at this stage we are trying to keep everything as simple as possible. Does L-glutamine have other benefits? Yes, but we aren't looking to write a product review here, we only need to understand our own thinking. Once this becomes a daily habit you can always expand on it by adding side notes etc.

Any supplemental gaps in between we can (and should) fill with nutrition. This will be covered in more detail later. With the right approach, a large portion of these vitamins and minerals can be obtained from foods grown in *nutrient dense soils.* In simple speak, this means YOU AREN'T GOING TO FIND THEM IN PROCESSED FOODS.

To those in the supplement industry, I know this idea of popping *fewer* pills is making me about as popular as a fart in a space suit. But before you leave me scathing reviews pointing out that I failed to include important compounds like selenium, magnesium, calcium, glutathione, Zinc, NAC, A, B, C, D and E, yada, yada, yada let me again remind you that this is an example ONLY which we will be building on later.

I didn't decide to write this chapter to make myself unpopular; I wrote it because it's important for anyone looking to avoid or overcome chronic illness to know this information. There is often a fine line between the *benefits* of taking supplements X, Y, and Z and the potential imbalance that comes with blindly taking supplements.

Again, the aim of this chapter is not to discourage, as some supplements can and *do* bring relief – its aim is to illustrate that to solve a problem we first need to understand it.

For the moment, that problem is failing to take into account that the kidneys and liver are already pushed into working overtime as they struggle to keep up with the daily demands we place on them. As we move through later sections of this book, practical solutions will become more apparent.

SUPPLEMENT CONTRADICTIONS

Before we explore those solutions in detail, let us first explore a few contradictions. These may serve to better highlight the larger point I am striving to make which is **balance is important.** As Newton famously said, "For every action there is an equal and opposite reaction."

THYROID MADNESS

It's easy to lose count of the number of contradictions that exist for every supplement out there. For example, a simple Google search reveals that iodine is essential for good thyroid health, and while this may be true, it's not the whole story.

Any thyroid that isn't functioning optimally is typically classified as either *hyperthyroid* or *hypothyroid*. The latter being the more prevalent of the two. There is a popular school of thought that suggests that giving iodine to a person with hypothyroid can, on occasion, be like pouring gasoline on an open flame.

Why?

A *hypo*thyroid patient has a 90% chance of having an autoimmune condition by the name of Hashimoto's. During a flare up, the body attacks its own thyroid. Adding unregulated iodine either as a standalone supplement (or as a mega dose multivitamin) has the potential to magnify and intensify the problem.

Given that Hashimoto's was the *first* ever autoimmune condition to be discovered way back in 1934, you would have thought that supplement manufacturers have had ample time to understand this basic concept. Hashimoto's name is taken from the Japanese physician, Hakaru Hashimoto. The iodine contradiction is one reason why taking a blanket multivitamin can send some people into a tail spin.

If we know that the thyroid *needs* iodine, what's the solution to stop it from destroying itself? The short answer lies in a selenium supplement. And here's where we begin to see the beauty of things working together *synergistically,* but even then it's a delicate see-saw balancing act that needs careful consideration. It's worth noting that selenium should always be taken with Vitamin E

Now we are off to the races, taking iodine (in the right dose) with selenium and Vitamin E has been shown to have an impact on thyroid-specific autoimmune disease such as Hashimoto's. *Why?*

Selenium *significantly* reduces TPO and TgAb antibodies; up to 55-86% and 35-92% respectively.

But the devil is once again in the details; too HIGH a dose of selenium can easily accelerate the problem if iodine is deficient. *I know, right? Let's think before we act.* The reverse is also true and each needs to remain *in balance.* If either is too low (or too high) symptoms will become much worse. Both must be addressed *simultaneously and in direct proportion to each other.* Even this is an overly simplified version of events, but it serves to make the point ... there is always more to supplementation than meets the eye!

Autoimmune conditions are *always* a complicated business so it pays to keep an open mind. Some Hashimoto's patients may even respond better *without* the use of any iodine and instead may do better by simply supporting the thyroid with supplements such as B12, Selenium and Iron. Soy products can have an adverse effect on the thyroid, as can gluten, rest assured, this is covered in more detail later in the book.

Thyroid problems are on the rise and, as I mentioned earlier, if you suspect that you have any type of a thyroid issue it pays to insist that your doctor goes beyond having the standard TSH test done. The TSH test is capable of doing a great disservice to the patient because it only looks at 20% of the problem.

If you have any type of thyroid issue you might find the work of Dr. Izabella Wentz, Pharm.D., FASCP interesting. Dr. Izabella Wentz is a passionate, innovative, and solution-focused clinical pharmacist. What Mrs. Wentz *doesn't* know about the thyroid wouldn't take up any space on the back of a postage stamp. To fully understand all these interactions and combinations it seems we might all benefit from a PhD in chemistry such as Dr. Wentz has. Yet all too often we go along to the pharmacy and take the advice of the first person we can find.

VITAMIN D

Let's not limit this problem to iodine; the same argument can be put forth with just about any vitamin, dare I say even vitamin D? While it's true that vitamin D is critical to good health, it's also worth noting that vitamin D isn't a vitamin at all, it's actually a hormone.

Vitamin D is fat soluble, which means taking too much of it can build up and cause toxicity. Taking vitamin D in pill form can be harsh on the kidneys. If you have a known vitamin D deficiency, a "sublingual" version of vitamin D is far less damaging. Taking sublingual vitamin D simply means you allow it to dissolve slowly on the tongue which is much easier for the kidneys to process.

We should also note that vitamin D works best with calcium, the two go hand in hand and both are needed for absorption. But once again there is a little more to this story and here's where it gets a little bumpy so you might want to hold onto your hat. Ready?
If calcium is aided in absorption by vitamin D3 then K2 is also needed for it to do so effectively. *Huh?* But wait there's more; vitamin D is good friends with other vitamins (like vitamin A) and cooperates synergistically with minerals like magnesium and zinc. Many of the proteins involved in vitamin A metabolism (and the receptors for both vitamins A and D) only function correctly in the presence of zinc. *I know, right? It seems easier to get this wrong than it is to get it right, but don't lose faith, a solution is coming.*

Surely there must be an easier way to get our vitamin D safely and in the right amount? Yes there is, and it's usually just above your head – and free...but here's the kicker: we have been conditioned over the years to cover up our living, breathing skin with sunscreen. Yet, when done *sensibly,* the best way to get your vitamin D is directly from the sun – in small doses.
Exposing the skin to direct sunlight for 30 mins a day in the morning can be a much safer alternative to popping vitamin D pills. As with all things, *moderation is key* and getting your vitamin D this way beats anything you can buy in the store by a royal mile.

Not everyone has access to sunshine year round, which makes the whole sublingual vitamin D lesson here all the more important.

DON'T DO IT

This next pitfall is one I have fallen into myself more times than I care to remember. Let's say you managed to get the correct X-Y-Z supplement and even began to feel some noticeable benefit. There is a new danger lurking in our own thinking – any guesses what it is? Top marks if you said, "Hey, if one is good – two must be better, right?"

With a family to support and bills to pay the obvious temptation is to see a small benefit and then rush forward with haste. *I get it* – we need to get back on our feet ASAP but the *more* we take the more we run the risk of increasing our chances of a setback.

If ever there was a time to use the phrase, less is more, this is it. You are ill in part because your liver and kidneys couldn't keep up with your toxic exposure, so blindly slamming them with mega doses of vitamins isn't helping the situation.

Note to self

It is of little consequence if flawed logic is grounded in either desperation or greed, for both will take you on a fool's errand.
– James Lilley

Let's go back to that set of scales in our mind's eye. When we blindly put multiple isolated compounds on the scale it becomes harder to keep the body in balance, for this was never the way we humans were designed to digest our nutrients. We know the body strives for equilibrium so we also know that taking mega doses of ANYTHING only makes the recovering body work harder.

Tip- *If you find yourself constantly shooting yourself in the foot by pill popping (either out of desperation or a lack of understanding) then it's a good idea to box up all those supplements and put them out of reach for* *the next 30 days. This can help remove temptation and bring your body back into balance.*

So what's the solution? If you are trying to correct a deficiency with vitamins, then *food based* supplementation is generally the better way to go. Known as "whole food supplements" or "plant based supplements," there are several good brands on the market that can be found in your local health food store. The golden rule is everything in moderation, for every action causes a reaction. And this reaction can sometimes involve the immune system.

The immune system gets complicated which is why it's covered in a separate chapter, but while we are here there is an important point I'd like you to remember. Your immune system can be stimulated or suppressed by certain supplements and herbs; this is why some people feel *worse* after taking supplements. *Hmm, I see.*

Any supplement that has the potential to cause an imbalance in the body will almost certainly rub the immune system the wrong way. And with more than a 100 autoimmune conditions primed to attack from within, creating such an imbalance can be a costly mistake to make. Most people with an autoimmune condition spend years being misdiagnosed. At this stage let's *not* rule out the possibility that you could *absolutely* be one of those people.
Without a basic understanding of your Th1 and Th2 cells, it's never a good idea to provoke any type of immune reaction. Happily, this topic is broken down and made easy to understand later in the book.

BUT HOW DID WE GET HERE?

For sure our early ancestors weren't wandering around with their pockets filled with pills, so why is it that we now feel the need to supplement? The short answer to that question is relatively more straightforward than you may think. Today, much of the commercially grown food arriving on our plate is devoid of minerals because the soil is so overworked and weak – essentially it's been exhausted of its nutrients. Adding a handful of fertilizers to already depleted soil only adds to the problem and it's a far cry from the 90 essential nutrients our body needs to thrive.

The bottom line is this: if the foods, we choose to eat have a mineral deficiency, then *we* have a mineral deficiency. And from that came man's solution: supplements! But surely this is twisted logic.

While it might be reassuring to believe in a supplement that's going to take away all our problems, without a clear understanding of the subject of nutrition your health problems aren't going away any time soon. **You simply can't supplement your way out of a bad diet, and with a good diet you don't need to.**

Healthy vibrant food grown in nutrient dense soil has been shown to contain more essential minerals and it naturally repels bugs. Weaker crops, however, are more prone to infestation; they then have the added burden of being exposed to heavy chemical spraying. *I know, right? Spraying the food with poison, what could possibly go wrong?*
Think of soil as a bank account, if you take too much out you have to deposit some back in or the soil becomes bankrupt. This is *not* the way our Victorian ancestors grew food. They grew food in *nutrient dense* soils that had just about every mineral you could ever need. This is common sense farming rather than simply farming for profit. Alas, as my-old-mum used to say, "Common sense isn't always that common."

Since the beginning of time, the preferred fuel to power the human body has been whole foods found in their natural state. Foods grown in nutrient dense soils are superior in every way to commercially grown foods.

Today so many of the foods we choose to eat are heavily processed and far removed from that concept. *Are you getting this? It's kinda important.*

Understanding supplements and the way they affect the body takes time and discipline. Periodically it might be a good idea to re-read the instructions on the supplement box, there are some supplements that are best taken with food, others are best not taken with food, etc. There is also an element of trial and error. You should remain aware that the risk of getting it wrong is ever present. The good news is that even if you totally mess up you can help the body come back into balance on its own by simply refraining from taking ANY supplements for seven days.

THE OTHER WAY

Taking *selective* supplements that work synergistically has obvious advantages, but the take-home message here is the body likes harmony. Supplements are one way to get your nutrients, but they are not the only way.

For sensitive individuals, bone broths, juicing, and even sprouting all pack a nutritional punch. (These topics, along with many others, are covered in more detail later.) For some, *boosting* nutritional intake this way is a safer alternative.

What did we learn from this chapter?

Controlling pain and, to some degree, suffering is as easy as popping a pill. However, this simple rationale serves only to mask symptoms and rarely gets to the root cause. The notion that you can simply swallow a pill and have all your problems go away is an appealing one, but it's fraught with complications and contradictions.

During any prolonged illness the liver and kidneys are already working overtime. This is important to remember because certain medications and even supplements can force these stressed organs to work even harder. If you live in an area where natural sunlight is limited then *sublingual* forms of vitamin D can be easier on the kidneys.

If your system is a little on the sensitive side, you will not respond well to either mega doses or synthetic supplements. Quality **food based** supplements are usually found in good health food stores and may be better tolerated. Keep in mind that taking any supplement out of blind panic can take you on a counterproductive downward spiral.

Homework: anyone with a suspected thyroid issue should immediately check out the insightful work of Dr. Izabella Wentz, she can be found with a simple Google search.

E-book readers may find this short video 4-minute interesting.
https://www.youtube.com/watch?v=7MvJpE80mc8

Side note:

At the moment, very few people know that this book exists. If you find any of these contacts helpful, please feel free to mention where you found their information. Thanks.

Chapter 14

THE CARDBOARD DIET, WTF?

When you stop and really think about it, it's quite remarkable that food has changed more in the last 30 years than it has in the last 3000. Chickens no longer roam free to eat bugs; cows no longer eat grass; fruits are being restructured by genetic modification; vegetables are now grown in water by means of hydroponics; and 90% of grains are being sprayed with harsh chemicals.

Food has become such a loosely defined term it now includes unnatural preservatives, excessive sugars, artificial colorings, high fructose corn syrup, corn starch, MSG, and just about any other toxic additive you can think of. *Gee, I wonder if any of this could have an impact on how we feel?*

The vast majority of foods found on supermarket shelves have been processed. Processed "foods" might have started off as real food, but somewhere on the way to market (and to you) they took a wrong turn and ended up on a production line having "stuff" added to them.

Once they'd been added to, these "food" products were put in a box, a can, or a packet and passed on to you through a third party with the sole purpose of making a profit. While I am not in any way opposed to anyone making a tidy profit, I can't help feeling this style of production works best in the automotive industry rather than in the food industry.

A conglomerate of these new "foods" roll off production lines with added (and excess) sugars mixed into them which ensures that customers will keep coming back for more (sugar has a way about it). Once food becomes a mish-mash of things it can become the root cause of food sensitivities and allergies.
Many of these heavily processed foods have been linked to obesity, depression, heart disease, joint pain, and diabetes. And while processed food is, admittedly, convenient – *illness certainly is not.*

As mentioned, the digestive system plays a pivotal role in our health and consuming these types of foods won't flood your cells with key nutrients, it will only add to the toxic burden. In short, it's the wrong fuel for your engine.

Since the beginning of time, the human body has been designed to run on clean water and whole food. It's always been our *preferred* fuel. *Whole* foods are easy to identify because they are made from only one ingredient and rarely (like never) grow in boxes or cans. Once we begin to understand that eating a heavily processed diet provides the wrong fuel, the solution is always going to be the same: *we need to stop eating processed foods. Am I right?*

We could go around in circles all day long to make this same point sound more intelligent or complicated than it needs to be, but essentially the time is coming for you to take greater responsibility for your health and, ultimately, everything that goes onto your plate.

As any recovering drug addict will tell you, *it's far easier to avoid temptation than it is to resist it.* Food manufacturers do everything they can to keep you coming back for their products again and again. And often, quitting unhealthy foods is easier said than done. With that in mind, what we need is a plan to *exclude* these toxic foods from your diet. In this chapter you will find such a plan.

Let's not forget that sugar is both addictive and deceptive. It can be found in every type of processed food from crackers to salad dressing, making the standard American diet (SAD) extremely *high* in calories but *low* in actual nutritional content. In short, it's Frankenfood.
Fortunately for us, this makes the whole transition process really quite simple.

Heavily processed food = bad.
Whole food = good.
Processed foods = more than one ingredient.
Whole foods = have only one ingredient.

Unfortunately, things like that "all natural" golden crispy organic granola bar needs a rethink. Yup, if it's been on a production line then it's still processed. This is *not* how your robust ancestors ate, and we really don't have to go that far back in history to see it. If they could only see some of the things we buy today, I'm sure they would be like, WTF? (Who's-The-Farmer?)

Here's your rule of thumb: if it came from a plant eat it, if it was made in a plant then *don't.* Okay, there is no easy way to do this. What say we rip the band aid off right now and get right to the solution? *I just know you are going to love this!*

CARDBOARD

First, go to the store and buy several medium sized cardboard boxes. Fear not, the nutritional content of cardboard is of little value to us here, the boxes are needed to put stuff in. Up until this point you have gotten off pretty light, but now the oven mitts are coming off! You wanted to get well and I'm about to show you the best way to do it.

Once you have your boxes stand them in front of your pantry. Now, open up the cupboard doors and begin placing **every** single edible item directly into the boxes. *I know right, this guy is crazy, but keep reading anyway; I promise it gets better.* As Carl Jung once said, "Show me a sane man and I will cure him for you."
Okay, I know what you are thinking. You're looking at that can of black beans and wondering why in the world you can't keep them. If the label says: Organic Black Beans, Water, Sea Salt, you can. If after "Black Beans" there are a bunch of ingredients listed that do not sound like anything you'd eat as a snack by itself (e.g., dextrose, glucono delta-lactone, high fructose corn syrup), then in the box it goes.

If there is someone on your street, maybe an underweight elderly neighbor with a dog that barks all night (or any other person against whom you hold a grudge) simply gift the box to them. If not, draw a skull and crossbones on it and put the damned box out for the garbage man.

I realize that this is a bold move and for some it might be a bridge too far. If this is you, I'd like to assure you that what we have just done is absolutely critical to your success.

Here's why.

- All temptation is removed
- There are no more labels to read
- No more calories to count
- Food sensitivities, be gone
- No complicated diet to follow. *Hoorah!*

Still not convinced, huh?

Maybe you are fighting me on this because times are hard. If that's the case, let's calculate the cost of the food in your cupboard and then approximate how much money you stand to lose if you have to spend weeks, months, or years going to doctors, getting tests, taking medications, and missing time from work. Got the figure? Perfect, now stand back and ask yourself, is that all your health is worth to you?

What do we have? Maybe a couple of hundred bucks of toxic food? I'd bet the farm that any illness costs more in weekly medications alone. Look at it this way, if I'm right, you get your health back, if I'm wrong you lose a little money.

Sacrifice something else if you have to, sell your hat or sell the cat. Then take another hard look at the stuff we cram into our garden sheds and wardrobes. If you *really* stop and think about it, when we have no peace in our lives, we don't own any of these things, they own us!

Perhaps it's time to stop sleep walking into illness and let this bold, decisive call to action serve as your wake up call. It's time to bite the bullet, *not the biscuits.* If you want me to liberate your health, help me help you do it. We both know if heavily processed foods remain in the house you are going to eat them, so banish anything with a toxic element to it into the cardboard boxes.

Making poor food choices can either contribute to your illness or *keep* you in illness. Think of it this way, you live *inside* a body, if you don't take care of it, may I ask where you are going to live?
Just as a car runs on gasoline, food is the essential fuel that runs a body. If you have been listening to the standard mainstream nutritional mantra everything you *think* you know about food is probably wrong. Keep reading and I'll show you why.

Once you clear out all that junk food, all those hidden food additives and deceptive sugars are no longer a threat to you (or to your colon). The flip side of that also holds true; once we have *real* food in the house *this* is what you will eat when you are hungry, it's a WIN-WIN.

I get it, new challenges bring resistance, if frozen pizza has been working for you, then more power to you, if not, maybe we need to try something different. If you need motivation maybe find an earlier photo of yourself looking healthy and pin it to the fridge. The photo needs to represent something bigger than your temptation, it could be a photo of your spouse, or if applicable, your kids. Find something deep inside that matters more to you than a couple hundred bucks' worth of toxic food. Do that and the rest is easy.

> *The food you eat can be either the safest and most powerful*
> *form of medicine, or the slowest form of poison.*
> – Ann Wigmore

The idea here is that we are looking for a clean slate to work with, *new habits bring new results.* Old habits got you into this mess! If you want your health back you have to fight for it, so yes, this step is important and we don't want you to be even an eenie-weenie little bit tempted.

Think about it: alcoholics who successfully recover don't sit in a house full of booze. I'm not doing this to be mean, I *really* do want you to succeed.

Done right, this is going to work for you because this is a plan like none other you have tried.

The trick to your success is planning ahead. Keep applying these simple steps and in a very short space of time good health can be yours for the taking.

HOW TO FAIL IN THREE STAGES

1. Keep processed food in the house.
2. Don't have a plan.
3. Repeat step one.

You might be asking, "Hey, does this also include all those condiments?" Yes, remember it's do or die, and the "do" part always seems like a much better option to me, so please, while you are at it, box that bleached iodized salt, *the replacement I have coming for you is better beyond comparison.* This is a whole fresh start, with *fresh* food.

MILK FROM A COW

I've had to do this a few times in my life and it really is much easier to do *without* thinking too much, just keep putting that "food" into those cardboard boxes and this *will* be a breath of fresh air to your health, I promise. Now take a deep breath as we take one of those cardboard boxes and approach the fridge. *I know, right? Not the fridge too!*

Yes, obviously, this includes that block of mucus forming cheese, yes that sugar spiking organic orange juice that's probably owned by one of the cola giants, and yes that carton of milk even if it is "fortified" with vitamin D. (D for Don't get me started.)

Now you dunnit! Milk is absolutely packed with wonderful nutrients if you happen to be a cow. Are we a cow? I think not. We are humans and the *only* mammals on this planet that drink a different mammal's milk. *What's up with that?*

But, seeing as we humans are so much smarter than the cow we have to take it a step further by taking their milk and heating it up and killing all the beneficial enzymes in the process. We then add sweeteners, and to top it all off, we stick it in a toxic BPA plastic container for its 1500 mile ride to the store. It's only use now is to make the mind boggle … and the food manufactures call this healthy.

Of course, just as with your pantry clean-out, the same principle holds true here in your fridge and freezer. If those eggs are free-range then yes you can obviously keep them, ditto to any grass-fed beef you may have. And no, don't toss the broccoli if you recently brought it home from the farmer's market. Use your head – by this point you know what real food is and what just isn't. As for that bottled salad dressing with 19 unpronounceable ingredients? Nope out it must go.

MILK FROM A GOAT

Consider this, a farmer living close by has a wife who keeps goats; they are obviously her pride and joy and it's easy to see that the goats are well cared for, clean, healthy, and happy. When she recently had raw goat's milk for sale, you can bet I was first in line.

Goat's milk differs from cow's milk in that it has thirty-five percent fatty acids, making it *more* nutritionally wholesome than cow's milk by a country mile. It's also easier to digest and can even be helpful to those who are lactose intolerant.

Buying it locally also cuts out the middleman, which benefits the farmer, the local economy, and me. Having it poured directly into my *glass* jar by someone I know is for me just as important as the rich creamy taste. For many, goat's milk is a WIN/WIN. But here's the kicker…. when I bought the goat's milk I was asked to comply with a state mandated law that required me to sign a two-page disclaimer, enforced at the request of the FDA. The irony is that in the U.S. it's easier to buy an AK47 assault rifle than it is to buy raw milk. *I know, right? You can't make this stuff up.*

Yet by comparison, the supermarket two miles up the road is selling cow's milk that comes from stressed-out cows that have probably been fed antibiotics and growth hormones and are milked by robots. Supermarket milk has only seventeen percent fatty acids making it less nutritious than goat's milk, and it tastes like a watered down imposter.

So *yes,* the cow's milk too must go into the box. If you know ahead of time that you have an issue with self-discipline but simply can't throw food out, then seal the box and have someone save it for you for thirty days. Your fridge should now look just like it did the day you bought it. Empty!

FAMILY

If you happen to share a fridge, I accept this step may be more challenging, so you now have two options. First, get the whole family on board, maybe even give them a copy of this book to read (hello family member) this way they know where you are coming from.

It wouldn't kill *them* to eat healthy, whereas eating toxic food certainly might! **In the history of mankind there has never been a recorded illness relating to a *deficiency* of toxic food additives.** *Seriously, never.*

Getting family members on board would be an ideal solution. But if you are feeling a certain amount of pushback from the family, or they refuse to cooperate, simply unplug the freezer for a few hours and say, "Hey guys, we lost power and I had no choice but to throw all the food out!" The point is this: if you are determined, you will find a way, if not you will find an excuse.

Okay, almost there, just one last important thing to know in advance. Whenever you set about to change your life, people will inadvertently attempt to derail your attempts. It's just the way it is.

As sure as night follows day, the second you remove all temptation from your home someone is going to knock on your door and offer you cake. Remember the rule, accept the cake, but do not *eat* the cake.

Knowing that people are going to try to tempt you in advance *gives the power back to you.* This power comes from within *and you should not count on the support of others for your success.*

At this stage you may be forgiven for saying, "Gee, after I do all this cleaning out, what the heck am I going to eat?" I'm so glad you asked. By the time this book ends your nutritional options will be clearly spelled out and you will also have a better understanding of what good food is and what it isn't. It's actually so simple even a fat burning caveman could do it, so don't despair, more is coming.

What did we learn from this chapter?

When faced with illness treat anything that comes in a box, a can, or a packet with suspicion for a minimum of thirty days. Removing all processed foods from your cupboards not only removes temptation *it takes all the guesswork away.*

Homework: pick up some cardboard packing boxes...you know the rest.

Chapter 15

HIT THE RESET BUTTON

As we move through this book together, I'd again like to remind you that an open mind is an extremely helpful tool. To some, many of these ideas may at first seem a little extreme or even odd. The challenge is to simply keep reading to the end of each chapter. By that time, you should have a very different perspective and hopefully this will all make sense.

Okay, here we go.

Your body is smart. Ever notice the first thing our bodies do when we become ill? We lose our appetite and our body shuts itself down, essentially forcing us into fasting mode. Fasting gives the digestive system the green light to rest; it's actually a tried and tested principle that dates back to pre-biblical times. Whoa! Hear me out on this one, what if I also told you there was a way to tap into the benefits of fasting **without** feeling hungry (true story).

In a very short space of time, fasting can be a highly effective way to lift brain fog, clean out toxins, and increase energy, as well as help reveal a list of hidden food sensitivities. But wait, there's more.

Over a lifetime we ask an awful lot of our digestive system, we bombard it day in and day out with foods *that even the bugs won't eat.* Throw into the mix handfuls of pills, excessive amounts of sugar, bread, sugar, pretzels, sugar, tinned foods, more sugar, chips, even more sugar, processed foods, sugar in the form of soda, and carbohydrates (carbs for short) that all turn to sugar along with a whole bunch of food additives with unpronounceable names! Make no mistake, digesting food is a labor intense process that takes valuable energy *away* from the body.
Now we are *really* asking our digestive system to go to work without ever giving it the opportunity it needs to take a break. Imagine if your boss pushed you that hard all week and then wouldn't let you take the weekend off, or any weekend – I wonder how *you* would feel. Perhaps tired, depressed, lethargic, or even chronically fatigued? Hmm, I see.

Look at it this way, today more than ever we are constantly bombarded with messages telling us to do this or that with our health. With so much conflicting information wouldn't it be nice if just once all those health experts could find a way to fix a whole bunch of ailments quickly in one swoop so we didn't have to worry the details.

Why do we have to do all the hard work, like avoiding toxic food additives and putting the right nutrients into the body yada, yada, yada? Why can't we just have a *simple* plan to help get the toxins out and give our *overworked* digestive systems a well-earned rest?

Be careful what you wish for, *someone already did!*

Maybe you missed it while you were distracted; it was discovered way back in the 1940s. Jared Leto has found it, so have Gwyneth Paltrow, Anne Hathaway, and Beyoncé to name but a few.

If you do this step right, and use the tips offered in this chapter, you won't just have clearer thinking and more energy, you'll sail through the whole process without feeling hungry. I know what you are thinking because I thought it too. Anything that sounds too good to be true usually is – or there is money (yours) involved. Okay, let's get down to the money part. Here it comes ….

Actually, I *loathe* the whole notion of expensive fixes. The following information is available to you *free* of charge and the raw materials needed to pull this off can be found in your local grocery store *for less than the price of junk food and your daily coffee!*

Okay, there is one *small* catch, but I'll get to that in a moment. On the *plus* side, let me remind you that the rewards can be nothing short of astounding *and* for some it can feel like you have just hit the reset button. Welcome to THE MASTER CLEANSE! *I know, right? That really deserved a drum roll.*

THE MASTER CLEANSE

The master cleanse is not a new fad, it's the brainchild of Stanley Burroughs and has over the years been successfully completed by more people than you can shake a hairy stick at. It remains popular today (even with the Hollywood set) because it's easy to do and it works really, really well.

To pull this off it may take a couple of attempts and a disciplined mindset, or simply a strong desire to get well. While the master cleanse is not for airy-fairy types, those who successfully complete it *will* automatically come to crave clean foods over junk foods, *no question about it.*

But, the master cleanse isn't recommended for anyone taking medications (or mega doses of vitamins) because the two simply don't mix. If this is you, keep reading because I have another tip just for you. And who knows? Perhaps down the road your circumstances may even change. If at some point you decide to try the full master cleanse it's important to work with your own doctor and scale down any medication first, and *gradually* over time.

Mr. Stanley Burroughs published a small booklet on the "master cleanse" which is available as a **free** download online. It's well-written and very easy to understand. A hard copy is still in print and you can find that at Amazon.com. I could easily pad the rest of this chapter with the exact protocol, but seeing as the information is available for *free*, I believe *it's always better* coming direct from the source. (Details can be found in today's homework section.)

The master cleanse is one of the many things I've done that helped my health leap forward and it's a great tool to have in your toolbox. The purpose of this chapter is to explain some of the benefits of the master cleanse and then give you some helpful tips on how to do it.

Before attempting any type of cleanse, it's important to know that the first four days can be the most challenging, after that your body enters a fat burning mode and things get a whole lot easier.

169

There are two parts to the master cleanse, the first is the salt-water-flush (*say what now?*) first thing in the morning. If you can get your head around that, the rest is a stroll in the park.

The master cleanse also helps clean out the liver *and* kidneys, while at the same time giving the digestive system time to rest and repair. Once the burden of food sensitivities is lifted from the body, batteries are quickly recharged and key nutrients flow into the cells.

PART 1

The salt-water-flush (*huh?*) helps facilitate digestion by **cleaning** the entire digestive system from top to bottom. Over the years it can become impacted with rancid fats, proteins, and impacted fecal matter. *I know, right? Gross. But once you remove this thick slimy coating digestion improves along with health.*

You may have heard of colonic irrigation which has become a recent trend that's not without merit, but for my money the salt-water-flush (geez, he just keeps saying it) does the job *much* better because it works in the correct direction, from the top down as opposed to colonic irrigation which works from the bottom up (pun intended). *The master cleanse* can also be done in the comfort of your home for a *fraction* of the cost of colonic irrigation.

It may take a couple of attempts to get things moving, and the first attempt at a salt-water-flush (he said it *again*) may be a little uncomfortable because all the junk in the trunk slowly becomes dislodged. Hang in there because once things get kick-started it will move through much easier and faster next time. If digestion has been a problem for you then this step is going to be more challenging. Drinking Smooth Move tea at night may prove helpful.

A while ago I reached the point where I no longer cared what anything tasted (or looked) like *so long as it gave positive results.* And for me, this step, along with several others, brought results.

As well as the **free** master cleanse booklet, there is a mountain of YouTube clips to assist you if you have unanswered questions. If you don't manage to "flush" the first time, you may need to check that you have the correct dose before trying to drink more salt water. There, I said it. Busted. Yup, it's true, the first part of the master cleanse includes drinking salt water in the morning on an empty stomach which helps to flush the colon, but please keep reading, there is an upside and it's coming ….

Done right, per the exact Stanley Burroughs protocol, the salt-water-flush helps force out toxins that have become trapped inside you and that contribute to sluggishness and constipation.

I know we have all been conditioned to think salt is bad for us, and certainly we were taught (probably in a sea disaster movie) that you should certainly not drink salt water, but there is actually a lot of science behind this cleanse and the salt isn't going to be in your system for very long (*if you catch my drift*).

To do the salt water flush, the trick is to give yourself a dedicated hour in the morning and a definite need to stay close to a bathroom – so plan ahead. Once the flush is complete, you can go about your day as usual, feeling lighter and refreshed.

Psychologically you need to be up for this and it's important to understand that to succeed you will need to use *good water* and you absolutely CANNOT use regular table salt. It may help to mix the salt-water-flush the night before so that (a) it is room temperature in the morning, and (b) the salt is properly dissolved in the water.

PART 2

The second part of the master cleanse is actually quite pleasant. It's another drink but this time it tastes much better than it sounds. *No really.* It also does a great job at ensuring your cells get what they need while keeping hunger at bay.

The master cleanse drink should be made fresh each day using the following: *organic* lemons, *grade B* maple syrup, and a pinch of cayenne pepper. Any time you manage to try the salt-water-flush (*oh come on*) you will find you crave the lemons.

While you can certainly *reduce* the amount of maple syrup in each drink, you really can't skimp on the *quality* of these three key ingredients which are critical for success. Keep in mind, the additional cost of going organic is relatively easy to justify because you aren't buying food. If you stop and do the math, buying fast food and soda would actually cost more over the course of a week.

When doing the master cleanse, Grade B maple syrup is the preferred choice. Because it's produced later in the season, it's darker and more maple flavored and it's also higher in minerals than standard maple syrup. In some areas the term "Grade B" has been replaced with the term "Grade A Very Dark" *or* "Extra Dark." This isn't done to confuse people; it's done to comply with new international standards for labeling maple syrup.

These past few weeks I've reluctantly found myself on the road and living out of a suitcase, which (a) makes it notoriously difficult to write, and (b) not always easy to keep to a clean diet.

I was feeling tired and sluggish so I've just completed a ten-day master cleanse and come back to this chapter to give it an updated tweak. This time around I found it really helped to clear my thinking as well as helping with a minor stomach issue I'd picked up.

I find that starting a master cleanse entails far more effort than finishing it. This time I told myself that it all sounded like more work than I was prepared to do, but by the end of the cleanse, things always look and feel very different and I feel better for having done it.

I'd also like to point out the first couple of times I tried the master cleanse I failed miserably. But after researching the master cleanse in some detail, I soon understood why some people find it so beneficial. Long story short,

I persisted and the aim of this chapter is first to encourage you to try it and then to offer some tips that I've found helpful.

The key to succeeding with the master cleanse is preparation. Have everything you need ahead of time because running out of lemons is a great excuse to quit halfway through. Mix up a batch of drinks *before* you leave the house and take them with you in a small cooler.

Stanley Burroughs believed that *a toxic body that is not eliminating properly is the root of all illness.* I guess another way of saying it is *toxins out, nutrients in.*

The master cleanse might not be for everyone, but those looking to fix a multitude of sins in one swoop may find it very helpful. The upside of this is it allows the digestive system time to regroup and regenerate itself.

The master cleanse can last however long you like but typically it's a 10 day cleanse. And, depending on your levels of toxicity, you may hit a few bumps on the way. Sometimes this can happen during the first few days or it might happen somewhere in the middle. Either way, try to stick to it because once you get past the fourth day things can feel very different.

If this all sounds too intense then all is not lost, you can still tap into the master cleanse by totally missing out the salt water flush part and going straight to the second part. Will the results be the same? Perhaps not, but there are still some benefits to doing a mini master cleanse each morning.

THE MINI CLEANSE

For some, the full master cleanse is simply too much too quick – I get it. If this is you, hang in there and don't be discouraged. This mini cleanse is actually easy-peasy to do, it's *not* an exact science; it's more about giving yourself a trial run *without* feeling under pressure or deprived of food. If at any point you feel worse you can simply stop.

Okay, here's how to make the juice.

Use a 16oz glass mason jar and fill it with clean, *room temperature* water (it's easier on digestion). It's best to make the drink first thing in the morning. Add three tablespoons of freshly squeezed lemon juice into the glass jar, bonus points for using organic lemons, then add one teaspoon of maple syrup and a pinch of cayenne pepper to taste.

If you are trying to get into ketosis (more on this later) you could skip the maple syrup. The pinch of cayenne helps with digestion, boosts metabolism, and gives detox support. When you mix these three key ingredients together it has a surprisingly nice kick to it.

Try this drink for a few days as a replacement for breakfast and see how you do. Don't be surprised if it holds you over as much as any breakfast meal would. For the rest of the day eat as normal. The idea here is to build confidence that you *can* do this for longer periods.

When you feel ready, try cranking it up a little, maybe the next day instead of making just one drink for breakfast try making two and see if you can through lunch time until dinner. As your confidence grows, keep stretching out the time until you can do a full day, and so on.

My wife doesn't care too much for the cayenne taste so she takes less, but I actually like it. She also prefers more maple syrup and I prefer less. *My point?* Find what works for you.

The important part of the master cleanse is obviously the healing power of the lemons. *Here's why*:

- Room temp lemon water helps detoxify the liver and kidneys
- It encourages the production of bile
- It's a great source of citric acid, potassium, calcium, phosphorus, and magnesium
- Despite being acidic, lemons help keep your pH balance in check
- Lemons are an excellent and rich source of vitamin C
- Vitamin C helps boost the immune system so that your body can fight off illness

- Lemon water is great for your colon and digestive health
- Lemon juice can aid in the treatment of urinary tract infections
- Lemons contain pectin fiber, which serves as a powerful antibacterial
- Warm lemon water helps flush out toxins and it helps reduce pain and inflammation in the joints and knees
- Gives the body a break from food sensitivities

The last bullet point is *especially* helpful because so many people today have become sensitive to foods. Food sensitivities can result in anything from debilitating migraines to chronic fatigue.

To add to the complication, there is often a total disconnect in the time it takes to eat something and the time it takes the body to react negatively to it. Not everyone with a food sensitivity turns blue and immediately rolls around on the floor. The master cleanse allows us to spot borderline food sensitivities much more easily.

The beauty of the master cleanse is that it consists of only three simple ingredients, organic lemon, a pinch of cayenne, and extra dark maple syrup. Once allergic triggers are removed from the body, good things begin to happen. Any time we lift the burden, it helps the body heal.

It's important **not** to substitute standard maple syrup for grade B maple syrup (sometimes called *grade A extra dark*). It might surprise you to know extra dark maple syrup contains calcium, iron, magnesium, phosphorus, sodium, potassium, and zinc, as well as vitamins such as thiamin, riboflavin, niacin, and B6.

Grade B or Grade A Extra Dark maple syrup is the preferred choice because it's lower on the glycemic index score than regular cane sugar, and the lower the score the less of an impact it has on blood sugar levels. Maple syrup also has a certain antioxidant value to it, which regular sugar does *not*.

Tip, if you get any form of tooth sensitivity from juice you can get around this by drinking through a straw.

The master cleanse has been tried and tested by thousands of people with positive results. Again, let me remind you that many of those **success** stories can be found via YouTube. Ultimately, you are a unique individual and, as with anything new, it pays to take some time to play around with this idea to ensure it is a good fit for you.

Whenever toxins are removed from the body, it's always best to do it slowly. The more toxic your liver is, the slower you will want to go. If you are currently ill, I suspect food will be at the bottom of your priority list and perhaps trying the gentle *mini*-master cleanse will help you slowly recover at a pace that's right for you.

Whichever route you take, be aware that any time you fast sufficient temptation will be sent along the way via your friends and family – it's just the way life is. Being aware of this ahead of time gives you ample opportunity to find a coping strategy.

For those contemplating the full master cleanse, you may find the following tips for ending the fast helpful.

TIPS FOR ENDING A 10-DAY, FULL ON, HARDCORE FAST

The reward for getting to this point is food will now smell and taste very different and your body will automatically crave clean food. However, it's important to *ease* yourself back into eating solid food to avoid the risk of digestive upsets. Mentally it may help to think of the full master cleanse as a fifteen-day event. *I know, right? No harm in just thinking.* Stanley Burroughs recommends ending the fast in the following way.

Day 1 – At the end of the 10-day fast, drink one 8 oz. glass of freshly squeezed organic orange juice, if you experience any digestive upsets you can dilute the juice with clean/filtered water. (Whereas normally I am not in favor of drinking juice, freshly squeezed or not, in this case its purpose is to prepare your digestive system for the reintroduction of food and is part of the master cleanse protocol.)

By the time your fast ends you may feel the urge to gulp the orange juice down. Try to resist this temptation. It's always best to sip slowly for the first 24 hours. This helps to prepare the digestive system to properly digest and assimilate regular food, doing this right will help give digestion a blank slate to work up from.

Not too much orange juice mind you; we don't want to flood the body with a form of liquid sugar. And after ten days of fasting this is something to be mindful of.

Step 2.

Day 2 – The next morning again gently sip a little freshly squeezed organic orange juice, adding extra water if needed. In the afternoon begin preparing a vegetable soup (not from a can) and make enough soup for two meals using organic vegetables. This doesn't have to be bland in anyway shape or form, you can add celery, carrot, onion, kale, potato, greens, okra, tomato, squash, zucchini, green peppers, and two kinds of organic legumes, beans, split peas, and lentils – but for today *don't add any meat.*

Cut the vegetables into small pieces to aid digestion. Add sea salt for taste and let the soup simmer. Once cooked, first try sipping a cup of the broth because it's loaded with nutrients and will aid digestion. Then take the soup as your first evening meal.

After 10 days of fasting, this will be the best tasting soup you've ever had! Don't waste all your hard work by cramming bread and crackers back into your diet – you *are in the process of earning your health back, don't blow it now!* Store the remaining soup in the fridge for tomorrow.

Step 3.

Day 3 – Drink fresh-squeezed orange juice again in the morning, at lunchtime have the vegetable soup leftover from the previous day. For your evening meal, use any leftover vegetables to make a salad.

At this point stay away from the big four: **bread, milk, cheese, and eggs.**

Keeping things simple will really help you to highlight any sensitivities. If you want to do this, it's worth doing right, then for the rest of today also refrain away from fish, meat, pastries, sugar, coffee, and alcohol.

Step 4.

Days 4 and 5 – Congratulations, you are almost there. Continue to ease back into eating clean foods such as soups, salads, freshly sprouted seeds, and a small amount of fruit.

Over the next few days, *slowly* begin adding in grass-fed meats, but again remember to **stay away from bread, milk, eggs, and cheese**. As you *slowly* introduce solid foods back into your diet, be aware of how they make you feel. Keeping a food journal may prove helpful.
The master cleanse is an ideal way to clean up your diet after being on the road or overindulging during the holidays. With that in mind, I'd like to challenge you to make a habit of doing this once a year as part of your annual spring cleaning. But obviously, this is subject to you not taking any medications and having your own doctor be happy with your not doing so.

If you are still sitting on the fence, that's okay. It's important to do things at your own pace.

The next few chapters have some really interesting topics so just keep reading as we are just beginning to get warmed up. Rest assured, there are plenty more suggestions waiting ahead of us

Ironically, as I end this chapter a new movie has just come out starring Kyle Gallner, Anjelica Huston, and Anna Friel. The title of the movie is *The Master Cleanse*. If you have the ability **not** to take yourself too seriously, this might be something worth taking a look at.

What did we learn from this chapter?

The first four days of any cleanse can be the most challenging; after that your body enters a fat burning mode and your thinking will naturally become much clearer.

The master cleanse replaces food while gently easing the body into fasting mode. Done *correctly, you really don't feel hungry while you are doing it*. If you can't get your head around the salt water flush (huh?) simply skip that step because there are still benefits to doing the mini cleanse.

The master cleanse helps the body shed toxins while flooding the body with key nutrients. It also allows the gut to rest and repair. This in turn creates a solid base for us to work from.

Often there is a disconnect between food sensitivities. For some, the master cleanse can help identify these sensitivities as foods are *gradually* reintroduced back into the diet.

Homework: find a copy of *The Master Cleanse* by Mr. Stanley Burroughs online. It's available as a *free* download or you can purchase a hardcopy through Amazon (ISBN 9781607966074)

Chapter 16

HEAVY METALS

If the phrase heavy metal has you immediately thinking of Metallica, then unfortunately I am the bearer of bad news. Heavy metals are to you what kryptonite is to Superman. In this chapter we switch gears and begin to explore what is classically referred to as any relatively dense metal that negatively affects a person's health. Welcome to the world of heavy metals!

We now live on a toxic planet where it's inevitable that you will come into contact with a toxic heavy metal at some point. Heavy metals have the potential to cause a wide variety of health problems ranging from acute to chronic. How well the body handles this toxic exposure depends on the following three things.

1. The substance

2. The amount of time we spend coming into contact with it

3. An individual's ability to detoxify it

Trying to unravel the mystery of any illness steeped in heavy metals can be a hideously complex process not least because symptoms have the potential to present themselves in so many different forms. And a susceptibility to one heavy metal can lead to the increased risk of accumulating another. Bottom line: getting heavy metals *into* the system is the easy part, getting them out presents more of a challenge – but it is doable.

When faced with any toxic burden, we rely heavily on our filtering organs to keep the body running smoothly. These filters include the liver, kidneys, lungs, and skin which are all doing their absolute best to keep toxins from building up. When the burden becomes too great, these organs can quickly become clogged up and generally less effective. If you have ever changed an air filter in your car or vacuum cleaner, then you get the picture of how a filtering system works. Once the kidneys become less effective, a wide range of health problems can quickly follow.

The brain works a little differently because it has a protective barrier to prevent most toxins from entering; it's commonly known as the blood-brain barrier. However effective the blood-brain barrier is at keeping out certain toxins, mercury has the ability to cross that barrier with ease.

The pituitary gland, which is located deep inside the brain, is known to play an important part in the endocrine system. Some believe it also plays a role in our intuition (I had a feeling about that). Once heavy metals cross the blood-brain barrier, this essential gland is left exposed and our very thoughts can become polluted.

THE WEAKEST LINK

It seems that toxic heavy metals can land anywhere they like and once they get settled in their new home they do a first class job of messing up your body chemistry. It's highly probable that these heavy metals will tend to settle in the place of least resistance. Essentially, once they have breached the security of your body they seek out the weakest link.

Keep in mind a buildup of heavy metals has the ability to mimic disorders of the cardiovascular system, the gastrointestinal system, as well as the lungs, kidneys, liver, endocrine glands, and even bones! Unfortunately, the list goes on and on and on. More worrisome, heavy metals have the potential to affect the central nervous system, which obviously contains the brain. For that reason, heavy metals can play a significant role in mental health.

Make no mistake, heavy metals are mental assassins and clearly the human mind can't cope with them. When they are present in the body even rational thinking can become an unachievable skill. At best, foggy thinking becomes the new norm; at worst a person is capable of lashing out in frustration. Perhaps both consequences are a result of a mind that is slowly being poisoned. For many, that road can lead to incarceration. Although I have no available data to support this claim, I speculate that, if tested, a high percentage of people who make regrettable choices would have a higher than average reading if they were tested for heavy metal toxicity.

The negative effects heavy metals can have on the mind can be found in the term "mad as a hatter." This is a reference to English hat makers who, once upon a time, used mercury as part of their hat-making process. These craftsmen were well known for their mental instability, confused speech, and irrational outbursts. *Guess I'll not be buying a hat from that store anytime soon.*

These symptoms were often attributed to the toxic heavy metal used in finishing a top hat. Once the mercury entered the bloodstream it easily crossed the blood-brain barrier. Other undesirable traits of these 19th century hat makers included being quick to anger and a tendency toward violence.

To be clear, mercury isn't the only heavy metal that causes mental anguish. According to the New York University Langone Medical Center, symptoms of aluminum toxicity can include serious mental health problems, including slurred speech or speech problems and nervous system problems that may cause involuntary tics and confusion.

Lead is yet another well-known and researched neurotoxin that has been scientifically associated with major depression, reduced IQ, and anxiety disorders. It was even speculated that the fall of the mighty Roman Empire was due in part to the introduction of lead plumbing.

The CDC also reports that exposure to gaseous metallic mercury over a long period of time may cause irritability, sleep disturbances, excessive shyness, coordination problems, tremors, memory problems, and mood swings.

Let's not forget copper. Doctor Lawrence Wilson writes extensively about what he calls copper toxicity syndrome. This condition is believed to cause a number of mental health symptoms, including depression, feeling spacey, detachment, learning disorders, and Alzheimer's disease.

Bottom line: when the burden of heavy metals overwhelms the body's ability to detoxify them, these kinds of problems start to intensify.

Heavy metals can also disrupt minerals found in the body. Cadmium can compete with and displace zinc from proteins and enzymes; lead is chemically similar to calcium which can leech into the bones; and thallium mimics potassium which can affect nerves and even the cardiovascular system!

Because of their high degree of toxicity, arsenic, cadmium, chromium, lead, and mercury all rank among the priority metals that are of particular significance to our health, although this is by no means a complete list. So yup, any heavy metal (or groups of heavy metals) can adversely affect our health. Heavy metals may also compete with essential metallic cofactors for entry into the cells.

I had the privilege of speaking at great length on this subject with Dr. Alan Greenberg who is a leading expert in the field. At the time of this writing, Dr. Greenberg is an eighty-plus year old retired physician and what he *doesn't* know about heavy metal toxicity really isn't worth knowing. Standard testing for heavy metals is usually done by taking blood and urine samples, but Dr. Greenberg holds firm in the belief that the only accurate way to test a person's toxicity level is by conducting a *comprehensive* hair sample.

Establishing a toxicity level BEFORE attempting to treat a heavy metal issue is both helpful and insightful. Without knowing the cause of *your* toxicity you are running in a long race with only one shoe on. Once you have the results of a hair test, a baseline can be established.

As with our earlier chapter relating to household toxins, the most obvious first step must be to reduce any further exposure. With humans now *consistently* polluting our rivers, seas, and skies this is sometimes easier said than done. It should come as no surprise that high readings of heavy metals can be found in our rivers and streams.

Methylmercury is found in many fish supplies. This news should be of immediate concern for anyone taking fish oil supplements, although there are some highly reputable companies who offer third party testing. Third party testing basically means someone who is perceived to be independent checks the fish for excessive levels of heavy metals.

SILVER/MERCURY

Heavy metals interest me personally because I had to deal with my own exposure to mercury, arsenic, uranium, and lead. This led me to Dr. Chris Shade, PhD, whose lectures I have studied at length online. A few years ago, when my mind couldn't put these pieces of the puzzle together for myself, Dr. Shade was kind enough to talk briefly with me by telephone.

As both Dr. Shade and Dr. Greenberg pointed out, silver dental fillings contain an element of mercury, which has the potential to leach into the mouth and, therefore, the rest of the body.

Both these leading experts in their fields assure me that once these types of "silver" dental fillings become an integral part of the body, they cause a multitude of health problems. When these kinds of fillings are present, a form of mercury vapor leaches into the system, around the clock, 365 days a year. Over time this buildup has the potential to compound.

Removal of these dangerous fillings is the **only** way to prevent further exposure. In the wrong hands, however, unsafe removal adds to the problem. *Been there done that, and now have the damned tooth extraction to prove it.*

Working with a dentist who *fully* understands the dangers of this form of mercury is critical. Sadly, most don't. In Dr. Greenberg's opinion, these types of fillings should have been banned years ago. But in a complete display of either ignorance or arrogance (or both), some dentists are still putting these silver fillings into the mouths of children *despite* a mountain of evidence alerting them to the dangers!

As a child I actually went through this myself; a dentist put *seven* of these large silver fillings in my mouth. When I look back on my school days I can still recall how my ability to absorb information was greatly hindered. My

185

reading level was so bad that I was often ridiculed when asked to read out loud; my math teacher totally gave up on me, I can seriously remember being almost eleven years old before I could tell time and yet here I am writing this book, a testament to how the human body can recover.

Sadly, my problems didn't stop inside the school. Once outside, I'd often find myself doing battle with anyone who looked at me a certain way. On the whole, I was a pretty messed up angry kid. *I know, right? Why would they put mercury in kids' teeth?*

Thankfully I have since had them all removed. It was only *after* removal of those toxic silver fillings (along with a chelation process) that I began to better understand that I was actually capable of thinking clearly. Today I might have fewer teeth, but to be honest I'm enjoying getting more use out of my brain.

Unfortunately, heavy metals aren't confined to teeth. They can come to you in anything from the water you drink to the environment you work in. Trying to figure out *where* the most prolific toxic offender is coming from is sometimes easier than trying to source the less obvious.

Heavy metals are an extremely complicated riddle to solve and trying to work it out on your own as I did can be a real source of frustration, *especially* if you aren't feeling well to begin with. I found having a hair sample done helped take away some of the guesswork which then allowed me to target my research in a more specific direction.

This was a simple matter of sending away a sample to a laboratory that later returned a full color-coded print-out of my exposure to heavy metals, many of which had built up over years.

(See diagram)

TOXIC METALS		RESULT µg/g	REFERENCE INTERVAL	PERCENTILE 68th 95th
Aluminum	(Al)	9.0	< 8.0	
Antimony	(Sb)	0.088	< 0.066	
Arsenic	(As)	0.14	< 0.080	
Barium	(Ba)	0.30	< 0.75	
Beryllium	(Be)	< 0.01	< 0.020	
Bismuth	(Bi)	0.13	< 2.0	
Cadmium	(Cd)	0.025	< 0.070	
Lead	(Pb)	0.92	< 1.0	
Mercury	(Hg)	1.1	< 0.40	
Platinum	(Pt)	< 0.003	< 0.005	
Thallium	(Tl)	< 0.001	< 0.002	
Thorium	(Th)	< 0.001	< 0.002	
Uranium	(U)	0.010	< 0.060	
Nickel	(Ni)	0.13	< 0.20	
Silver	(Ag)	0.14	< 0.14	
Tin	(Sn)	0.32	< 0.30	
Titanium	(Ti)	0.51	< 0.70	
Total Toxic Representation				

In some states you may need a licensed practitioner to order the test for you, but once you have it, the test can be carried out at home and mailed back in a prepaid envelope. The company I used for the hair sample was Doctorsdata and I believe they still have a website by the same name.

Once you know what you are up against there are numerous ways to chelate (remove) heavy metals from the body. Given that it is easier to get this wrong than it is to get it right I urge anyone with a heavy metal issue to work with a *knowledgeable* practitioner who has a clear understanding of this issue.

Once you have your hair sample test results, solving the puzzle of which heavy metals may be affecting you and how to get rid of them becomes much more doable.

Different heavy metal toxicities require different chelation methods depending largely on your unique individual needs. If your hair sample comes back with a high reading showing uranium, try not to freak yourself out. Uranium can easily come up from the bedrock if you are drinking water from a well. In most people, when the liver and kidneys are working optimally, uranium passes through the body without too much of an issue. However, there is something that hinders this process, *any guesses what it is?*
According to Dr. Alan Greenberg silver/mercury fillings have the potential to contribute to the buildup of uranium in the cells. This can be quite an

issue if there is a lot of granite deep down in the bedrock. Once again those metal fillings are going to come back to bite you.

Given my own personal exposure to silver/mercury fillings, it was no great surprise to see uranium levels reflected in my hair sample. But some months later, a follow-up hair sample showed a reduction. I believe this was achieved by adding a small amount of sodium bicarbonate to my drinking water every morning, although I have yet to see this idea anywhere else in print so my thoughts on this are purely speculative.

Heavy metals are masters of disruption and can affect the whole physiology of the body; *they can also mimic many of the minerals the body readily uses.* For example, lead is mistaken for calcium by the body and both are easily absorbed into the bones.

To have a better understanding of this fascinating subject let's dig a little deeper before we peel away and begin looking at a few practical solutions. Don't let the science bit scare you away, by the time this chapter ends it should all make sense.

Messing with the body's enzymes is what heavy metals appear to do best. Enzymes are designed to help regulate different processes and make certain chemical reactions happen. Enzymes do this by tying together things like sulfhydryl groups, which are basically a certain kind of sulfur.

Keep in mind that enzymes are proteins built of amino acids, and inside the amino acid cysteine groups is the sulfhydryl group. *Okay, so why is this important to know?*

Sulfhydryl groups are great at moving electrons around and holding the good metals in place, such as copper and zinc. Unfortunately, the thing that also likes to link up with sulfhydryl groups is mercury. Once mercury gets attached, it displaces the copper or the zinc that was *supposed* to be there. Bottom line: *these heavy metals, particularly mercury, block essential minerals like copper and zinc from doing their job.*

Heavy metals have the potential to disrupt just about any of the essential minerals needed by the body, but for the moment let's stay with copper and zinc.

Zinc, as you may already know, is required for the catalytic activity of more than 300 enzymes; it's involved in the synthesis and metabolism of carbohydrates, fats, proteins, nucleic acids, and other micronutrients. To understand the importance of this, know that mercury totally messes up how these enzymes work.

Copper and zinc are a team that likes to work together. Copper is important for a healthy heart, bones, and brain development. Zinc is an immune-system booster that helps the body stay healthy. But once again it's a delicate **balance**. Copper and zinc have an interesting relationship where the intake of one of these elements causes the other element to decrease in your body.

Taking too much zinc can be dangerous; it can result in irreversible neurological ailments often associated with copper deficiency. A **balance** between the two is critically important to prevent a buildup of toxicity in the body while ensuring both the functions of these two minerals is preserved. Now throw in the mix a destructive heavy metal and the fine balance soon becomes unglued.

Are we there yet? Heavy metals have the potential to disrupt just about every mineral in the body. Yes, copper and zinc are important but so are all the other minerals that also need to be kept in balance. Can you imagine the confusion that happens in the mind? *Hmm, I see.*

But it doesn't stop there; this blocking of essential minerals also takes place in the mitochondria. Now we are really off to the races. Mitochondria are the energy factory of the body and when these bad boys go down so too does your energy. *Hello again chronic fatigue.*

Heavy metals are not only destructive; they can be very difficult to remove. The term for removing heavy metals from the body is described as "chelation" and here's the golden rule. Whenever an attempt is made to remove heavy metals, don't be greedy. This simply means that *chelation* needs to be done slowly by someone who understands the dangers. Any attempt to do this too quickly will cause you to crash and burn. Trust me, I've been there and you don't want to go there.

Although my persistence eventually paid off, I went through a heck of a lot of trial and error and some of the error was extremely unpleasant. For this very reason I recommended you work with an expert in this field; the information presented here is offered only as a basic research tool.

Why go slow?

If your body has a buildup of heavy metals there is a very good chance your liver and kidneys aren't performing optimally (this was mentioned in an earlier chapter). Trying to force out toxic heavy metals *quickly* will inevitably cause a huge *bottleneck* and when the heavy metals can't get out fast enough they are reabsorbed. *Why is this a problem?*

Think about it, many of these heavy metals may have been stored away for years in separate parts of the body in the hope that they could be processed at a later date.

This storing of these heavy metals could happen anywhere from the muscles to the brain. Along comes your well-meaning natural doctor who then tries to get them out a little too quickly and now the heavy metals are suddenly back circulating the blood stream. The trick to pulling this off is to (a) first help the liver and kidneys with an effective protocol, and (b) go slow.

In case you were wondering how it feels to get it wrong, say hello to your new apocalyptic zombie self. Been there, done that. *Please* don't make the same mistake; luckily I also had a few emergency tools in the box to help pull myself out of it again.

If you are looking to do this safely, *then this isn't a process you can rush.* Think of chelation as a marathon, not a sprint. Make sure that whoever is treating you has a clear understanding of why it's important to start small and go slow. It might be someone else's treatment you are tapping into, *but ultimately it is your life.*

When working with your own practitioner they will inevitably have their own protocol for removing heavy metals based on YOUR individual circumstance. This is good. They may look to use natural supplements like glutathione (GSH) vitamin C, and methylsulfonylmethane (MSM) because all three of these work synergistically.

Both vitamin C and MSM are precursors to glutathione, which is a substance produced naturally by the liver and is also helpful in chelation.

Tip – MSM is widely available in powder form. To check the quality of the product add it to a clear glass of water. Pure MSM will sink straight to the bottom; whatever is left floating on the top of the water is being used as a filler.

GLUTATHIONE

Glutathione (or GSH) is an antioxidant most people have probably never heard of but it's important to help keep everything in balance. Glutathione is considered the mother of all antioxidants and the master detoxifier. It's deemed so important that your body decided it needed to be able to make its own, but poor diet, toxins, stress, and too many ongoing infections all help to deplete the body's glutathione stores.

Taking glutathione in pill form can be tricky because it's easily broken down and lost in digestion. Some of the better quality products may offer Liposomal Glutathione which has the advantage of being protected from the stomach due to the manufacturing process used. Glutathione can also be given intravenously by your doctor and there is a lot of data to support the idea that this may be helpful for people with Parkinson's disease.

Low glutathione would also be suspected in a body that is simply feeling run down. Instead of paying for treatment, another way to increase your glutathione levels naturally is to eat more avocados. *Yes, really.*
For a super quick, super healthy meal, simply mix avocado with blueberries, add the juice from a freshly squeezed lime and a pinch of sea salt and hey, presto, you just made a good fat snack in under two minutes.

Sulfur also increases glutathione, which means garlic and onions are good sources. Sulfur is a sticky, smelly molecule that sticks to bad things like free radicals, toxins, and heavy metals with almost magnetic strength and then ships them out of the body.

Glutathione is actually a very simple molecule, a combination of three simple building blocks of protein or amino acids — cysteine, glycine, and glutamine. The secret of its power is the sulfur. **Bottom line: glutathione is critical to our overall health and that of the immune system.**

Another gentle tool to assist in removing heavy metals is dark leafy greens. Do you see why nutrition is so important? Maybe the reason some mainstream doctors fail to fully grasp the concept of chelation is that most of them receive virtually no nutritional training. *A little odd don't you think?*

As with glutathione, the body also has a small reserve of vitamin C, which can quickly become exhausted as toxicity levels increase. These are not the only healing tools at your disposal and you could also target some of your research toward activated charcoal, which may also be helpful in removing certain heavy metals. Activated charcoal can also be helpful for stomach aches.

The following information is good to have in your toolbox – however, rather than see you get this wrong, I've been intentionally vague about doses.

In some circles of natural chelation there is something known as a "healing triangle." This triangle consists of Chlorella, Alpha Lipoic Acid (ALA), and Cilantro. It's really a three-part trick and if you have a known heavy metal issue, then FFS go easy with the cilantro part. *Cilantro should be consumed in absolute moderation and never on its own. Here's why.*

In this triangle, the role of cilantro is to stir up heavy metals in the body. This only becomes helpful when used with the other two parts of the healing triangle. Think of a clear bowl of water with a thin layer dirt at the bottom. The dirt is representative of the heavy metals. Now take a spoon and stir the water. Think of the action of the spoon as cilantro.

That's a pretty neat trick but remember that this trick comes in three parts. Using too much cilantro on its own can (and will) make you wish you had not been in such a rush to have a wave toxic heavy metals flowing through your bloodstream.

Why?

When you stirred up the heavy metals you didn't offer the heavy metals a way out. With nothing in place to catch them, it's like stirring up a hornet's nest. Thanks to the cilantro, heavy metals are now racing through your bloodstream and no doubt making you feel worse than when you started. *Had you known about the second part of the triangle, however, all would not have been lost.*

Again I'd like to stress the purpose of this information is to help guide you toward making better research choices and ultimately your best option is to work with a well-versed doctor who understands these basic principles. *Got it? I'm trying to do you a solid here.*

The next part of the trick requires chlorella. Chlorella is freshwater algae that has been shown to be helpful in detoxifying low levels of heavy metals. Once the cilantro has stirred up all those heavy metals, chlorella collects them from the gut. So far so good, but there's a problem, *can you see it?*

Remember I said that some heavy metals have the ability to cross the blood brain barrier? As useful as chlorella is at collecting heavy metals in the gut, it's doing nothing to help remove those deeper set heavy metals now circulating in the brain. This is where the third part of the trick comes in.

ALA (Alpha Lipoic Acid) *is* known to cross into the blood-brain barrier and in doing so binds to heavy metals; hence the triangle is now complete **when all are used in conjunction with each other.** But the devil is in the details and your individual circumstance will vary greatly. Keep in mind that trying to force heavy metals out of a body that isn't working properly is simply asking for more problems, hence my reluctance to supply you with exact doses.

However, if circumstances allow, you could try the least invasive option first, which is adding chlorella to the diet. You can buy this in supplement form in any health food store. Chlorella is a source of Chlorophyll, Protein, Iron, Magnesium, and amino acids, but it is primarily known as a detoxifying supplement. Simply sprinkle a small amount onto your food or you can dip a sliced apple into it which also carries the benefit of pectin and can help remove lead.

Also be sure not to underestimate the value of green leafy vegetables. You may have noticed that food keeps emerging as a common thread; there are some foods that are helpful and some that are more destructive. Green leafy vegetables have been shown to help the body detoxify and should be eaten in abundance (and then some). Sooner or later I'm hoping the penny will drop that the food you choose to put into your mouth plays a strong role in linking all of this all together.

A good quality vitamin C may also be helpful in the detoxification process but be smart, don't try too many new things at once; maybe keep a diary to plot your progress. Whenever you try something new challenge yourself to find three benefits for taking it, and then balance it out by making yourself aware of at least three potential side effects. This will prevent you from getting carried away by the often euphoric claims made online.

Sweating can help you detoxify heavy metals and this process can be assisted with the use of a sauna. If you have access to a local gym make a point of asking if they have an infrared sauna, these types of saunas are superior as they reach deeper into the cells. And as a bonus they are more comfortable to sit in.

Lastly, if you find yourself in a heavy metal bind with no way out then you could always check out a product by the name of Zeolite. It's something I have used on occasion but it's super important to get the *right* quality. Be sure to do your homework, a good starting point would be to Google Dr. Garry Gordon / ZeoGold.

What did we learn from this chapter?

To some degree we all have trace amounts of heavy metals in our bodies – it's the price of modern living. When the burden becomes too great, a wide range of symptoms can manifest as physical, mental, or both. Essential minerals like zinc can be blocked by mercury.

There is no getting away from heavy metals. Some of their effects are subtle and others are profoundly destructive. This is often an under-reported problem that can have serious health implications. Heavy metals can settle ANYWHERE in the body with a tendency to go for the weakest link in your chain.

Don't try to remove heavy metals yourself. Find someone to work *with*. This doesn't necessarily mean you can't still be active in your own recovery. You can start by educating yourself on the subject. Remember the golden rule: don't get greedy and try to remove heavy metals too quickly. Always start with the smallest dose and go slow.

Homework: consider getting tested for heavy metals by using a respected hair sample company. To better understand this chapter, please be sure to watch this short video clip.

https://www.youtube.com/watch?v=9ylnQ-T7oiA

Chapter 17

STALK A SENIOR

When attempting to move through my local supermarket at speed, I can't help noticing that my flow is interrupted by a six foot wall of soda stacked on pallets. One sugar spike side-stepped, and I'm immediately presented with another. Brightly colored cakes, cookies, and pastries are all lined up to whisper sweet nothings in my ear. Making a hard left, it's hard to miss a whole aisle that has been turned into something of a candy store. As you cruise past the boxed cereals, you just know that all those unnatural colors are heavily laced with even more sugar.

Full speed ahead and I'm walking through the freezer section and its row after row after row of sugar spiking ice cream and popsicles. Finally, as I am forced to wait in line at the checkout, I'm confronted with a glass doored refrigerator to my right that's brimming with fruit juice and even more soda. I avert my gaze, and it's a full-on sales pitch from the bubble gum and candy companies on the left. I place my carefully planned purchase of a dozen pencils on the conveyor belt and the checkout lady looks up at me and with a totally straight face and asks if I'd like to donate a dollar to diabetes research? *I know, right? You can't make this stuff up!*

Whether we realize it or not, most of our dietary information comes from the people we should trust the least: *those with a product to sell us!* At best this can form a conflict of interest, at worst it can be a real challenge to see past those slick commercials that fool us all into buying more of those hidden sugars, food additives, and preservatives.

Let's strive to keep this simple. There are only two types of foods of interest to us, *those foods that keep us healthy and those foods that keep us sick.* Those on the fringe of ill health may get away with faking it for a while, but the sicker you are the more relevant this chapter becomes.

Something in your diet obviously sucks or you wouldn't be feeling ill. Here's the rub. Ask most people if *they* eat healthy and you will usually get this response, "Yup, I eat fairly healthy." Now we see the problem for what it is. A *fairly healthy diet* is a **perception** or a belief system that's built on the back of misinformation. Okay, but where the heck did this misinformation come from?

This idea that we have *"a fairly good diet"* is a dangerous one. I already know that you *don't* have a good diet because you told me so when you picked up this book.

Until we find the answer, it pays to keep an open mind. When we view our diet as good, three times a day we unintentionally shoot ourselves in the foot. Few people think, *hmm, best I nip myself down to the shop and load up on some toxic anti-nutrients.* Nope that idea is often gifted to us by the people selling us our food in the form of subliminal advertising.

As mentioned earlier, processed foods started off in life as one ingredient and then quickly ended up on someone's production line to maximize profit. This isn't how our ancestors ate. I think we can safely say illness *isn't* due to a deficiency in processed foods. Fortunately, your solutions are now coming.

First, we have to give credit where it's due. Supermarkets *really* do know how to sell us a product, and all too often we don't even realize that we are being sold to! Supermarket floor plans are not laid out by accident but are purposefully arranged to make you go wherever *they* want you to go. Once we enter the store we are unwittingly influenced to buy products we didn't even know we needed. Colors and labels are arranged not by chance but in a calculated bid to grab our attention. *I know, right? Why would we listen to them?*

Well, for starters, the food industry is profitable and as such it can afford to run marketing campaigns at peak meal times. The timing of these commercials is slick and their effectiveness can stretch across generations. I suspect if we dug a little deeper, we'd learn that some of the nutritional advice we own today was handed down to us by our well-meaning parents. *Drink your milk up, it's good for your bones.* Right? If only it were that easy.

To be clear, the food industry is in business to make a profit. This is good for the economy and provides countless jobs. I have no problem with commerce and good luck to anyone making an *honest* buck, but it's important to understand the laws of business do not allow for cheap and quality to coexist in the same product.

Supermarkets are constantly trying to undercut their competition on price and while this might seem like a good deal for the consumer, this price cutting can result in a race to the bottom. *Maybe it's time we stopped asking why healthy food is so expensive and start asking why junk food is so cheap?*

Discount supermarkets are missing out on a unique opportunity. A strong undercurrent of better informed consumers is now developing. People are waking up to the idea that food preservatives are conveniently solving one problem but causing another of much greater magnitude in the process.

If supermarkets took the bold move to slant their own brands toward health rather than price, I suspect loyal customers would line up to support those markets that appear to have their backs. Alas, rather than employ a health guru, the food industry has seen fit to employ top psychologists as a way help tempt your hard-earned money away. *Whoa! Why would a supermarket want to hire someone that studies human emotions and behavior?*

THE BRAIN REWARD SYSTEM

The answer is simple: supermarkets want to find the best way to tap into your *brain-reward-system* to help them sell more products. The *brain-reward-system* is well documented and involves several parts of the brain.

Originally this system was designed for *survival* eating rather than *pleasure* eating. When the *brain-reward-system* is tricked by certain foods (particularly fats and sweets) it changes brain chemistry in a way that drives people to over consume.

Once the *brain-reward-system* is hacked, these types of foods are able to provide a hit of pleasure in the form of dopamine. This is good news for food industry profits, but not so good for anyone trying to break the junk food cycle.

Dopamine is a neurotransmitter. It's also a chemical messenger that helps with brain signals and makes us feel good; hence overindulgence has an **addictive** quality to it. It's the reason you can't eat just one cookie.

The word "addiction" is derived from a Latin term for "enslaved by" or "bound to." Anyone struggling to overcome a sugar addiction will understand the challenge this brings. According to USDA Economic Research Service, the average child under twelve is now *addicted* to consuming, on average, forty-nine pounds of sugar per year. *I know, right? Who the heck is running the food industry, Montgomery Burns?*

THE SUGAR DECEPTION

With one in four kids now thought to be diabetic or pre-diabetic you might wonder how adding sugar to the food supply (as a way to increase profits) is even legal. But I digress.

A brief walk around any supermarket highlights the scope of the problem. Whether you recognize it or not, sugar is in just about every product. But you can't rely on the food manufacturers to call it sugar. According to sugarscience.org, sugar comes in many guises.

There are currently at least *sixty-one* different names for sugar listed on food labels! These include common names such as barley malt, dextrose, maltose, sucrose, high-fructose corn syrup, and rice syrup – to name just a few.

> *It's easier to fool people than to convince*
> *them that they have been fooled.*
> – Mark Twain

Run from any food whose label boasts "All Natural" for this is the cruelest con of all. It preys on the very people that are *trying* to make better choices. Sadly, neither the FDA nor the USDA seem keen to police these "all-natural" labels.

As a result, food manufacturers are free to place a "natural" label on foods that could potentially contain any number of processed ingredients. It may help to think of it this way: 100 years ago, 80% of the food found on supermarket shelves didn't even exist. *What's up with that?* As you walk the food aisle, keep in mind that the average vegetable now travels approximately 1500 miles to get to your dinner plate and then compare it to the food found at your local farmer's market. To our ancestors, this would have seemed like wasteful folly because they would have walked less than fifty feet to pluck a full basket of *clean*, ripe produce from the garden.

Our ancestors understood the value of eating *real* food and *not* what today we perceive as food. We could argue that the hand that stirs the cooking pot is the one that rules the world. With an epidemic of childhood pre-diabetes rates now spiraling out of control, awareness becomes key. Back in the day, owning a garden would have been a normal, everyday occurrence with zero options for buying chemically sprayed food.

Still not convinced?

Unless you have spent the past few years living in a creepy apartment with the curtains closed, you might have also noticed the rest of the outside world is experiencing an upsurge in food allergies. Maybe it's not food that is the problem, but what's been done *to* the food.

We are so preoccupied with counting calories that we fail to count the number of additives and pesticides in our food. If the bugs won't go near it with a 12ft pole, why are we rushing to fill our carts with it? What do the bugs know that we don't? *Let's take a closer look.*

GMO

The food industry is quick to tell us that GMO crops are safe. While this might even be true, this technology is still in its infancy and as yet nobody has conducted any *long-term* studies to back that bold statement up.

As it stands, what we do know is that companies have begun splicing animal bacteria and viral genes with our raw vegetables and fruit, something that has never been done before in our history. *I know, right? Man messing with our food, what could possibly go wrong?*

A rock solid good idea will usually stand the test of time. Who hasn't heard the now famous quote, "Let food be thy medicine and medicine be thy food."? If we are still quoting Hippocrates almost 2500 years later, maybe he knew a thing or two after all. Hippocrates did not say, *"Spray thy food with chemicals and then splice it with the bacteria of an animal."* Surely that would be utter nonsense.

STANDING IN LINE

Slowly we are moving toward exploring the idea that there are foods that heal, and foods that absolutely don't. How do we find the foods that heal?

One way to find a diet that works for you is to keep reading. Another is to find a senior over the age of sixty who still looks healthy and politely ask them what it is they eat. Think about it, the body can't take six decades of eating junk food and still work so they *must* be doing something right. Young people can get away with it and still look good because, as Bernard Shaw once said, "Youth is wasted on the young."

Typically, anyone who's over 60 and is still active has to be doing something right, *right?* If you approach people in the right way, most will be glad to share what it is that keeps them healthy. Be **respectful** and some may even be flattered that you've noticed. If you want to see what a healthy 60+ person looks like without a shirt on, be sure to check out today's homework section.

Maybe the next time you are standing in line at the supermarket, be on the lookout for anyone who's over sixty and still looks to have radiant health. Don't be stalking now, just smile and take a discreet glance at the things they are buying. You may be surprised to see a lack of processed foods in their shopping carts.

The most heavily processed foods are pre-made meals – obviously these include things like frozen pizza and microwaveable dinners. These foods are high in calories and **low** in actual nutritional content.

Microwave meals are cheap and quick to make, but there really is no such thing as cheap food if, in the process, it fails to restore health.

> *The microwave is the consolation prize*
> *in our struggle to understand physics.*
> –Jason Love

Now, back in the supermarket line, do you also see that *other* person, yup, you know the one I'm talking about, the guy whose kids are bouncing off the walls high on sugar. How does his cart look? If discretion is a new tool to you, please refrain from pointing or, God forbid, giving in to the urge to start prodding with your organic cucumber ... *it happens.*

Making poor choices in the supermarket all but guarantees that poor choices will be made in the kitchen. Astonishingly enough, there is a strong connection between whatever we put into the shopping cart and what ends up in our mouths.
Let's cut to the chase – our ancestors got a lot of things right. For them, cooking real food at home with whole food ingredients was an everyday event. Keep in mind the Roman army marched on its stomach, *not* Captain Crunchy.

What did we learn from this chapter?

Supermarkets are designed to conspire against our subconscious and have become masters of distraction. Sugar is now routinely added to lots of foods, but it's not always called sugar.

The *perception* of what is healthy can dramatically vary from one person to another. For some a healthy choice might be a vegetarian version of only eating pizza and French fries twice a week.

Homework: to see what a healthy 60+ man looks like with no shirt on check out a blog by the name of "Mark's Daily Apple" or click on the link below.

http://www.marksdailyapple.com/

Chapter 18

MEET THE TOXIC FUNGI

Fungi is the plural of *fungus*. Fungi have many forms and they have been a part of this world since the beginning of time. Fungi can be found in nature and they can also be found inside you. In a healthy, well balanced body, fungi often coexist with little disruption to the host, but fungi are an opportunistic organism. Once they gain the upper hand they can cause a wide range of health problems.

Fungi are also persistent and adaptable; they can mimic parts of your body and even send out confusing signals to evade detection. Left unchecked, fungi can become quite the formidable foe. Some reports even suggest there is a strong a connection between fungus and cancer, although Nobel peace prize winner Otto Warburg believed that fungus was *not* a cancer, but it certainly acted like one.

It's fair to say that fungi are extremely effective at what they do, although attempting to eradicate all fungi from the body is probably not the right way to look at this challenging problem. Like so many battles, this isn't one you can win, *it has to be managed.*

We humans often like to think in terms of waging war on a disease, but fungi, bacteria, viruses and even cancerous cells are all in relatively healthy people. *So what does that mean?*

Any one of the above conditions can lead to a disease but they are not necessarily the problem. It might be more helpful to ask, "Is my body effectively managing these potential threats?

A stressed, malnourished body will always result in an imbalance *somewhere* in the body, usually in the form of a wakened immune system. Throw in a few manmade sugars and fungi are presented with the ideal opportunity to gain the upper hand; we have now come full circle.

The body's preferred state is to be in balance. Remembering this profoundly simple concept will serve you well as we continue moving forward. You could call it being in a state of equilibrium.

For the body to maintain a sense of balance, the body keeps fungi in-check by crowding them out with good bacteria. It's a case of having more good guys than bad guys in your system. Unfortunately, the bad guys in your system have an affinity for junk food. So, a smart first step in the right direction is obviously limiting their preferred food supply (manmade sugar). Getting this part of the puzzle right is important because so many of the other techniques rely on it.

Fungal infections can spread quickly or slowly, they can be either superficial or systemic, they can range in severity from acute to chronic, and they can even turn deadly! The word systemic simply refers to something that's affecting the entire body rather than a single organ or body part.

Superficial infections are far more annoying than problematic as they grow on the *outside* of the body, affecting the nails and surface of the skin. Fungal infections can pop up just about anywhere, but mostly occur in moist areas, such as between the toes, in the crotch, or in the mouth. Ever seen that thick white coating on the tongue?

Systemic fungal infections become more of a concern because they develop slowly, taking weeks or months to become an issue and eventually targeting internal organs. Problems often start in the lungs, but in severe cases can spread to the blood, heart, brain, kidneys, and liver. These toxic organisms know how to wait for balance to tip in their favor – and when it does, they are prepared to act quickly. And they have the potential to cause a variety of *serious* illnesses.

At this point, you should be asking yourself, what the hell would tip the balance in their favor? *Are* you asking that?

The answer is twofold. The first is sugar (well hello again!). Fungi thrives on the stuff. Make no mistake, sugar isn't always what you think it is. All

206

those carbohydrates you eat quickly turn to sugar. It might also surprise you to know that fruit adds to the problem – fruit juice in particular. Once the fiber is removed from fruit it's essentially turned into liquid sugar. Oh, but the fun doesn't stop there.

Make no mistake, sugar can be found in abundance even BEFORE we start in with all those manmade sugars. And let's not forget the glycemic table where you will find that certain vegetables, such as carrots and beets, have a naturally high sugar contents – even protein turns to sugar.

Why am I telling you all this? Think about it; sugar is now hidden in everything from frozen yogurt to baked beans, from bread to soup, from salad dressing to sushi, it's even added to some bacon. *Are you catching all this? Sugar isn't just cookies, candy, and soda!*

Processed foods are heavily laden with sugar often you won't even know it. Walk down any aisle in the supermarket and you will find sugar, sugar, and more sugar. To make matters worse, you can't even count on the food manufacturer calling it sugar. *I know, right? But wait till you hear this.*
When the amount of sugar overshadows the body's ability to regulate it, the balance is tipped. This really isn't that difficult to do when you stop to think that on average, a single soft drink contains the equivalent of seven teaspoons of sugar!
For now, let's go back to those fungi – you know, the ones already inside you. Think of them as small groups of dangerous rebels who like to feed on sugar. In a healthy body they are surrounded by an army of *good* bacteria so the threat remains pretty low.

But, the fungi have aspirations to one day overthrow the government (that's *you*) so this battle plays out daily in the gut. So long as fungi remain vastly outnumbered by the good guys, the body can keep them at a manageable level.

Once the right opportunity presents itself, fungi can spring into action and quickly develop a stronghold. *Be warned, getting the genie back in the bottle is no easy process.* As their numbers begin to swell, they leave behind a trail of lingering illness and destruction with the potential to tear down the whole system (unfortunately, you again).

Let's see who's paying attention.

Is sugar bad for you?

If you said yes, then you would be wrong. Sugar isn't the problem; it's the *amount* of sugar that causes the problem. Let's not forget that the body actually makes its own sugar by converting simple and complex carbohydrates, hence it really doesn't need any more from you in the form of those *hidden* manmade sugars.

ANTI-LIFE

The standard American diet has now been exported around the world. Sadly for everyone this diet has way too many *hidden* sugars for the body to cope with. Keeping fungi in check is a challenge at the best of times — when we add a **second** part into this problem all bets are off. Any guesses what that second part is?

Statistically speaking it's probably already happened to you. Hands up anyone who's ever taken antibiotics. Antibiotics are now so ***over-prescribed*** that it's helping the bad guys get that firmer foothold they've been waiting for.

Antibiotics work by helping kill off the bad bacteria (that's good), but antibiotics also kill indiscriminately (not so good). Any potential infection treated by antibiotics is essentially wiping out many of the good guys along with the bad.

The fear of many is that each prescription for stronger antibiotics will eventually create super-strength bacteria (and in many cases, already has). This new, super-bacteria will in turn become resistant to *all forms* of antibiotics. Worse, even if *you* choose *not* to take antibiotics, the problem isn't entirely eliminated. *Why is that?*

Antibiotics are now heavily used in the food supply (oh come on) and if the animals we eat consume antibiotics, so do we. If we already know that it's the job of the good bacteria to keep fungi in check, then it is logical to conclude that **antibiotic overuse has the potential to solve one problem but create another.**

Let's look at it this way. The word "anti" means against, biotic pertains to life, in this context we could think of antibiotics as being anti-life. Earlier we suggested that the gut was the cornerstone of our health. Once we decide to disproportionately kill off large groups of gut bacteria, our overall health suffers. *Are you beginning to see how this sugar thing keeps coming back into play?*

Antibiotic overuse can be a recipe for disaster, a constant craving for sugar may be an indicator that an imbalance has already begun. Pathogenic bacteria, parasites, and yeast, such as candida feed off sugar. The more sugar you eat, the more inviting you make your gut for these "bad guys."

Some have suggested that during this critical window when rebel fungi gain the upper hand fungi may even have strong links with cancer. While this may be speculative, what we do know for sure is that both cancer and fungi seem to have a love for sugar. Feeling hungry all the time makes cutting out junk foods a *real* challenge. This obstacle has the potential to derail all attempts to change. To add to the problem, your average doctor receives very little training on this subject. The good news is, when you learn to pay attention, fungus becomes an excellent teacher. Usually, a body with a fungal infection that's gained the upper hand will itch, almost to the point where you could scratch through the skin whenever excess sugar is consumed. *Are you getting this? Your body is so smart it's telling you when you get it wrong.*

PROBIOTICS

While it's unfortunate that antibiotics wreak havoc on our delicate ecosystem it may be possible to readjust the balance in the favor of the good guys again by consuming *fermented foods* or taking a *quality* probiotic – but it does take time. Probiotics can be found in most good health food stores and come in pill form. Once swallowed, they may help to repopulate the good bacteria. As with most things, you get what you pay for, so don't be too surprised if that "bargain" brand probiotic at the box store doesn't do it for you.

Buy the *best* probiotics you can afford rather than what's on sale. *This is your health and as such it needs to have a value.* Some probiotics can be heat or moisture sensitive, and some may need refrigeration. With that in mind it's a good idea not to leave probiotics sitting inside your hot car or out on the kitchen counter.

CANDIDA

All fungus types are masters of survival but if they have one quality above all others it is this: *they know how to adapt.* Put simply, yeast cells aren't going to just roll over and die for you while your sugar levels are elevated.

The one you may have heard most about is candida – and *it's already living inside you.* It may surprise you to learn that a certain level of candida helps you to digest your food, but candida can easily get out of control, especially with the overuse of antibiotics and/or excessive sugars. When this happens, watch out!

Candida is a fungus that comes in the form of yeast that lives in the intestines. When it's kept in check its *primary* function is to assist with digestion and the absorption of nutrients. It coexists with good bacteria and, all things being equal, the two live happily together. But it's a delicate balance and problems start when candida gets a little too big for its boots.

If presented with the right opportunity, candida can quickly become invasive. Once it has the upper hand, a cascade of problems usually follows. Out of control candida becomes destructive and can even break down the wall of the intestine releasing toxic byproducts into your bloodstream in the process. *Well, hello again to you, cheeky-leaky gut.*

A diet that's high in processed foods and sugar and then loaded with carbohydrates will favor candida, as can sustained levels of stress, antibiotics, alcohol consumption, and oral contraceptives (and hello again to you, estrogen disruptor).

I previously mentioned that fermented foods could help to repopulate gut flora. However, with an outbreak of candida, the situation becomes more of a challenge and fermented foods should be restricted until candida is under control. This is due in part to an increased Herxheimer reaction, sometimes called a "die-off" reaction.

When a die-off occurs, metabolic by-products are released into the body. When the candida yeast cells die, they release 79 different toxins, including ethanol and acetaldehyde. Die-off symptoms can include the following.

- Nausea
- Headache, fatigue, dizziness
- Swollen glands
- Bloating, gas, constipation, or diarrhea
- Increased joint or muscle pain
- Elevated heart rate
- Chills, cold feeling in your extremities
- Body itchiness, hives, or rashes
- Sweating
- Fever
- Skin breakouts
- Recurring vaginal, prostate, and sinus infections

The point when the die-off symptoms begin is the time when many people prematurely abandon their candida diet. It might surprise you to know that the health drink kombucha, favored by many health freaks, can *add* to the problem. *Why?*

Kombucha contains wild strains of yeast and, due to the activity of the yeast, is also slightly alcoholic. The immune system of someone struggling with Candida overgrowth may find it a challenge to deal with these wild strains of yeast. Once candida is back under control, however, drinking kombucha in moderation can be a good thing.

For sure, sugar has an addictive quality much the same as any ugly street drug, but frequent strong cravings for cookies, candy, and bread can be a sign that something else is going on. If you find yourself constantly heading to the food cupboard I need to ask, *how is your brain fog and energy?*

If you have strong sugar cravings, brain fog, and low energy it could be a sign of a candida overgrowth. Happily, by the time you finish this very chapter you will have a way to test yourself for candida in the comfort of your own home without it costing you a penny. It is estimated that **70% of us** live with a candida overgrowth and contrary to popular belief it affects **both** men and women. Some of the typical symptoms are:

- *Strong* cravings for sugar and refined carbohydrates
- Frequent brain fog and inability to concentrate
- Digestive issues such as bloating, constipation, or diarrhea
- Feeling tired and worn out all the time
- A white coat on tongue
- Difficulty concentrating, poor memory, lack of focus, ADD, ADHD
- Skin issues like eczema, psoriasis, hives, and rashes
- Irritability, mood swings
- Anxiety or depression
- Severe seasonal allergies or itchy ears
- Fibromyalgia
- Athlete's foot or toenail fungus
- Bad breath
- Hormone imbalance
- Joint pain
- Loss of sex drive

- Chronic sinus and allergy issues
- Urinary tract infections, rectal itching, or vaginal itching
- Weakened immune system
- Autoimmune diseases such as Hashimoto's thyroiditis, rheumatoid arthritis, ulcerative colitis, lupus, psoriasis, or multiple sclerosis

Phew, that's quite a list! That white coating on the tongue is a particular giveaway that something funky is going, on or that something is out of balance. If you suspect candida might be an issue, here's that simple self-test I promised you.

CANDIDA SELF TEST

Before going to bed fill a clear glass with water, allow it to stand overnight *at room temperature,* then pin a note to your bathroom mirror to remind you to spit into the glass first thing in the morning BEFORE you eat, drink, or brush your teeth.

The trick is to accumulate enough saliva in your mouth and then with the glass held close to your mouth *gently* spit the saliva into the glass of water. *I know, gross,* but watch carefully, the sample saliva is then going to do one of three things.

(1) Float on the top of the water

(2) Sink to the bottom

(3) Slowly make its way downward and begin looking like it's growing jellyfish type legs

So far so good, now give it five minutes and then hold the glass up to the daylight from the bathroom window. This will help you see the result more clearly. If the spit remains floating on the top, then the spit test suggests you are free of candida.

If it's sinking or growing jellyfish-type legs, it suggests a candida presence. This test needs to be carried out for six consecutive mornings in a row to be accurate. If candida is confirmed after the sixth day, then you could also ask your doctor to double check for candida by running a blood test to check your levels of antibodies called IgG, IgA, and IgM. **At this point DON'T get too freaked out if you test positive, most of us do and it's totally manageable. Cutting out sugar is ALWAYS a smart first step in the right direction.**

Treating fungi is a marathon race not a sprint, *it takes time and effort* but the rewards for getting this step right are real. Here's the part that you have to contribute to. Fungus thrives on manmade sugar, so for the next six weeks your sugar intake has to be kept to an absolute minimum. Keep in mind that even fruit, which is perceived as being healthy, is loaded with natural sugars. To do this right, you will find it helpful to also cut out those other sugars that are perceived as healthy such as honey, agave syrup, and even our old friend maple syrup.

By now you should be noticing there is a systematic order to everything in this book hence the master cleanse came *before* this chapter. With that in mind, the *coming* chapter is equally important because the two topics overlap seamlessly. And they can also exist together at the same time.

For now, we are looking to starve the candida primarily with diet; this will not only benefit your gut but also your immune system, thyroid, and adrenal glands. Once you have the amount of sugar reduced, treating candida with specific **pro**biotics may also prove helpful. To do this correctly, you will need a brand that contains a strain of Saccharomyces Boulardii.

Often it is labeled simply as S Boulardii. Saccharomyces Boulardii (to use its full name) is a friendly yeast that binds to the same sites on the intestinal wall lining as candida does, effectively crowding it out. S. Boulardii has also been shown to be helpful in the treatment of diarrhea, IBS, and IBD.

Heed the warning, however; eradicating a candida overgrowth too quickly will cause die-off, the side effect we discussed earlier.

When candida albicans are destroyed they start to breakdown in the body, and as they do they release toxins into the bloodstream. The key here is to do things **gradually** by slowly building up the dose of S. Boulardii. This will help keep any unpleasant symptoms of die-off to a minimum.

As always, start with a small dose and go slow. By this I mean don't take a mega dose, and whenever you take any form of probiotic supplements, be sure to space out the times.

Candida can also be fought with the help of *food grade* diatomaceous earth and bentonite red clay. Both of these will prove themselves to be useful allies and are discussed in more detail later. Typically, I'm not a fan of using too many things at the same time, as we mentioned earlier, because it can cause the body to go out of balance.

As with any new supplement, some people will do better than others, which is why I'll always give you several options to try. When used sensibly, GSE (grape seed extract) is another powerful tool and can be helpful at killing sugar cravings. GSE also has other benefits. The brand of GSE I personally like is made by Pure Encapsulations. *Are there other products you can successfully use? You betcha.*

Whenever problems in the gut are addressed, it might also be a good idea to stay close to the bathroom, especially if you have a sensitive system. This should work itself out and the bigger picture can lead to a drastic improvement.

I could spend a large portion of this book covering candida in more specific detail and in the process lose valuable time for covering *other* important topics. The whole idea of this book is to raise awareness to potential health problems and then encourage **you** to play a bigger role in your own health by following up with your own research.

Obviously, I'll guide you to extremely knowledgeable people to take away any guesswork. This time around I'd like to tip my hat to a lady with an effective candida protocol that is well thought out and easy to implement.

Christa Orecchio is a clinical and holistic nutritionist dedicated to helping individuals use food as medicine to heal from the root cause. Her details can be found in today's homework assignment below.

What did we learn from this chapter?

Fungi come in many different forms, they can be helpful, invasive, destructive, and when left unchecked some can become life threatening! It takes a sustained effort to rid the body of the worst of them, but once fungi are in check, good health will flourish. Cutting out sugar and restricting antibiotic use is a great start in the fight against candida as well as all other bodily fungi.

Fungi are single-celled or multicellular organisms. They can be true pathogens which cause infections in healthy people, or they can be opportunistic pathogens.

A spit test is a tool that can be backed up with a blood test to confirm a candida overgrowth. However, it's important to know that your average doctor receives very little training on this subject which is why many of their patients go on the pill popping merry-go-round without ever seeing any positive results.
In order for the body to deal with fungi, it needs to be in balance. Too much or too little of anything can be a bad thing. This is something we will continue to explore in more detail.

Homework: Google Christa Orecchio for an effective candida protocol, or click on the link below

https://www.youtube.com/watch?v=HjymtezoWH8

Chapter 19

THE P-CLEANSE, PLEASE

As we learned in the last chapter, fungi can have far reaching detrimental effects on our health. Fungi also have a bunch of toxic cousins and *already* I just know you aren't going to like the sound of them. A quirk of human nature is that when we're told something that makes us feel uncomfortable, we pretend we didn't hear it. This presents a unique challenge for me as I attempt to convey this important message to you.

Hmm...okay, let's try this.

The book market is a highly competitive place, I'm very aware of that. As a realist, I'm also aware that I'm a first time author with no social media following. As such, there's a pretty good chance this book could drown in a sea of other books. *For me to know this in advance,* but to carry on typing in such detail really makes no financial sense, but I do so in the hope that the information I am attempting to convey here has a value beyond money. Rest assured, if I didn't think this subject was so important I wouldn't be wasting our time.

This next step is going to help you get the toxins out and allow the nutrients to flood in. And the issue I'm about to address may form *part* of an overlapping problem that has made your illness difficult to detect or diagnose.

You are not going to like what I'm about to say. In fact, I've already anticipated that your mind will shut off mid-sentence and you'll say something to yourself like, "*Eww that* does *not* apply to me," or, "That only happens to *other* people." And you would be wrong. In fact, statistically speaking, there is a 90% chance that you are wrong, and with odds like that this is something we should cover, *just because.*

The problem I am about to make you aware of is *hugely* underreported and can come to you through food or water, it can even be airborne! It affects all races, rich and poor alike – even that health freak you see every morning jogging in the park; it can impact everyone from adorable little babies to reliable old grandpas.

At worst it kills by the *millions* and at best it steals vital nutrients. I hate to be the one to tell you this, but a large portion of those valuable nutrients are stolen by parasites and worms. WAIT, there's more – don't take my word for it. Let's ask a doctor who's considered *totally mainstream.* Keep reading and I'll tell you his name.

Parasites come in all shapes and sizes; some are so microscopic that you wouldn't even know if you had them. The largest is the Diphyllobothrium latum species. It can grow up to 82 feet (25m) long. I guess something that size would need feeding at least three times a day ... *just sayin'.* Thankfully anything that long is quite rare and a lot more noticeable than those microscopic guys. But smaller ones*? Meh, not so rare.* If you have ever swam in a stream, kept a dog, been on holiday abroad, eaten meat, or even had a glass of water, your risk increases – *no, seriously it's true.*

Once inside us, parasites not only steal our nutrients they weaken our immune system. This *consequence by itself is perfectly capable of being the cause of so much fatigue, brain fog, or junk food cravings.* You can watch a one-minute clip of Dr. Oz actually holding one of these things on YouTube (Google, Dr. Oz, Tapeworm). I only use Dr. Oz as an example here because he is such a household name, *but so you know, I could have made the same point with a hundred other examples.*

Parasites can come to us from a whole bunch of different places. Today the animals we eat are often kept in filthy overpopulated conditions. To help control disease they are fed antibiotics, but antibiotics don't kill every species of parasite – and let's not forget we could be looking for something the size of a pinhead!

Make no mistake, commercial farming can be a *barbaric* practice and far removed from the way our ancestors raised livestock. It's widely thought that *undercooked* pork is particularly susceptible to parasites, although when cooked properly, local bacon from pasture- raised pigs can be a source of "good fat."

Strangely enough, pork in *any* form is considered unclean by three of the world's largest religions, I wonder if this has anything to do with those tapeworms Dr. Oz was holding? *I know, right? Why would you do that?*

It's worth remembering that parasites are *not* confined to meat. Most of us have heard of malaria, but did you know that the spread of this deadly infection is caused by a parasite?

According to the World Health Organization (WHO), malaria killed 438,000 people in 2015 alone. You might think parasites are a third world problem, but today the world is a much smaller place than it once was. What makes parasite detection such a challenge is that once it enters the body it can live there for years. This creates a real disconnect between having been on vacation one year and feeling unwell a year later (or even two).

Milwaukee USA

It's not a prerequisite for you to visit a third world country. Food is now regularly flown and shipped here from around the world. Parasites now come to us, and thanks to more efficient travel and transportation, they don't even need a visa to do so.

Still not convinced?

Two decades ago in the U.S. a parasite entered Milwaukee drinking water and killed 69 people and sickened 400,000. More recently, in 2015, a potentially deadly amoeba was found in the water supply of a parish outside New Orleans for the second time in two years. This is real, and it can happen in *any* town or city across the globe.

The good news is there *is* a solution for you, but first I'd really like for you to see what I am talking about. They say a picture is worth a thousand words, so be sure to check out this chapter's homework assignment. This time it's a short Discovery documentary that should help us both get on the same page. It also mentions a U.S. city water infection. Clearly this is a problem that can happen anywhere.

Fortunately, a parasite and worm cleanse is easy enough to do, *getting you to do it is the hard part*. One of the better cleanses is sold by a company called Grandma's Herbs but you could also check out your local health food store. The cleanse sold by Grandma's comes in capsule form and is taken for twenty-one days straight, then stopped for fourteen days, then taken for another twenty-one days.

The reason for this 21on-14off-21on protocol is that the eggs aren't always killed; hence, the fourteen days allows the larva to hatch and then be swept aside with the *next* round of twenty-one days. It's very easy to get lost counting days so it's best to mark it on a calendar. If discretion is an issue, simply write P-Cleanse on the dates.

Doses of P-Cleanse will vary for children; if you have any further questions the Grandma's Herbs people are extremely helpful and knowledgeable, they also sell a lot of other products and personally I've always found them to be effective.

To complete the course, you will need three bottles. By my math it's a pretty cost effective solution for less than fifty bucks. There are plenty of other cleanses out there that you can use; this is just one of many.

If, like me, you like to be double sure of things you may also want to look into "Zapping." This is a curious little device but *unlike* the name suggests, it's perfectly harmless to you but not so much to parasites. Trust me, *you* won't feel a thing. It works by emitting a very low range frequency onto the skin which then disrupts parasite cycles.

There are some expensive zapping units out there but I'm often suspicious of any product if large sums of money are involved, so I was pleasantly surprised to see a basic one being offered at just $35, and mid-range one around $130. *Combining* the zapper with the parasite cleanse is more effective. You can find out more information at A World without Parasites.com, as with anything that has the potential to cause a die-off reaction, start small and go slow.

If your budget is running a little tight you could also check out *food grade* diatomaceous earth. This was also mentioned in the previous chapter and it works for both fungi and parasites. It's as cheap as chips to buy and a 1lb bag through Amazon sells for around 10 bucks.

The upside is this low cost option also has a whole range of other health benefits. When buying diatomaceous earth, it's imperative to order FOOD GRADE. Diatomaceous earth is best when taken on an empty stomach and first thing in the morning with water. The dose will vary *so always consult the company you buy it from*. As an added bonus, doing any type of parasite cleanse is great at helping curb junk food cravings!

Diatomaceous earth is a white, porous, sedimentary rock, naturally-made from the fossilized remains of diatoms. Diatoms are one of the types of unicellular phytoplankton that are surrounded by silica-rich cell walls. The silica found in diatomaceous earth is an essential mineral needed by plants, animals, and humans to grow and remain healthy. As diatomaceous earth passes through the body it can help eliminate harmful organisms and even heavy metals. Diatomaceous earth can also help with bowel movements; some people say they "just feel better" after consuming it.

Depending on how congested you are, it may take a week or so before you begin to see more regular bowel movements. If you decide to try diatomaceous earth, remember that it needs to be taken on an empty stomach each morning. If things are super congested we may need to also tweak your diet a little, but for now, just relax, the answers you need are coming.

Again, I wouldn't try too many new products at the same time. Diatomaceous earth and the parasite cleanse sold by Grandma's Herbs are two totally separate protocols; I'm just making sure you have plenty of affordable options at your disposal.

ORDER PLEASE

Doing things with a certain sense of order typically renders better results. The P-Cleanse, zapper, and diatomaceous earth are great tools to have at our disposal because pretty soon we are going to start talking about your diet.

As we are working our way through this book we have lightly touched on a few nutritional choices. As yet, however, we haven't covered the subject of diet in any great detail. The justification for this should by now be obvious: having the information from this chapter first ensures that our chances of success increase. *Are you getting this? These tools will help you with those junk food cravings!*

Food manufacturers have a very clear understanding of your food cravings and they know how to exploit them. We talked about this earlier and by now know that the brain has pleasure sensors that are rewarded when certain nutrients hit the spot. This is a calculated and premeditated attempt to get you to want more. *Having P-Cleanse on our side can only be viewed as helpful.*

The good news is that the P-Cleanse is something you can start today, right now even if your current diet isn't quite up to scratch and you'll still see a benefit! I try to do a P-Cleanse once a year and always feel better for having done it. **If you only try one thing out of this book, let it be the P-Cleanse.**

Keep in mind that the full 21-14-21 Grandma's Herbs protocol takes time to complete (56 days, to be precise). Also, most P-Cleanses have to be taken two hours BEFORE food.

If you decide to try this, it makes sense to order the P-Cleanse early. This will give you a head start and time to finish the protocol while still reading this book. If you order it from Grandma's Herbs, please feel free to mention where you found their information.

What did we learn from this chapter?

Estimates are that parasites affect 90% of us. That's pretty good odds that this unpleasant topic is forming at least part of your problem, if you only complete one step in this book, please make it this one!

We might not like the idea of sharing our nutrients with these tiny critters. This makes doing the P-Cleanse all the more important. The P-Cleanse is something you can start right now even if you don't yet have a good diet.

Homework: watch a short Discovery documentary called *Parasites Eating Us Alive.* You can find it on YouTube or click on the link below.

https://www.youtube.com/watch?v=w_D6yPVrYjo

Chapter 20

12 ESSENTIAL FOOD CONCEPTS
YOU NEED TO KNOW

To pull my own health out of the ditch I had to learn, apply, and understand many of the nutritional concepts found in this chapter. It really didn't take me very long to realize that the subject of nutrition can be ridiculously complicated to navigate. However, it really doesn't have to be this way if we first learn to break our meals down into basic food groups.

To help us better understand this concept, let's go over some important basics to give us a better understanding of what nutrition *is* and *isn't*. On the surface, terms such as fats, fiber, fruit, starch, carbohydrates, and protein all seem pretty straightforward and yet they are often confused with the intended meaning behind them. As a result, our health is then taken down the wrong road.

Before we get into this chapter, let's first remind ourselves that rather than applying a clumsy one-size-fits-all, the needs of each individual body should be closely listened to. With that in mind, I'm not advocating any one particular diet other than saying stop eating out of cans and boxes. The only thing healthy in *that* arrangement is the profit margin for the supermarkets selling to you.

Once you learn to listen to your body it will almost certainly guide you to what it needs. To help you find your feet, I'll be making a few dietary suggestions later in the book, for now just hang in there because finding the best fit for you requires a little trial and error. It also pays to know that our dietary needs may fluctuate from season to season. Solving this riddle often involves a little tweaking on your part. And just to be clear, I said tweaking *not* twerking.

Okay, let's explore all the things you need to know about these basic terms but were afraid to ask. Shall we kick off with fruitsandvegetables?

FRUITS and VEGETABLES

"Fruitsandvegetables" wasn't a typo. It's written that way because most people incorrectly refer to them as if they are one thing. To be clear, fruit gets people into trouble much faster than vegetables do because of their higher sugar content, and even more so when it comes to *dried* fruit.

Once the water is removed, the sugar levels of dried food become more concentrated which causes a spike in sugar. To avoid sugar spikes, reduce your fruit intake to a single small portion per day, preferably after dinner. It might help if you think of a piece of fruit as a watery bag of sugar best enjoyed as a dessert. *We wouldn't eat dessert for breakfast, right?*

Hexose sugar found in fruit and honey is also known as fructose. In some people, fructose malabsorption causes a wide range of digestive upsets.

Keep in mind the old saying, "An apple a day keeps the doctor away," was a reference to dentists who, back in the day, were often called doctors.

Melons digest pretty quickly because of their high liquid content. For that reason, they are best eaten by themselves and not in combination with any other food. It may help to remember this expression, "Eat melons alone or leave them alone." When melon is eaten with other foods it can no longer pass through your digestive system quickly. In effect, it gets trapped as it waits for other foods to catch up and this can lead to bloating, gas, or other digestive issues.

Fruit juice is really liquid sugar because all the fiber has been taken out. If you are looking to give yourself a sugar spike, even "organic" fruit juice is the perfect way to do it. Some experts maintain that fructose fools our brains into thinking we are still hungry causing us to crave more which in turn causes us to overeat.

Today, fruits are *over-consumed* and vegetables are being *under-consumed.* While it makes sense to view fruit as an occasional treat, vegetables can be added to *any* meal (and every meal) with benefits. As you look at vegetables, pay particular attention to their bold colors. Ideally you want to get a good variety of these colors on every plate. A great expression to remember is "eat the rainbow" For those who can handle them, think purple cabbage and red carrots next to the vibrant green of kale and yellow peppers. Vegetables can be viewed as an alkalizing food, but more important many of the uncooked *clean* leafy greens help the body detoxify. Don't worry, more detailed info is coming.

FATS AND OILS

Using the word "fat" as a blanket term does a great disservice to this important nutrient. Not all fats are the same; there are **good fats** and there are bad fats. From the get-go, let's also put it out there that your brain is made up of approximately 60% fat. **Good fat** is important because vitamins A, E, D and K are all fat soluble – in other words, you *need* good fats to help absorb those important vitamins. This is probably why Mother Nature hides fat in breast milk. *Hmm, I see.*

Fats can be split into groups containing saturated fat and unsaturated fat, but to keep this from getting complicated let's stick with using the term's good and bad. What we **don't** need are those manmade fats such as trans-fats or partially hydrogenated vegetable oils. The foods you get in fast food restaurants and the junk foods you find on supermarket shelves are cooked in this kind of fat – it's cheaper and has a much longer shelf life than the good fats. These types of bad-fats can also be found in some margarines and vegetable shortening.

You can get **good** fats by eating certain fish, especially wild caught salmon, or sardines if you are on a tight budget. Good fat can also be found in raw nuts such as the macadamia nut, and in fatty meats, olives, eggs, and yup, let's not forget avocados. One medium avocado has approximately 23 grams of fat. If you find yourself in a bind, coconut cream sold in a can typically has 14g of good fat and if mixed with berries, nuts, and a little imagination (along with a bit of time in the freezer), can almost taste like ice cream.

I'm going to go off the deep end here and break with the standard mantra and call butter made from *pasture-raised* cows a beneficial fat. I'll explain the logic of this in a later chapter. Those who are lactose intolerant might

227

find that this type of butter is better tolerated. Cheese from pasture-raised cows also has good fat, but those with dairy sensitivities should still avoid it.

Another source of **good** fat is found in a concentrated version of MCT coconut oil (Medium-Chain-Triglycerides) which may prove helpful with mental clarity.

More good fat comes in the form of omega-3 fatty acids, which our bodies cannot produce. The two crucial ones are EPA and DHA, also well-known for their anti-inflammatory benefits. If you are trying to limit the amount of fish products in your diet because you have concerns about heavy metal toxicity, a good source of essential DHA and EPA omega-3 fatty acids is krill oil.

Omega-3s can also be found in chia seeds, flax seeds, and walnuts. Eggs from free range chickens have been shown to contain *more* Omega-3 fatty acids and vitamin-A than regular factory farmed eggs.

A healthy balance of omega-3 and omega-6 is something that needs to be addressed because an incorrect balance can increase inflammation in the body. As a rule of thumb, strive for a balance of 1:1 which is better than an excessive imbalance. Good luck getting there, though, because today's typical western diet has waaaay too many omega-6s and not enough omega-3s. Some estimates put the imbalance as far out as 40:1 in favor of omega-6s.

Eating more good fat also helps you feel fuller longer; it slows down the absorption of carbohydrates which can help keep blood sugar levels under control. Perhaps in the past we were all a little quick to follow a *low fat* diet. Some nutrition experts suggest that the current food pyramid would actually be more beneficial if it were turned upside down. Make no mistake, good fat is important to your health.

Many of those on the absolute cutting edge of good nutrition now suggest that we should be getting as much as 70% of our daily caloric intake from **good** fats, only 20% from protein, and as little as 10% from carbohydrates.

Again this should serve as a reminder that perhaps the current food pyramid has it all twisted (or upside down).

Am I suggesting this ratio is a good fit for you? Nope, we all have different needs and, for some, consuming too much good fat when the body isn't used to it can present a new problem – a stressed gallbladder. The correct way to increase the amount of good fat in your diet is *gradually*. As with anything new, always start small and go slow.

PROTEIN

Humans and gorillas are genetically very similar; we share 98% of our genes with them. An adult silverback gorilla can weigh 500+ pounds and is estimated to be twenty times stronger than an adult man, yet gorillas don't eat chickens or cows. Gorillas are composed mostly of muscle with a fat content of just 3%. Their muscle building protein comes from the sixteen pounds of plants and leaves they eat every single day. Yup, protein can absolutely be found in vegetation. *I know, right? Who knew?*

This point is being made early on because it's a common misconception that protein = meat and vegetables = weak. Again let me remind you that a gorilla is twenty times stronger than a human.

Am I saying you should become a vegetarian? *Nope, never did say that.* However the perception that any diet consisting of vegetables is somehow inferior needs to be challenged. Think about it, muscle that powers a racehorse is formed without consuming any meat. As any vegan bodybuilder will tell you, meat is not the only way to get protein.

Often the word "protein" is inaccurately used to describe meat, and even then is applied with an enormously liberal brush.

Technically speaking, deep fried chicken is a protein but let's not forget that it's usually fried in rancid oils (bad fat) which can be an instant hit of inflammation-forming free radicals.

Again, I'm not attempting to convert meat eaters into vegetarians or vegetarians into meat eaters, I'm simply *challenging* your perception of what protein is. We can then look to finding something that works for *you.*

Bottom line: protein can be found in meat, but not all meats are the same. Keep this in mind as we move through the rest of these food groups. There is always going to be a junk version and a healthy version and they really are as different as chalk and cheese.

FIBER AND STARCH

Even though both starch and fiber are complex carbs, they act very differently in your body. If you are looking for something to give you energy, a starchy food may help. If you want something filling that isn't loaded with calories, opt for something high in fiber. Enzymes in your body can easily break the bonds that form starches, turning them into sugars for energy. You can't make the enzymes break down fiber, so fiber isn't digested – but it does have health benefits, including lowering your risk for heart disease, high blood pressure, obesity, and digestive problems like constipation.

FIBER is important, not least to aid in good digestion. Unfortunately, much of the standard dietary advice often lists breakfast cereal and whole grain bread as good forms of fiber. It may be true that the fiber content in these foods is high, so too is the possibility of a reaction, particularly from gluten. There are lots of alternative sources of fiber. Quinoa is gluten free, high in fiber, and has a higher nutrient content than most grains. Oatmeal made from gluten free oats also has fiber, but be aware that many of the "instant" brands can be loaded with additives and sugar. While standard oats may take a few minutes longer to prepare, they are generally better tolerated. Soaking oats overnight can help turn them into instant oats. In the morning simply strain out the water and replace with warm almond milk.

The value of fiber shouldn't be underestimated because it is super important to your microbiome. Fiber can also be found in plant foods like vegetables, cooked turnip greens, spinach, beans, chickpeas, lentils, and nuts. For those who can tolerate it, brown rice has more fiber than white rice.

230

Fruits high in fiber also include avocado, pears, apples, blueberries, and raspberries.

STARCHES are found in vegetables like potatoes, broccoli, Brussels sprouts, peas, parsnips, green beans, dried beans, and corn. Be aware, however, that today most corn is genetically modified and for some people it can be notoriously harsh on the digestive system. Vegetables high in starches are also generally higher in calories.

SUGAR AND SPICE

SUGAR is a tricky one because it is eight times more addictive than cocaine! Food manufacturers know this, which is perhaps why sugar is added to everyday items like milk, bacon, bread, and even salad dressing. To make matters worse, you can't even rely on sugar to be called sugar by the people whose job it is to write the labels. *I know, right? What's up with that?*

Here are a few of the common bait and switch terms used for sugar – but be warned there are plenty more!

- Cane juice
- Corn sweetener
- Corn syrup
- Dextrose
- Fructose
- High-fructose corn syrup
- Invert sugar
- Maltose
- Lactose
- Sucrose
- White sugar
- Corn syrup solids
- Malt syrup
- Anhydrous dextrose

Make no mistake, sugar is as deceptive as it is destructive, and as mentioned earlier, it's not confined to manmade sugars. Fruit comes loaded with natural sugars, which quickly gets people into trouble because it's perceived as being healthy. Am I saying don't eat fruit? Yup. For the next thirty days think about giving fruit the boot, along with all those manmade sugary snacks, cakes, and sodas.

The problem is nature never intended for us to find ripe fruit every day of the week. Historically speaking, most of us only found ripe fruit in the fall. This would have allowed us to quickly load calories in preparation for a long winter. Today we wander around the supermarket picking low hanging fruit 365 days a year. *Are we there yet?*

If you aren't paying attention, all this sugar quickly adds up to a body that can no longer cope. The medical term for that is diabetes. Remember, carbs and protein are also broken down into sugar and even some vegetables also have a high sugar count.

Vegetables such as beets and corn are at the higher end of the scale as are fruits such as dried bananas, figs, and grapes. You can find a FULL list of the sugar content of foods in the glycemic index table. The glycemic index table is a value assigned to foods based on how slowly or how quickly those foods cause increases in blood glucose levels, also known as "blood sugar" levels.

Spice –Turmeric is arguably one of the most studied and powerful spices on the planet. Turmeric has been used in cooking for thousands of years. It has a warm, peppery, and bitter flavor and a mild fragrance slightly reminiscent of orange and ginger. The main active ingredient in turmeric is curcumin which has powerful anti-inflammatory effects and is a very strong antioxidant. Adding turmeric to your food is easy to do and is thought to have wide ranging beneficial effects.
Turmeric/curcumin has even been studied for its cancer preventative properties. Turmeric is fat-soluble – this simply means if you want to get the benefit of turmeric you need to take it with food that has a certain level of fat content. This will allow the turmeric to be absorbed.

Other useful spices known to have health benefits are garlic, cinnamon, ginseng, and ginger. Ginger has an astounding number of health benefits that range from everything to aiding digestion to speeding up metabolism. It's also antibacterial, anti-parasitic (as is garlic) and because of its sulfur content garlic aids in detoxification. Be aware it's also a potent lectin which you will soon learn can be a problem in some individuals.

SIMPLE AND COMPLEX CARBOHYDRATES

Simply put, we could think of carbs as one or more sugar molecules bound together and then broken down by the body to be used as fuel. I'm going to keep saying it: ALL carbs turn to sugar, some faster than others. The root of the problem here isn't *sugar*; it's the *amount* and *type* of sugar that causes so many complicating issues.
But what does this mean?

The bigger problem lies in the body's inability to process sugar at the rate we currently consume it. This can happen by eating too many complicated manmade sugars, too much fruit, or a combination of both. Carbs are found in lots of different foods including fruits, grains, vegetables, pastries, potatoes, bread, and even milk, candy, and soda. Carbs can be split into two basic groups, either simple or complex. *Shall we take a look?*

Simple carbs are easily absorbed into the bloodstream because of their *simple* molecular structure. Think fruit, milk, table sugar, etc. Simple carbs can be thought of as giving you a faster hit of sugar.
Complex carbs have a more *complex* molecular structure that can take longer for the body to break down into sugar. Think grains, vegetables, potatoes, etc. Complex carbs can be thought of as giving you a slower hit of sugar.

The subject of carbohydrates is sometimes misunderstood and conjures up all sorts of images in our minds, but really it's just a question of splitting things into different groups. So far we have **simple** carbs and **complex** carbs, now we need to split them once again into **good** carbs and **bad** carbs.

In the interest of simplicity, let us think of **bad carbs** as those that have been heavily processed such as cereals, crackers, pastries, white bread, soda, etc. Bad carbs are high in calories but essentially *low* in nutrients.

This now gets easier because it only leaves **good carbs**. Good carbs are the *unprocessed* foods such as fruits, vegetables, beans, etc., and are always found in their *natural state.*

If you are trying to reduce the amount of sugar in your diet, it's worth remembering that both simple and complex carbohydrates will turn into sugar, and as such, anything that appears high on the glycemic table should be reduced, along with *bad* carbohydrates.

Eating too many carbohydrates in the form of processed, starchy, or sugary foods can cause an increase in total calories and weight gain. For now, the goal isn't to eliminate all carbs but it will prove helpful to begin cutting out all the bad ones.

So much of the standard American diet is top heavy with carbs. Later we will explore the idea of switching out a portion of these and replacing them with an alternative fuel – like good fats.

Severely restricting carbohydrates puts the body in a state of ketosis. This will be explained in more detail down the road, but for now, think of it as the body using fat stores for energy whenever there are not enough carbohydrates from food. Ketosis is a natural state and should not be confused with ketoacidosis. They sound the same but are as different as cats and cars.

MEAT

Meat is another term that is often applied with a broad brush. Not all meat is raised to the same standard, so it's incorrect to define meat simply as meat. Some animals are raised in filthy, inhumane conditions and as a result of overcrowding and disease must be fed antibiotics. Let's not forget, when the animal you eat consumes antibiotics, so do you.

Grass-fed meat is a term used to describe the way an animal has been raised and essentially means it's been left to graze as nature intended. When it comes to buying meat, try to support local farmers who allow their animals to be raised on open pastures and look to buy meat that has come from a single animal rather than meat that has been through a processing plant and turned into sausage.

Question – How many animals go into making a single sausage? Answer- *Once it leaves the meat factory it's anybody's guess!* That's a scary thought right? It could be ten, it could be a hundred. Compare that to buying a single steak or lamb chop, which comes from only **one** animal.

If you can't afford the sticker price of a farmer doing his job right, then simply eat less meat. *That's okay too.* Buying grass-fed meat can work out cheaper in the long run compared to the heavy cost of medications. This isn't simply a change in diet; it's more of a whole new way of life. Okay, last point I want to make on meat: don't waste quality meat by deep frying it, this will result in lots free radicals.

***Tip* –**
Always keep meat on the bottom shelf of your fridge, that way if it leaks for any reason it's not going to drip on your vegetables and make you sick.

FISH

Try to limit your fish consumption to those kinds that are known to be lower in mercury. Wild caught salmon from Alaska is a good choice, although any fish with a high selenium content can be consumed in moderation.

Selenium plays a role in counteracting mercury toxicity, something we have known about for more than forty-five years. Sardines fall in the high selenium category, but avoid fish such as swordfish, shark, king mackerel, and tilefish. To be on the safe side, limit tuna to once every two weeks or less.

If you take away only one thing from this chapter, let it be the healing power of raw apple-cider-vinegar (sometimes called ACV) which has **a** wide range of health benefits.

The healing properties of vinegar dates back thousands of years and was used by the Egyptians and Greeks; even Hippocrates used it. Apple cider vinegar is said to contain vitamins A, B6, C, and E, as well as thiamin, riboflavin, niacin, pantothenic acid, beta-carotene, lycopene, and soluble fiber in the form of pectin. That's not all – it also contains minerals such as sodium, phosphorus, potassium, calcium, iron, and magnesium.

Apple cider vinegar is great for helping food taste better, but it's also a powerful tonic to keep in the cupboard. Acetate is a molecule found in apple cider vinegar that has been shown to increase metabolism. Acetate is made by good bacteria in the gut and science is just discovering its use in calming down an overactive immune system.

Many of these claims are backed up with legitimate scientific studies and data can be found on sites such as PubMed. From asthma to migraines (and a whole lot of stuff in between), some people report remarkable improvements after taking a therapeutic dose of ACV.

Apple cider vinegar can also be helpful for detoxing the body and fighting infection. It's also believed that apple cider vinegar helps the process of digestion become more effective.

Personally, I've found ACV helpful with seasonal allergies. Simply add two tablespoons in a small (16oz) BPA-free bottle of water and keep sipping on it. To some I'm sure it's not going to taste that great, but if you catch allergies early in the season it's far better than itching eyes and sneezing all summer long, *am I right?*

Some people report improvement with arthritis, high cholesterol, and even regulating blood pressure. Apple cider vinegar is best diluted in water and drunk on an empty stomach. A good starting point would be a tablespoon in 8 oz. of water

For a complete list of effective home remedies (including apple cider vinegar) check out a website by the name of earthclinic.com, I used this site often as it's packed with helpful tips and it's also very easy to navigate.

SALT

Salt is often demonized but salt isn't the problem, very often it's the **type** of salt that creates the problem. Regular table salt is heavily processed and usually contains numerous additives to prevent clumping. Regular table salt has fewer natural minerals than other, natural salts and was the first thing I threw out of my own diet. Himalayan salt, by comparison, not only tastes better it has many health benefits that come in the form of natural minerals.

NUTS AND SEEDS

Be mindful not to consume too many nuts in one sitting because doing so might throw your balance of omega-3 and omega-6 fats into a bad ratio. Anthropological research suggests that our hunter-gatherer ancestors consumed omega-6 and omega-3 fats in a ratio of roughly 1.1.

When it comes to eating nuts, moderation may serve you better than excess. Think how long it would have taken our ancestors to crack open a single nut. Today it's possible to consume large amounts of nuts because all the hard work of removing the shell has been done for us. Also, peanuts and pistachios are both prone to molds.

Sprouted seeds are less problematic that un-sprouted seeds. If you are looking for an economical way to bring an abundance of minerals and live enzymes into your diet, be sure to add sprouted seeds which can act as tiny nutritional dynamos. Sprouted seeds meet paleo standards and, if done right, are the essence of *clean* nutrition.

FERMENTED FOODS

Some estimates put the weight of the tiny gut microorganisms at approximately three pounds per person! Given the extraordinary ability of the gut to affect both our physical *and* mental health, any attempts to influence the gut flora could produce a certain amount of unpredictability.

It's no easy task to estimate how a large and sudden shift in gut flora will impact a person's mental state. The words "unpredictability" and "mental health" in the same sentence rarely bode well. Even though fermented foods have obvious benefits, it's best to start small and slow. Once you have a handle on them you can certainly up your daily intake.

Fermented foods are packed with *good* probiotics and can help boost the amount of *good* bacteria found in your gut. Fermented foods also have the ability to positively influence the immune system, but it's better to gradually work your way up. As in the case of candida, too many fermented foods *too quickly* could hasten a die-off reaction.

CALORIES

Looking at food as a number is too much of a one dimensional approach to nutrition. Calorie counting fails to take into account the **quality** of the food because it focuses instead on a measurement of energy.

While it's obviously important to have enough calories coming into the diet, the obsession with calorie counting will have no effect on trigger foods such as those found in the nightshade family, gluten, or lectins. For this reason, counting calories has the potential to become counterproductive. ***Stop counting calories and start counting quality!***

THE DIRTY DOZEN

When buying fresh fruits and vegetables, be aware that some foods absorb *more* pesticides than others. These are known as the "dirty dozen." It's a fact that inferior crops are cheaper to grow than nutrient-dense ones, thus making more money for the corporations selling them, but not helping you at all.

If you are on a limited budget, try to save money elsewhere first – for example with unnecessary impulse buys. Lord knows supermarkets are masters of distraction and these places keep adding more and more products that invite us to keep spending. *Ever go into a store for salad and leave with socks?*

If you can't yet see the logic in buying quality clean food, then at least steer away from the dirty dozen. These are twelve foods *known* to have a higher pesticide count due to their absorbent skin. Think strawberries, which act like sponges when absorbing pesticides. This also applies to any products where these foods are mixed into them.

The 12 most contaminated foods (The Dirty Dozen)

- Peaches
- Apples (always peel)
- Sweet Bell Peppers
- Celery
- Nectarines
- Strawberries
- Cherries
- Pears
- Grapes (imported)
- Spinach
- Lettuce
- Potatoes

The 12 least contaminated

- Onions
- Avocado
- Sweet Corn (Frozen)

- Pineapples
- Mango
- Asparagus
- Sweet Peas (Frozen)
- Papaya
- Kiwi Fruit
- Bananas
- Cabbage
- Broccoli

RICE AND GRAINS

Rice is a borderline trigger food that some people do okay with and in others can prove reactive. If you have any type of stomach issue, try white rice over brown. If that doesn't resolve the issue, try giving rice a vacation for thirty days, and then gradually reintroduce it back into your diet. Brown rice has more fiber than white rice which, **for those who can handle it**, might be helpful for constipation – although eating in moderation is key.

Grains – Nope, no grains. The ones used in today's food simply aren't the same quality they were even thirty years ago. In some parts of old Europe you might get away with it, but for the rest of us grains have become an ugly form of kryptonite.

WHAT TO BUY

You now have literally hundreds of food combinations at your disposal, you can choose to keep it simple or incorporate the help of a gazillion cookbooks. While paleo and keto seem to have become new buzzwords, try to think of it as simply food that doesn't come out of a box, a can, or a packet. We'll obvious be looking more into this as we move along.

It's easy to lose patience with some of the more complicated cookbooks so I have a few of my own simplified suggestions coming up to help get you started. Below is a suggested list of **basic** raw materials. What you do with them is up to you. FREEDOM!

Unless you have any *known* allergies,
here's your new shopping list:

- Grass-fed meats – if possible pick a local farmer; it can be less expensive and better quality and also helps the community
- Eggs from free-range chickens – they have more vitamin A and omega-3 fatty acids
- *Wild* caught salmon – mercury levels in many other fish are just too high
- Nuts – no peanuts or pistachios because both are prone to molds
- Seeds – sprouted seeds *really* pack a nutritional punch
- Fresh vegetables – preferably free of pesticides
- Milk – raw goat's milk would be awesome
- Bone broth – preferably made from grass-fed meats which are super healthy and filling
- Himalayan sea salt and apple cider vinegar – add as desired for taste
- Fresh fruits – in moderation, and be mindful of the dirty dozen mentioned earlier; go for the *thicker*-skinned fruits.
- Drink lots of water – your own filtered water can be better than BPA bottled *provided* that the filter is a good standard

TRY TO STAY AWAY FROM:

- Processed foods – if it comes in a box, a can, or a packet remember that someone, somewhere processed it on a production line
- Dairy products – milk, cheese, yogurts
- Grains – including breads, pasta, crackers, cakes, cereals, etc.
- Gluten free products that come in a box, can, or packet

- Soda – it's loaded with sugar and your kidneys won't like the carbonation
- No fruit juice even if it carries the label "all natural"

Take a moment to stop and look at the food on the average plate. Today it's not uncommon to find most plates stacked with a disproportionate amount of bad carbs, grains, dairy, or excessive amounts of fructose in the form of fruit. *I know, right? WTF? (Where's The Fat?)*

Try to think of foods in the groups they belong to, remembering that some foods will obviously belong to more than one group. As a very basic rule of thumb, if this is all new to you then try to fill half your plate with leafy green vegetables and split the other half of the plate between good fats, proteins, agreeable forms carbohydrates, starch, and fiber, leaving room for just a small amount of fruit for dessert.

Finally, keep in mind that all food spoils, so whenever you find yourself asking another family member to smell something to see if it *smells funny,* remember the rule: if in doubt, throw it out.

What did we learn from this chapter?

Food is divided into different groups and each has the potential to affect the body in one way or another. The topic of nutrition forms an important base for us to build on. The important take-home message is that sugar comes to us in many forms, all of which we need to dial down. Good fats, however, are like a long lost friend to be welcomed through the door.

Homework: to help cement what we have just learned, there's a super helpful video on YouTube called "Gut reaction part 1." It is well worth watching because it makes understanding this whole chapter so much easier.

Chapter 21

HALF TIME

As we now find ourselves at the halfway point in the book, what-say we take a left turn here and see where it takes us. This short chapter shouldn't be at all hard to read because you will not be asked to learn anything new. For now, just take it easy as we ponder this life together.

Getting this book to the point where I'm okay to share it with you took me far longer than I ever expected – a little over a year to be precise. A lot can happen in a year and during this time my dad died.

Dad was a genuinely decent man and I miss him terribly. It's fair to say that the day we buried him I also buried a part of myself.

Over the years, Dad's life had been anything but easy. To his credit, *I never heard him complain about anything,* he simply wasn't wired that way. As a teenager he broke his back and spent six months in a cast. He was lucky to walk again, but as a result of that early injury he spent the rest of his life in a great deal of pain. He absolutely point-blank refused to complain about it or even let it stop him from being active. He often used humor as a way to cope with his pain.
Some of his jokes were so bad they were actually quite funny. I once asked him how much it cost to get married and without missing a beat he said, "I'm really not too sure son, I'm still paying for it." He'd been married to my mom for more than sixty years and with some degree of predictability he always joked that the first fifty-nine were the hardest.

To celebrate our parents' sixtieth wedding anniversary, my sister contacted the Queen of England who actually sent back a *signed* congratulations card!
Mom cooked and cleaned for him and she loved him. In all their time together, they never spent a night apart. Mom and Dad were inseparable, so the day Dad complained of chest pain they even went off to the doctor *together.* The doctor shook her head and immediately sent them to the

hospital for more testing. My parents rode in the ambulance together, holding hands.

Once there, Dad was put through a pretty intense examination and it was deemed necessary to keep him for observation. Now separated from each other, Dad quickly found himself being prodded and poked by a team of eager medical students. The following morning I managed to call him while he was still on the ward. When I asked how he was doing, he told me that of all the procedures they were putting him through, the one that hurt the most was having a large needle plunged into his left lung to see if they could drain out any fluid. Because he so rarely complained, I knew this must have hurt him even more than he was saying.

Dad was then told to drink Barium. If you haven't heard of this before, Barium is used in medicine to highlight any defects during an X-ray. It's also used as an insoluble additive in oil well drilling and is even added to fireworks to make that bright green color. One of the known side effects of drinking Barium is it can cause a hiatal hernia (an internal defect that causes the stomach to slide partially into the chest).

Despite the risks (and that he was eighty years old), Dad was asked to drink a *second* batch so that the doctors could carry out yet another round of high radiation x-rays. Then they stuck a needle in his arm and drew blood for a standard panel of bloodwork.

The next time I called him he asked me to pray for him, only this time there was no punchline. This struck me as very odd because neither of us was particularly religious. I could only guess that the tests they were now constantly running on him had become pretty intense.

Later that evening I called Dad again. His mind had *always* been as sharp as a tack so as we talked I struggled to understand why his thoughts kept wandering off track to subjects that had little relevance. As the conversation unfolded it became clear that he had been given heavy-duty painkillers that his liver and kidneys were now trying to cope with along with the liquid Barium sulfate.

A week later Dad was still in hospital and had by then seen six specialists. When all his test results were in, all six doctors sat in a semi-circle around him and each told him he was going to die. Dad had always been a very positive man and rarely expressed any outward sign of emotion that might cause others around him to worry. My sister told me that as he heard the doctors' damning news, his large square shoulders suddenly dropped. His heart was still beating but I believe *this* was the exact moment the doctors made sure he lost all **hope**. Following that damning diagnosis he was sent home. His beautiful, determined inner spirit had already begun to wither.

As if he hadn't been through enough already, a day nurse came to visit him at the house. She brought a signed order to inject him twice a day with warfarin; this was deemed necessary to prevent blood clots. It might surprise you to know that warfarin is the same product used in rat poison. My suggestion that Hawthorne would be a better fit for an eighty-year-old was immediately scoffed at. Emotion got the better of me and I found myself shouting into the phone that warfarin would kill him quicker than any blood clot. By the time I had booked my flight, the emergency services had already been called and a team of paramedics stood in Dad's living room desperately trying to resuscitate him. Before I could get on the plane, Dad's life had come to an abrupt end.
The paramedics packed up their bulky equipment and left. Mom, of course, instinctively went back to holding his hand, and only after the warmth left his lifeless body did she think to call me long distance to deliver the bad news. With a great deal of dignity in her voice, she uttered these words, *"I wanted to be the one to tell you that we lost Dad today."*

Given his situation, I was expecting that dreaded call but it was still a punch in the gut. A few days later I saw my mom standing without her best friend for the first time. She did what all good moms do in the face of adversity and simply smiled through her pain.

At the funeral, Mom looked like a butterfly trapped behind a glass window with no way out. And yet she somehow found the strength to go around and thank each and every person for coming. I now have a much deeper understanding of what the term *paying your last respects* really means.

Dad *was* ill and I accept that, and to be fair, everyone was doing the best they could in extremely difficult circumstances, but when six experts issue the verdict to a human spirit that it's about to die, I believe that is what it does.

Look, we all know this life isn't easy, even more so when we become ill. Trying to find answers when our world is falling apart can be a real challenge – *believe me, I get it.* But if you have made it this far in the book then you, like me, must have a knack for sticking with it and *that* takes guts, *especially* when you don't feel good to begin with.

If this is you, I can only imagine the circumstances that brought you here and I applaud you for playing an active role in your own recovery and health. Here's my question: *why are you still reading this book? What's driving you to keep going in the face of adversity?*

I may not know you personally, but I suspect that even in ill health your inner spirit burns brightly or quite simply you wouldn't still be reading. This is actually a *really* good sign. Regardless of what's happening to your body today, know that a month from now things could look very different. Without even realizing it you could be on the cusp of a unique turning point – so keep coming, don't quit.

At this point I'd like to sincerely thank you for allowing me to be a small part of your journey, **you are the reason I wrote this book.** It's never been about me, although I suspect by the time this book ends we will both have overcome much adversity *together.*

It seems the human spirit burns brightly *wherever there is hope.* Like a small pilot light inside every one of us, it can accomplish things far beyond our understanding.

> *Hope is independent of the apparatus of logic.*
> – Norman Cousins

So, the second half of this book is about to kick off and you can rest assured there are lots of fascinating new topics coming up. Rather than running out of steam, we are only just getting warmed up! As we move forward, I'll once again be recommending that you check out a small group of informed people in each of the homework sections. These are good people to have on your team and they absolutely helped me in my own recovery.

What did we learn from this chapter?

No matter what the world is throwing at you, your inner spirit appears to be intact. For anyone looking to overcome illness, this is an excellent sign.

Homework: check out Mike Mutzel. Mike often chooses to interview those who are on the absolute cutting edge of natural medicine. Mike has a degree in biology and has completed his M.S. in clinical nutrition from the University of Bridgeport making him a pretty smart guy. Mike is also one of the most genuine people I have come across. You can keep up to date by following him on Facebook. Here's the direct link for e-book users.

https://www.facebook.com/MikeMutzelMS/?hc_ref=ARQ1dAyhNhdQrzld pZm66eiJtydtv5qjc1dLkRcW6S_i3p2J1q8C2hug1gvWhkMeDg8

Chapter 22

THE GOOD THE BAD AND THE UGLY

It's fair to say that my own brush with the US medical system left room for improvement, although I refuse to be jaded by the whole experience. I don't believe any doctor goes to work with the intention of damaging a person's health. Certainly there are plenty of good doctors out there who go to great lengths to improve the quality of their patients' lives; we should all be thankful to have them at our disposal. But that's not to say *all* doctors hit the same high standard.

When it comes to broken bones, gaping wounds, heart attacks, or any type of sudden trauma the work a doctor does is nothing short of miraculous. These dedicated men and women deserve the highest credit and we should salute them for the brilliant work they do. Clearly, there *are* plenty of good doctors who listen to their patients and can swiftly bring about good results – so *hoorah to all the good doctors!*

However, when symptoms present themselves in a *vague* fashion the medical profession can at times fall short of our expectations. Diseases such as chronic fatigue, crippling anxiety, and devastating depression are examples of this. And cures for even the common cold and cancer remain elusive.

We could also include a whole bunch of debilitating autoimmune diseases whose root cause are often written off as either "unknown" or genetic. Once labeled, these types of illnesses remain shrouded in mystery – although, as you've probably surmised, I have my own theories on the subject.

So while it's fair to say that good people exist, the law of averages dictates that in *any* profession there will be a percentage of *average* people working right alongside the more excellent ones. Depending on the intensity of your desire to get well, you may find average results frustrating. The gold standard for finding a good doctor is simple: if you are getting good results then you have a good doctor. If you are getting average results, then you are being treated by an average doctor and a rethink is in order. If you are getting very poor results …well, that's not hard to figure out.

In a perfect world *all* doctors would be perfect, but doctors are not gods and with more than 400+ US doctors committing suicide every year let me assure you, they are just as human as you and I. Sometimes they get it right and, unfortunately, sometimes they get it wrong. If for any reason you feel *un*happy with the results you receive from your doctor, then for God's sake don't be afraid to speak up. It's also important to note that good doctors and nice doctors are *not* always the same thing. Here's a true story…

A friend of my family has been dealing with a health issue for the past year or so. She has worked in the medical industry most of her life and has a *great* relationship with the doctor treating her. It's obvious that she likes him *a lot* and she is now trusting him with her life. However, it's plain to see that twelve months into her illness, her progress has been *stagnant* at best. A more critical mind might suggest she has actually gotten worse.

Maybe we all see things differently, but to me, being treated by a "nice" doctor can become a real drawback because the only thing that really matters is *results.* Having been locked into a likeable doctor for almost a year, this lady has little more to show for it than polite conversation and a series of inconclusive blood tests. Given the current health of the nation, I fear this same scenario is being played out across the country.
Average doctors have become far better at public relations than they are at treating people. We would do well to keep *firmly* in our minds that any doctor we employ **is there to fix a problem.** As in this case, finding a doctor you *like* can be a real disadvantage. If your goal is to get well, you may need to look past the polite BS and cheery bedside manner and find someone with a proven track record of bringing solid results to the table. **Even if that means you don't necessarily like the person or their methods.**

BLOODWORK

Bloodwork certainly has a place in medicine and has been shown to uncover a whole range of potential problems, but this is just one tool and it should never override a patient's physical symptoms. Today we appear to have this seemingly obvious truth a little twisted. Medicine now relies heavily on computerized blood tests and apparently nobody has the time to listen to the patient describe his or her symptoms. During my own brush with illness my wife once pushed me into the doctor's office in a wheelchair to discuss my bloodwork. After several minutes the doctor looked up from the paperwork and with a smile and announced that my bloodwork had come back "fine."

Personally, I don't believe any doctor goes into medicine with the intention of making mistakes, but I was very obviously NOT fine. I felt like grabbing him by the lapels and screaming *"LOOK AT ME, I'm sitting in a wheelchair, you idiot! Do I look fine?"* To rely so heavily on bloodwork alone displays an absence of sound reasoning. It also begs the question, if blood tests are so effective why are so many people still plagued with illness?

In days gone by, old-school doctors leaned toward asking a series of probing questions and then listened *carefully* to the answers. Today a computer is quick to churn out numbers based on averages. Essentially, a blood sample is attempting to make a match with a patch of dry ink. This arrangement may work well for the computer, but let's not forget that we are humans, and our variables are often incalculable.

The number a computer spits out for a 6' 5" man with green eyes shouldn't be in the same range as for a 5' 2" man with only one eye. *You catching my drift?*

Am I saying blood tests have no place in medicine? Nope, never did say that. I'm saying *it is imperative* that you find a doctor who listens *to **you**.* Yes, blood tests are a useful tool but only when used in conjunction with a little common sense. If a patient looks unwell and *says* he is unwell then you would think that any blood test to the contrary should be questioned. But today we seem to have that basic concept all backwards.

Consider this: Addison's disease is a serious complaint relating to the adrenal glands. In order to diagnose it a doctor can order a blood test to measure levels of sodium, potassium, cortisol and ACTH. So far so good, and to be fair this test *is* effective at measuring these kinds of levels. If the blood test picks up the symptoms of Addison's, bravo to the blood test, you win.

However, *early* stages of the disease are often missed, especially if the patient isn't probed for information. While the blood test does well to pick up a full-blown case of Addison's, it does little to notify either the patient or the doctor *in advance*. According to the test's logic, one day you don't have it and the next day you. Voila!

For sure, all things must have a starting point and maybe the *symptoms* of adrenal fatigue are an early indication of adrenal dysfunction. But as with leaky gut mentioned earlier, the medical profession doesn't recognize adrenal fatigue, *so it doesn't have a conclusive blood test,* much in the same way that leaky gut doesn't.

The point I'm trying to drive home is that heavily relying on a blood test and *ignoring* the patient has the potential to bend all the laws of common sense, and in doing so does a great disservice to the patient.

Tip- *If you find that progress with your regular doctor is has become stagnant you may find it helpful to search for someone who practices "Functional Medicine." Functional Medicine leans toward addressing the whole person, as opposed to an isolated set of symptoms.*

LOOKING FOR A USED CAR?

When we're looking for a reliable used car we expect to do our homework. We may even cross-reference prices and like-for-like MPG ratings. Some of us may even bring into question the car dealer's past integrity. To find that perfect used car we may diligently pump our friends and family for recommendations, yet when a car breaks down the *only* thing we stand to lose is a little money. It would seem logical that whenever we seek the services of a doctor we should practice at least the same level of diligence we do when making a used car purchase.

If you have an illness, finding a good doctor is a smart first step in the right direction, but this shouldn't mean you are ready to hand over full responsibility after a brief fifteen-minute appointment. **A motivated, informed patient should be able to spot an average doctor from a mile away and that can mean that he or she will recover much faster.**

I'm rarely impressed with the bricks and mortar of a doctor's office, the fancy artwork and certificates on the wall or the pitch perfect classical music being piped into the waiting area. Rather, give me a doctor who can answer the "Why am I ill?" question.
We live in a digital age with information all around us. If you have a medical appointment coming up, use that time to educate yourself. Going into *any* new situation blind and expecting a positive outcome is nothing more than hopeful. Prior to your appointment take notes and have a series of questions on hand.

This is *your* life and if progress has been stagnant then you need to become an active player in your own recovery, if need be, fight your own corner, don't just sit there blindly following the instructions of others in the hope that it's all going to work out for you. *Come on now, deep down you know I'm right. If you want to get well stop being a tourist in your own recovery.* Now is a good time to *stop* taking a back seat with your health and instead slide into the driver's seat and grab the wheel.

DEATH

It's worth noting that the tools of a doctor's trade are often steeped in profit. For sure, medications and medical procedures have the potential to save lives but, as I've learned (to my detriment), *they are not without risks.* The term medical malpractice is one we should ALL *fear* because it is now a leading cause of death in the U.S. If we break down that statement it simply means this: we go to the doctor, he or she gives us something for our illness, we take it, and we die.

No?

Okay, check this out.

In 1999 the pharmaceutical giant Merck released a drug by the name of Vioxx. With a TV budget running into the millions, Vioxx quickly became one of Merck's bestsellers. Americans were prescribed Vioxx as an aspirin substitute because it was believed to produce fewer complications. *I know, right? What could possibly go wrong?*

By 2007, **thousands** of people had died and the class action suit that followed was eventually settled for $4.85 billion. Unfortunately, cashing a check from inside a casket is a trick I have yet to see done. *But wait, there's more.* By the time Merck paid its fine, it had technically made more profit from selling a deadly drug than it had paid in fines! Conservative figures suggest that Vioxx killed hundreds of people, if not thousands, and yet nobody went to jail. *What's up with that?*

> Our prime purpose in this life is to help others.
> And if you can't help them, at least don't hurt them.
> – The Dalai Lama

The real concern is that Vioxx was first put on the market in 1999. Despite early alarm bells ringing and vigorous claims that thousands of patients were experiencing *deadly* complications, Vioxx remained on the market right up until 2004!

"First do no harm" is a noble oath that *good* doctors aspire to; it's also the same one many of those doctors prescribing Vioxx took. Perhaps doctors' iconic white coats should be required to carry the names of their sponsors the way NASCAR drivers do. To expand on this point we could easily fill up the remaining chapters with other deadly examples of pharmaceuticals gone rogue, but I suspect you have already been conditioned to accept that side effects are a necessary evil. This is often done with great skill via the medium of television. *Shall we take a look?*

For the past decade or so I personally haven't owned a TV set *nor do I want one.* Whenever I happen to catch sight of someone else's TV set I am literally stunned at the misleading images some drug companies will use to bait and sell their products. The carefully staged *slick* image of a healthy looking fifty year old man running through a sun-drenched sprinkler system on a manicured golf course rarely suggests that the product being marketed to you has a list of potential side effects that include death. *How is death even a side effect?*

Even if you live to tell the tale, some of the side effects from these drugs can be darn right strange. Recently I overheard a legal commercial asking the following question, *"Have you or your son developed breasts from taking the drug Risperdal?"* Maybe a more accurate picture would be to have the same healthy looking fifty year old man running in slow motion through a sprinkler system while wearing a double D sports bra. *Just sayin'.*

The irony is this: had a vitamin company sold any type of supplement that suddenly gave fathers (or their sons) boobs, the FDA would surely have them hanging upside down in jail faster than you could say Wonderbra. For some pharmaceutical companies with a stock price shooting through the roof, this appears to be just the cost of doing business.

Maybe it's me, but if a prescription drug gave me *(or my sons)* boobs as per the legal commercial, I'm not sure I'd be sitting patiently around on my sofa waiting to be told my next step. Make no mistake, I'd be banging on the doctor's door and shouting, *"Come out and see what you've done, you idiot!"*

Is this a good time to mention that doctors used to promote cigarettes on TV?

Doctors were once so keen to have us smoke, they were happy to appear in TV commercials to help us understand the health "benefits" of cigarettes. You can still see some of these old commercials on YouTube.

Seriously, you kinda gotta see this level of arrogance to believe it. For "proof" of **no adverse effects,** check out this link:
https://www.youtube.com/watch?v=TOKc6TNwlj4

Today we can look back at their pro-smoking statements and ask, what the hell were they thinking? Ever wonder how future generations will judge *this* moment in history?

In the right hands, a good doctor can be a blessing, although it does seem a little bizarre that most of us will spend more time researching a vacation than we do a medical procedure. Unless we play an *active* role in our own health we are giving total responsibility to someone else.

Let us be clear, when it comes to dangerous side effects, *we* are the ones left to pick up the pieces. Most people who become ill go to the doctor to get healthy. In my case, it happened exactly in reverse. Then I had to fight long and hard to regain my health on my own. *A little backward, don't you think?*

So, if you already have a good doctor and effective medications I congratulate you; this isn't always an easy combination to find. If this route is working for you, I again urge you to continue. All that matters is that you find a way to get well, how you get there is of little consequence.

LEGS

Clearly things can and do go wrong with medical procedures, but for this next example imagine for a moment you woke one morning with serious pain in your *left* leg. Over time this pain worsened to the point where you began limping. As the pain intensified a friend *quite rightly* suggested that you see a doctor. The news you received from the doctor is damning; tragically the doctor informs you that amputation is the only course of action.

Despite reassurances that prosthetics have come a long way you are deeply reluctant to cut off your left leg. On the way home your leg is hurting like hell and deep inside you accept that the doctor is right – obviously that leg needs to come off.

A month or so later you find yourself back in the doctor's office flipping through a glossy prosthetic leg magazine. After filling out the paperwork you are relieved that a date has finally been set for the operation. Now imagine waking up from that same operation and seeing your idiot doctor holding up your right leg. Yes, he amputated the wrong leg. *True story.*

In 1995, Tempa surgeon Dr. Rolanda R. Sanchez of the University Community Hospital listed the wrong leg for amputation. He and his lawyer Michael Blazicek publicly presented their side of the story.

Personally, I would have thought it a difficult case to defend once exhibit "A" (the leg) was presented, technically leaving him without a leg to stand on, so to speak. *Whoa! I'm just telling it like it is.*

As for the patient, God only knows what he must have been thinking as he faced the unenviable decision of having to decide for a *second time* whether or not to have his left leg cut off.

But every cloud has a silver lining. The next time around we can safely assume that the chances our patient's correct leg will be cut off are as close to 100% as anyone could hope. *Easy now … or would you rather I just deliver your medical news in a dull format?*

You might think this is an isolated incident *and you would be wrong.* It is well documented that removing the wrong limb – and even the wrong organ – happens with disturbing regularity. During seemingly routine operations there have even been reports of medical instruments gone missing and turning up stitched inside the patient!
My point is this: don't settle for average, do your research, be informed, fight your own corner or live with the consequences. Rushing into a relationship with a very nice but "average" doctor allows for ample opportunity to repent at leisure – but that's not what you're after when you seek medical help. So please, if you are heading for a hospital, have

good people around you and remain vigilant; it's important to play an active role in your own recovery.

HAPPY NOW?

If cutting off the wrong leg reeks of incompetence, then this *final* example suggests arrogance. A former neighbor of mine takes care of her disabled son. She has done so lovingly and around the clock for more than eighteen years. One of the problems she frequently faces is that he goes into seizures. Her son has been on medication his whole life and after this many years, Mom has become quite proficient at understanding the benefits *and limitations* of his medication.

A new doctor came to town (always a red flag) and during a routine visit he suggested giving the boy a much higher dose than he'd been taking. Mom told him they'd tried this in the past and it only made the problem worse. The doctor totally ignored her and persisted and the mom, feeling pressured by the *expert*, finally caved in. Out of fear of getting into trouble herself, she followed the doctor's orders. Retelling the story with tears in her eyes, she told me that the same afternoon the poor kid went into one of the most violent seizures she had ever seen. She immediately called the doctor. Only this time it wasn't to seek more advice at this turn of events, it was to say, "*Happy* now?"

I'm sure a *good* doctor would have listened to her eighteen plus years of *first-hand* experience and employed a degree of common sense, but all too often we allow ourselves to be intimidated by a seemingly educated person. Deep down we all know when something doesn't feel right, but we allow ourselves to be swept along without questioning because nobody ever told us that it's okay to say no.

When faced with ANY invasive procedure *first do your homework,* speak to people who have been in your situation (and in this day and age that's easy to do). Then compare their results with your expectations. People are always in a hurry to recommend *nice* people, but we should remember that *we aren't looking for nice, we are looking for competence and results.*

Ultimately it's always going to be *your* health that's on the line. Hear me now, if something doesn't feel right with any procedure, speak up for yourself and politely but firmly say no. It's your body, which means you *don't* even have to explain yourself. You should never feel pressured to do something that makes you feel *un*comfortable just to make someone else feel comfortable.

HOW TO FIND GOOD PEOPLE

Going into ANY doctor's office lacking awareness will leave you with no way of knowing if you are being treated by a competent doctor or an average one because *both* will appear the same. Good doctors aren't always the most expensive, nor do they need to have the best bedside manner. They do, however, have to have one dead giveaway.

Good people are busy people, and that's okay if he or she brings results. Try to keep this in mind. If you can pick up the phone and see the doctor (or dentist) the same afternoon, that should immediately be a red flag. Most competent doctors will be booked solid as good news *always* travels fast. If you can get in to see your doctor at the drop of a hat, then perhaps you should wait for that *other* guy – obviously this is subject to your appointment not being an emergency. (And of course, if the receptionist says, "Wow, what luck, we just had a cancellation a few minutes ago – otherwise it would be three months before I could get you in" ... well, that too is a different story.)

This same logic can be applied to anyone who has the potential to adversely affect your health. Let's take dentists, for example. There are good dentists and there are average dentists. An average or not-so-great dentist can have a serious effect on your health with the potential to last a lifetime. These days most dental practices have more than one dentist on duty in the office. If you *really* want to know who the better dentist is, ask the receptionist *which dentist has the longest waiting list?* If your situation allows it, wait it out for *that* person. Visit the dentist twiddling his thumbs at your peril.

Had I had the benefit of my *own* advice earlier I could have saved myself an awful experience. In poor judgement I took the first available dentist appointment and my teeth have never fully recovered. The truth is that dentists have ample opportunity to cause lasting problems to your health. As mentioned in an earlier chapter, BPA (Bisphenol A) is the same stuff everyone is freaking out about in plastic bottles. It should, therefore, be on your radar when the dentist comes along and wants to put that white plastic filling in your mouth.

Remember earlier when we learned that silver fillings can be just as problematic. Yup, the name is a little deceptive as a percentage of that "silver filling" can be made of mercury. I know right WTF? (Why These Fillings?)

Once a silver/mercury filling becomes an integral part of your mouth, you can look forward to a **lifetime** of potential issues. Dr. Chris Shade Ph.D. has a substantial amount of time invested in this very subject. His findings are jaw dropping and I would *strongly* urge anyone with these types of metal fillings to listen to what he has to say in some of his free YouTube videos.

> *It is not often that nations learn from the past,*
> *even rarer that they draw the correct conclusions from it.*
> – Henry Kissinger

Sadly, it is still common practice for silver/ mercury fillings to be touted as harmless by some ignorant dentists. Remember, it wasn't that long ago that doctors were keen to have us line our kids up on the street and have them sprayed with DDT! (I am not kidding.) Today we know DDT to be a highly toxic substance and the practice is banned.

Root canals have been known to solve one problem (an abscessed tooth) but create another of equal complexity. Root canals can harbor insidious bacteria because once the inflected the tooth is sealed it's essentially shut off from the immune system. There are times when it might warrant removing the offending tooth altogether. **Bottom line:** research any and all medical procedures. If you are happy with what you found, then go for it.

> *The doctor of the future will give no medication,*
> *but will interest his patients in the care of the human frame, diet and in*
> *the cause and prevention of disease.* — Thomas Edison

If you find yourself looking for alternative ways to ease what ails you, remember the rule: good people usually stay busy. And this rule applies to naturopaths and/or chiropractors as well. When the spine is out, the whole body suffers and any good chiropractor knows this. Over the years I've met many chiropractors and it's been my experience that *most* do stellar work. Am I giving all chiropractors the green light? Hell no! I've met at least one who shouldn't be allowed anywhere near the human frame, so as always, if something doesn't seem right to you I urge you to always go with your gut instinct. Sadly, this is a *valuable* tool that we rarely employ.

A good chiropractor will *always* use his ears before his hands. If you are in good hands a trip to the chiropractor shouldn't be painful. A skilled chiropractor will fix your problem; a bad one can make it worse. Don't be shy about asking friends or family for their recommendations. Having spent the last ten years living in New England, here's mine.

If you find yourself in Northern New Hampshire, my recommendation would be Dr. Dean Powell of Powell Chiropractic. Dr. Powell is everything a good chiropractor should be. If you find yourself over the line in Vermont, you would do well to check out Lyndonville Chiropractic.

Tip *—For any guy who carries his wallet in his back pocket, here's a simple tip that might save you a chiropractic problem down the road. Know that each time you sit down your wallet causes your spine to be slightly out of line, over time this can become an issue especially if you are sitting for long periods during the day. A much better option is to carry your wallet in a front pocket, where it's also less likely to be stolen.*

Let's quickly recap. The goal of this chapter was to guide you into the hands of good people and perhaps even make you smile occasionally in the face of adversity. Before going for ANY medical procedure it's important to do your homework. As an *informed* patient you can then automatically look forward to a higher standard of care.

Whenever you meet your primary caregiver be polite and respectful but don't be afraid to ask probing questions. Pressing people for the *cause* of your illness allows you to evaluate that person's understanding of the problem. Without knowing the true *cause,* any treatment is speculative and has the potential to become detrimental.

This approach should be applied to anyone who comes into contact with your health, be it a doctor, dentist, chiropractor, or any type of naturopathic practitioner.

Finally, I'd just like to share that I'm often left in total awe at the intricacy of the human anatomy. I have a reverential respect for the fine detail and complexity of it all. However, it does seem to me at least, that the older we get the more likely we are to put something "out" as I did recently while working in the garden.

Now you dunnit.

Is it really me, or is the design of the spine perhaps a little *too* intricate? Don't get me wrong, if you are a thirteen year old gymnast looking to do a backbend then it's hard to improve upon the idea of lots of little bones all working together, *but for the rest of us? Meh, I think we could do away a whole bunch of them.*

Seems to me (as an avid gardener) that the spine is sometimes a little *too* fancy for its own good. I wonder if we could get away with having just one big bone, much as we have in the femur? As long as I could bend up and down when I'm planting my lettuce seeds, I really wouldn't even care if I looked like one of those wooden dipping duck toys. *I digress.*

What did we learn from this chapter?

The right doctor can be a godsend, but choose your new doctor/dentist with same care you would choose a new (or used) car, *and always do your homework.* A good doctor/dentist/chiropractor will never feel threatened by an informed patient. Ask questions and listen *carefully* to their answers. And make sure they are listening carefully to what you are telling *them.*

Homework: find a *good* doctor to have on your team. *If* your circumstances allow it, you may find it helpful to search for someone who practices "Functional Medicine." As always, do your research so that you are certain you are in good hands.

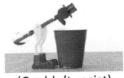

(Couldn't resist)

Chapter 23

THE IMMUNE SYSTEM

If you were to look at your immune system under a microscope (these days that's pretty easy to do online), you would quickly come to the conclusion that *this* system, above all others, is truly mind blowing. Once fired up, the immune system is an equal match for a wide range of would-be enemies.

Your immune system has at its disposal a boat-load of specialized weapons. It's also backed to the hilt by an army of eager foot soldiers and an elite squadron of Special Forces.

This formidable system can defend itself from multiple foreign invaders while at the same time launching a counter-attack with deadly precision. To be clear– your immune system comes well-equipped to deal with high level threats on a minute-to-minute basis. But there is a problem.

To keep it running at optimal performance the immune system requires key nutrients. Once found in abundance, today many of these key nutrients are missing from our diets – and in some cases, these nutrients have been replaced by toxic products.

For some, the immune system has become a nutritionally downgraded version of its former self making it far more susceptible to illness. Rather than first looking to *correct* the underlying nutritional deficiency, humans have taken the questionable step of propping up a weakened immune system by provoking it with pharmaceutical products.

For the past 100+ years, science has, with limited success, been locked in a bitter battle trying to rid the world of all infectious diseases. For the past fifteen years that goal has somewhat intensified and yet rates of serious illness continue to rise. *Hmm, I see.*

Given the current epidemic of diseases relating to a confused immune system, it could be argued that claims of success are being largely misaligned with actual results on the ground.

Science is quick to point out that it doesn't have an answer for this upsurge in autoimmune self-hacks, which opens the door for intelligent debate. In our relentless push to control diseases of an infectious nature, could it be that we have reduced the risk of one illness while *increasing the risk of another* in the process?

When the nutritional demands of the immune system are ignored, our quest to be disease-free has the potential to become a double-edged sword.

> *There's more than one way to skin a cat.*
> *But from the cat's perspective they all suck.*
> – Ze-Frank

This isn't a question *of being for or against* any particular ideology or approach; it's about exploring ways to achieve the *same goal* of fighting disease with an enhanced set of tools. I believe one of those tools is to remove anything of a toxic nature from the body and then flood the cells with peak nutrition, closely followed by thinking with an open mind.

As it stands, autoimmune conditions are skyrocketing and nobody seems to mind. The definition of an autoimmune condition can be thought of as an immune system that has become confused to the point where it now fails to recognize the difference between itself and extensions of itself.

Once triggered, a confused immune system can launch an attack on itself anywhere in the body. However, as we are about to see in this chapter, your immune system is anything but dumb.

Treat the immune system right and it becomes a formidable ally, treat it wrong and you now have a highly complex problem that few understand. For now, let's take a closer look at a normal functioning immune system.

PAC-MAN

The immune system essentially protects us three ways: by detecting, reflecting, and destroying. It's as if something is lurking deep inside us and playing a giant game of Pac-Man even as we sleep. The skin is our first line of defense and forms part of our *innate* defense system. It's a living barrier – like a wall built around a castle – and even a minor paper cut will allow you to see a miracle unfold right before your eyes. *No?*

While science is still patting itself on the back for splitting the atom, your immune system quietly gets on with completing far more complicated tasks every *second* of every day.

The last time you got a paper cut on your hand, do you remember healing it? Nope, of course you don't because an automatic chain reaction of events unfolded and did all the work for you. While you were wandering around with a flower in your hair your immune system went straight to work within a millisecond of the cut occurring.

Nerves quickly transported a signal directly to the brain that the skin had been breached, the brain then took that information and informed the immune system to be alert and ready. An immediate cascade of healing phases followed as tiny cell fragments sprang into action. Instantly, tiny capillaries contracted to reduce bleeding and platelets keenly meshed both sides of the cut together with speed and precision which helped stem blood loss.

THE MIRACLE CURE

Even though it was just a paper cut, inflammation flooded to the area as those tiny fragments worked diligently on your behalf. *But wait, there's more...*mast cells automatically joined the fight and began releasing histamine into action. This helped dilate blood cells and increased the flow of blood to the repair site.

Before long, here came the oddly named white blood cells neutrophils and macrophages, working as a kind of tag team to consume bacteria and

265

remove damaged tissue. Once the cleanup job was complete, a signal was sent back to the brain to let it know inflammation could stop.

Now fibroblast cells began to migrate from surrounding tissue secreting collagen and rapidly multiplying as they did. A week later, the scab fell away and you couldn't even see the repair. Your paper cut was fully cured *(and that's the only time I'm going to be using the C-word in this book).*

That was just a paper cut, and this remarkable chain of unfolding events I've just described is a massive over-simplification of the healing process. It might surprise you to know that the mind-blowing complexity of it all still isn't fully understood by science. Sure, science has given all the main players lots of fancy names like neutrophils and macrophages, but the exact nature of every single reaction remains a mystery.

This is the clearest signal yet that the medical system has underestimated the complexity of the immune system and yet it still continues to provoke it. When the only tool being used is a hammer, *everything* soon begins to look like a nail. I suspect there is more to this debate than meets the eye.

Sadly, humans have become quick to tamper with the immune system, once the immune system turns rogue on you, doctors are pretty quick to throw up their hands and have little to offer in the way of permanent solutions.

Autoimmune conditions can be notoriously difficult to diagnose and treat – although an autoimmune condition is actually pretty easy to spot. *So how do you know if you have one?*

First, take a look at your medical file. Have you seen five or more doctors? Is your file as thick as the US tax code and filled with bloodwork tests that have all come back "fine"? At home do you have a cupboard full of medicine, but still feel like crap? Do you have a second cupboard full of natural supplements that only seem to make things worse? Adding insult to injury, somewhere along the way has it been suggested that your suffering is all in your mind? And have you remained undiagnosed for at least two years? *If this is you, perfect, and welcome to the perplexing world of autoimmunity!*

An autoimmune condition can be like having an octopus on your back with its long tentacles reaching into every corner of your body. Whatever part of your body it comes in contact with, it attacks.

This now becomes your new autoimmune condition (or at least label). It's widely believed that once you have one autoimmune condition the chances of getting a second escalate. *So, there's the good news out of the way. And now for the bad.*

Once you have an autoimmune condition there is no cure for it; once the gene has been switched on it *can't* be switched off. However, before you throw yourself under a Number 52 bus, let me throw you a helpful lifeline. His name is Dr. Gundy and he is internationally recognized as being an inventor, researcher, author, and one of America's top *certified* doctors.

Dr. Gundy is also one of the early pioneers who have been able to demonstrate with statistical analysis that positive results can be experienced in patients with autoimmune conditions by reducing certain foods from their diet.

This is done in part by making drastic dietary changes that include restricting all grains, dairy (*didn't will already cover these?*), legumes, and foods belonging to the nightshade family which include foods like peppers, potatoes, and tomatoes. These groups of foods are collectively referred to here as lectins.

Maybe some of you are a little freaked out right now, running around your kitchen muttering random stuff to yourself about not eating **lectins.** *Try to take a deep breath; it's going to be okay, okay? This is all covered in another chapter.*

One way to reduce the lectin content of food is to cook those types of vegetables with a pressure cooker. So while there may not be a cure for autoimmune conditions, symptoms *can* be managed. And the good news is, *in the right circumstances this can be done almost to the point where symptoms cause an absolute minimum amount of disruption.*

Yes, it takes *effort* to get there, but what's the alternative, a life of pills and misery? I think we can do better than that. The human body is unlike anything else on our planet and the immune system is arguably the most complex, impressive, and effective system of all; it was put there to protect us. Let's work with it, not against it.

Anyone suffering from an autoimmune condition will typically experience a set of symptoms that reflect an immune system gone totally bonkers and out of balance. Once the immune system gets out of balance, a whole lot of things can go wrong at the same time. In an effort to *simplify* matters let us now split the immune system into two parts consisting of Th1 and Th2.

Please note, the following information is an oversimplified overview, the opinions in this chapter (as with all others) are for information purposes only, they are not intended to treat, diagnose, or prescribe for any illness or condition. For your specific diagnosis and treatment, consult with your own doctor or healthcare provider.

SO WHAT THE HECK ARE
Th1 and Th2 CELLS?

Th is an abbreviation for T-helper cells which form part of the immune system. Their job is to recognize and destroy any foreign microorganism that can cause disease. Th1 cells typically deal with infections by viruses and certain bacteria.

They are the body's first line of defense against any pathogen that gets inside our cells. Th1 cells tend to be pro-inflammatory. Th2 cells typically deal with bacteria, toxins, and allergens. They are responsible for stimulating the production of antibodies. Th2 cells tend *not* to be inflammatory. *But what does that mean?*

Well, it may sound complicated but it's really not, just keep in mind that both groups work together, sometimes Th1 may do more of the work and, depending on the threat level, Th2 may play a lesser role. As the threat changes, roles are quickly switched. Once the threat has been neutralized the two stand down and return to equal balance.

In an ideal situation neither one is displaying a more dominant position than the other. This is how a well-balanced immune system should work. However, in some people a prolonged pattern of either Th1 or Th2 dominance occurs. Each can then suppress the activity of the other and problems begin. *Why is this important to know?*

Think about it, knowing if your immune system is Th1 or Th2 dominant can be a hugely important part of the puzzle because knowing allows you to figure out which is the best course of action to take and which you should avoid. Rather than people identifying with certain diseases, perhaps it would be more helpful if patients had the knowledge to be able to say "hi my name is Joe, I'm Th1 dominant." ..... *just sayin.*

Remember some supplements have the potential to crank up the immune system. *So perhaps now it makes sense why that cupboard full of natural supplements made you feel worse.* Anything that boosts *one* side of the immune system tips the balance. If you have an autoimmune condition, then this has the potential to increase an attack. *So how do we know if we are Th1 or Th2 dominant?*

Well, as you might suspect there are a couple of clues that we can now explore. There is also a Th1, Th2 cytokine blood panel that your doctor can order.

Th1 cells are part of what's called cell-mediated immunity, which is an immune response that does *not* involve antibodies but *does* involve the release of various cytokines in response to foreign proteins. If this problem were a basic image, this is how it might look.

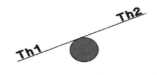

People who are typically Th1 dominant (but not all) may have *delayed* food sensitivities, increased brain fog, fatigue, increased likelihood of Type I diabetes, multiple sclerosis (although MS can be found in both Th1 and Th2 dominant types), Hashimoto's, Grave's disease, Crohn's Disease, psoriasis, Sjogren's syndrome, celiac disease, lichen planus, rheumatoid arthritis, and chronic viral infections. Again, these are generalizations and as with any autoimmune condition it can easily manifest itself in multiple ways. *Hmm, I see.*

Being Th1 dominant means the immune system is constantly amped up. Obviously balance is important, but another telltale sign of the Th1 dominant person may be a tendency to catch fewer colds and some reports even suggest lower cancer rates. The flip side is a higher incidence of autoimmune conditions.

Beware of any supplement that has the potential to boost the immune system which could, in theory, increase Th1 and add to the problem. For example, supplements like Echinacea, astragalus, olive leaf, elderberry, and any medicinal mushrooms that are immune boosting.

If you are Th1 dominant, be aware that lots of supplements have the potential to make you feel worse, so remain vigilant as this is by no means a complete list!

Th2 DOMINANCE

Having an immune system that is Th1 dominant is one thing but what happens when things swing the other way? Functionally, Th2 cytokines have effects on many cell types in the body because the cytokine receptors are widely expressed on numerous cell types.

Th2 cells stimulate and recruit specialized subsets of immune cells, such as eosinophils and basophils, to the site of infection or in response to allergens or toxins leading to tissue eosinophilia and mast cell hyperplasia. *I know, right? Who thinks this way? Let's look at an image of this instead. Ahhh, that's better.*

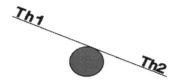

Th2 has some pretty beefy weapons called B cells and antibodies. These B cells are just totally fab to use in battle as they help produce even more antibodies whenever needed and they just keep going and never run out of ammo – cool, right? This is done to ensure there is always enough ammo on hand should any foreign invader ever try to sneak into the body. Also keep in mind that Th2 cells are **anti**-inflammatory.

Now can you see the importance of balance? Once a foreign invader enters the body it finds itself locked in mortal battle with BOTH elements of Th1 and Th2. As the battle rages, the pro-inflammatory process needs to be "cooled down" using anti-inflammatory cytokines; hence it's a team effort. It's really not helpful having one side that's always dominant because, left unchecked, systemic inflammation could easily occur throughout the body causing untold damage. When inflammation gets out of control you can sometimes smell it under the armpits as a more pungent type of BO. Before you shoot me down for being weird again just think back to the last time you felt really ill, your body had a totally different smell to it, *am I right?*

When Th2 gets to be the dominant one, we may be more inclined to get seasonal allergies, asthma, food and drug allergies, and anaphylactic reactions rather than systemic inflammation. Th2 dominance can also be caused by a variety of issues such as heavy metals like aluminum, mercury, and lead which are known to lower immune function. *Hello again, heavy metals – haven't we met before?*

When the immune system is shifted too much to the Th2 system, people generally have less inflammation but their potential to develop allergies to everything increases. It's the allergens that then begin causing problems.

Other possible diseases linked to Th2 dominant conditions may include Lupus, allergic dermatitis, atopic eczema, sinusitis, inflammatory bowel diseases, asthma, allergies, colitis, and multi chemical sensitivities. Some reports even suggest an elevated Th2 may increase the risk of certain cancers. Either way, once the immune system gets stuck out of balance, we lose. *I know, right? Let's not go there, let's instead focus on solutions. Agreed!*

Interestingly, Lyme disease has the ability to throw Th1 out of balance because Lyme disease creates a state of perpetual Th1 dominance; this unfortunately results in constant inflammation, causing an ongoing downward spiral of damage in the body.

Because Th1 dominance is pro-inflammatory, perhaps now we see the importance of eliminating all those foods that create inflammation. Foods like sugars, foods loaded with preservatives, refined and fried foods, and fast foods all contribute to complicating the problem.

Do you see how this is all beginning to fit together? Spices like curcumin, turmeric, and ginger along with omega 3 oils are thought to be helpful because they may help counteract inflammation imbalance.

Th17

In this chapter I've strived to keep the complex simple; however the immune system is a vast subject and we didn't even get chance to talk about Th17 cells. In case you are wondering why, it's because they are a subset of activated CD4+ T cells that are responsive to IL-1R1 and IL-23R signaling. *I know, right? Just thinking about it gave me a headache too.*

However, if the whole Th1, Th2, Th17 concept has piqued your interest then be sure to check out a website by the name of self-hacked.com. There you will find a *formidable* amount of solid information that you are unlikely to find anywhere else.

Autoimmune conditions are tricky and you may benefit from someone who thinks *outside the box.* Fortunately, the person behind the self-hacked blog (Joe) has the advantage of looking at the problem with fresh eyes. I greatly admire the good work Joe does and I read his blog often. If you visit his site, please tell him I said hi.

LYMPH

The design of the human body is as incredible as it is complicated and it's difficult to *fully* appreciate or cover every aspect of it in one book. However, I would like to briefly mention the lymphatic system which is a network of tissues and organs that help rid the body of toxins, waste, and other unwanted materials.

The primary function of the lymphatic system is to transport lymph, a fluid containing infection-fighting white blood cells, throughout the body. Under each of your armpits are more than twenty tiny lymph nodes.

These small but highly sensitive lumps act like checkpoints. If we know the lymphatic system's job is to help fight infection, you have to question the logic of squirting antiperspirant in such a delicate area. When you stop to look at the *loooong* list of toxic ingredients (which usually includes aluminum), it makes me wonder why some people *choose* to sleepwalk into illness this way.

As the name suggests, antiperspirant stops your skin from perspiring by literally clogging it up. Seeing how the skin is **alive** and needs to breathe, perhaps applying an antiperspirant isn't a smart idea for anyone looking to overcome illness. The irony is the more we overload the lymphatic system the worse B.O becomes.

Unlike the heart, the lymphatic system has no pump and requires *movement* to push lymphatic fluid around the body. This fluid moves best when *we* move, which is bad news if we happen to be sitting still most of the day with toxic chemicals under our armpits, but good news if we commit to moving more by either walking or jumping on a trampoline. Hippocrates said it this way: "Walking is man's **best** medicine."

007

I've never actually read any of the James Bond books or seen any of the movies but I do know plenty of people who have. Apparently, if you are fan you will already be aware of the "James Bond shower." Maybe Ian Fleming wrote about this technique to show Bond's brave Scottish ancestry, or maybe he was just trying to keep the character healthy. Either way, a James Bond shower is highly effective at moving lymph and pretty easy to do. *I know you are going to love this one!*
If you haven't been moving around too much then neither has your lymphatic fluid which is a shame as all that junk is now sitting in your trunk. However, all is not lost! Hop into a hot shower and relax – *feels good, right?*

Now at some point simply turn the water all the way to cold and count to thirty, longer if you can stand it. Repeat this three times and it will *really* help push the lymphatic fluid around the body. Doing this every day is no guarantee that you will live longer, *but by the end of the week it will seem as if you already have!*

What did we learn from this chapter?

When the immune system can no longer cope with the demands placed on it, the potential for it to spiral into the complex world of autoimmunity increases. The immune system is far from stupid – *perhaps we have inadvertently tricked it once too often.*

The human body is indeed a complex marvel, but we are *not* the grand masters of the universe we'd like to think we are, and yet we remain hell bent on trying to harness the complexities of the immune system. Too

274

often we fail or make things worse. Just sayin, perhaps there are better ways to enhance the immune system, for example by first removing the burdens we place on it and then flooding the cells with key nutrients. Personally, I also find an occasional teaspoon of colloidal silver is helpful to fight off infection, along with optimizing my Vitamin D levels.

Homework: if this chapter struck a chord with you, then take the time to research whether you are Th1 or Th2 dominant. You can do this with an initial scoping of symptoms followed up with a blood test.

You can also check out Joe at self-hacked, as always please feel free to mention where you found this information. Here's the direct link: https://selfhacked.com/

Chapter 24

A WALK ON THE DARK SIDE

We humans like to think that we are the one's running our own bodies and yet we have this strange system lurking inside us that has the power to shut us down without ever asking our permission. While it's true that we can override our need for sleep with stimulants, sooner or later the body will always have the last word. *No?*

Let's see, who's really in control, you or your body – ready? Try staying awake for seven nights in a row. Meh, didn't think so, perhaps we are being outsmarted by ourselves with good reason.

Sleep is essential to good health, no question about it, and better sleep quality equals better productivity. On the flip side, *lack* of sleep can adversely affect the way we act and feel. Reasoning quickly becomes impaired, attention to detail is lost, and even problem-solving skills decrease.

These are some pretty big clues that sleep is important to us, and yet so many of us try to fight going to bed at a reasonable time. The aim of this chapter is to help you appreciate the value of your sleep and also to help you improve it. Let's go take a look under the hood.

Make no mistake – your brain is a big fat an energy hog. Despite comprising only two percent of the body's weight, the brain gobbles up a whopping twenty percent of your daily energy intake! Each night when you go to sleep, a cleanup crew gets to work and literally washes the brain to ensure that everything is ready for the next day.

It does this by using cerebrospinal fluid which moves through the brain along a series of channels that surround blood vessels. Cerebrospinal fluid is a clear liquid that surrounds the brain and spinal cord.

This process is managed by the brain's glial cells. Science defines this as the "glymphatic system" which helps remove a toxic protein called beta-amyloid from brain tissue. *OMG are you getting this? Beta-amyloid is renowned for accumulating in the brains of patients with Alzheimer's disease!*

BRAIN DRAIN

From the moment your life began, your body has been using sleep to recharge and repair. We don't need to fully understand the mystery; we just need to understand that we can use sleep as yet another tool to assist in our recovery.

Think of it this way: we are quick to understand the importance of recharging our cell phones every night, yet we fight the same simple logic of getting enough sleep to recharge our bodies. The human brain is infinitely more complex than even an Apple iPhone, so it's hardly surprising that our brain fails to work when we suffer from lack of sleep

TICK-TOCK

Every evening when it begins to get dark outside, our brain begins increasing its production of the hormone melatonin which makes us feel sleepy. Melatonin production is designed to be switched off again upon sensing the morning blue sky. This is how we evolved. It's important to understand this because so much of our lives are now affected by the invention of the electric light bulb which gives off a blue light similar to the morning sky.

This manmade blue light can really throw our sleep into total chaos. Keep in mind that altered melatonin levels can lead to an increase in depression and irritability. Sabotaging your sleep with any form of blue light is easy to do. You can do it by playing video games, watching TV, or even looking at your computer screen. Your body is programmed to go to sleep when it gets dark outside and blue light totally messes up that whole process. I accept that I'm not your mom and you can go to bed at whatever the hell time you like, but it's smart to begin winding down at least two hours before bedtime rather than playing Grand Theft Auto V1 until the minute you're ready to close your eyes. *Just sayin'.*

If you want to succeed at this, challenge yourself to become a total blue light Nazi. Remember, *sleep is important,* otherwise the body wouldn't force us shut down and do it **every** night. Light streaming in through a bedroom window is something else to think about. Street lights, car headlights, and even the moon can all affect your sleep quality. For better sleep, quality black-out curtains are essential.

Waking in the middle of the night also poses an interesting problem because if your eyes see a bright light, your chances of going back to sleep are affected. Keep in mind those harsh bathroom lights will really disrupt melatonin, so wherever possible try to tone everything down by using small plug-in type night lights.

Tip- *You can limit the amount of blue light that's being emitted from your computer screen by installing a free download called F.lux. This tracks the time of day in your time zone and as evening comes on gradually reduces the amount of blue light on your computer screen. It may seem a little odd at first, but it can serve as a helpful reminder that really you should be winding down. If you decide you don't like it, simply uninstall it.*

HUNGER

If you find yourself waking up in the middle of the night because you are hungry it could be a sign that your blood sugar isn't being regulated properly. If this is you, try eating a bowl of rice an hour before bed as rice is pretty slow to digest. If rice isn't your thang, try a teaspoon of raw **local** honey at bedtime instead, why? As you sleep, the brain still uses energy and does so by tapping into glycogen which is a form of sugar stored in the liver. If you try this route be sure to use only quality honey. Much of the honey found in the supermarket is imported from China; it's simply not the same standard as raw local honey.

If you drink coffee, keep in mind that it can stay in the system for six or more hours, *even longer in sensitive people.* Try not to drink alcohol in the evening. Initially it may help you feel drowsy, but it will prevent you from entering the deeper stages of sleep which is where the body does most of its healing.

Many of us have heard that we need a standard eight hours of sleep, *but it's the quality of sleep that's important.* I'd like to suggest that we all have different needs, some of us may do better on six hours of sleep and others may need more. Ever wonder why teenagers always seem to need more sleep? The teenage years are a critical time for brain development so it's unfortunate that teenagers, who have the *most* need for sleep, are often the ones who don't get enough.

Perhaps we should be encouraging them to sleep in more, not less. If you are a teenager, show this book to Mom; if you are a mom, let your teenager know this isn't an excuse to stay in bed all afternoon, it's a suggestion that she or he should be going to bed at reasonable time. Somewhere, there is a compromise and a little give and take is sometimes helpful. Perhaps trade an early night off the computer for a few hours extra sleep in the morning…. just sayin'.

If you live to be seventy-five, you will have spent, on average, twenty-five years of your life asleep. *Ever wonder what happens in sleep?*

When we lie down and close our eyes our brain rests and our heart rate slows. This restorative and relaxing part of sleep helps induce the NREM (Non-Rapid-Eye-Movement) sleep cycle. NREM sleep is then followed by the REM cycle (Rapid-Eye-Movement). Research has shown that REM is the part of the sleep that helps consolidate our emotions. This is also the cycle where muscles relax but the brain is in full activity.

As the name suggests, REM sleep is where our eyes begin rapidly darting back and forth. In this state, brain waves are most similar to our waking hours. This is deep sleep, but in order to get there two things must happen. We need dark and we need quiet. Darkness helps with the production of melatonin and quiet just because I said so.

If sleep has been disrupted for any length of time, try not to take anything that might spook the system after 6 p.m. In sensitive people, certain medications **and even supplements can really throw the system off.**

I'm really not a fan of pharmaceutical sleeping pills as they can leave a person feeling groggy throughout the following day. Even worse, drug dependence can become a problem down the road. *If you need a little extra help to fall asleep try the following.*

MAGNESIUM

Sustained levels of stress will often deplete magnesium levels and if our goal is to experience better sleep then magnesium is your friend. Magnesium is used by the body as a currency for more than 300 enzymatic processes.

Today it's not uncommon for people to have a magnesium deficiency. When this important mineral becomes depleted it can produce a wide range of serious ailments ranging from anxiety to cardiovascular disease.

However, before you head off to the pharmacy to buy a bottle of magnesium pills know that magnesium isn't absorbed very well through the digestive system. The better way to get magnesium into the system is by combining both oral and transdermal methods. Transdermal simply means that it is absorbed through the skin.

SALT AND SODA BATH

To increase your magnesium level and help you sleep better, it may help to try a "salt and soda bath." To do this, simply pour two cups of a quality Epsom salts into a hot bath one hour before bedtime. The heat will allow the Epsom salts to be absorbed through the skin and thus flood the system with magnesium sulfate. Add the same amount of Arm & Hammer baking soda to the water and this may help drain the lymphatic system and balance your pH. Some reports suggest that a Salt and Soda bath may even be helpful to decrease radiation levels from x-rays – but that's a whole other story.

If salt and soda baths aren't your thing, you can also buy transdermal magnesium online and regularly apply to the skin throughout the day and then monitor how you feel. If the magnesium is of good quality, you can also expect to have more energy during the day and feel less stressed at night. *Yup, magnesium really is that cool.*

NIGHTMARE

If a lack of sleep has been an ongoing issue for any length of time a sense of bedtime anxiety may soon develop. *In more extreme cases, a set of recurring nightmares may set in. Yup, been there done that.*
While there could be many reasons for your recurring nightmare, I have at least one theory and a very simple way to test it. First, throw ALL your pillows in the garbage. *Why?*

In good health our immune system is able to deal with toxins quite well. When we are stressed/not sleeping properly the immune system becomes over-taxed and less efficient. Most pillows have fire retardant added into them, some more than others. Flame-retardant resembles the molecular structure of PCBs, which have been linked to reproductive problems, impaired fetal brain development, and even cancer! Is flame retardant enough to cause nightmares in those with a weakened immune system? I believe so. If nightmares have been a problem for you and you want to put my theory to the test, seek out a set of less toxic pillows. If you are on a tight budget, just try switching out your pillow for another brand and you might just get lucky.

Without wanting to sound like a hippy, you could also add a few drops of lavender oil directly to your **new** pillows. This will further aid relaxation and help reduce that nighttime sleep anxiety. This can be particularly helpful with kids, if you want to upgrade your sleep try buying an oil diffuser. These things work great, although it might take a couple of consecutive nights before you see the full effect.

CBD

If you are still struggling to sleep, here's another tip you can try. CBD oil may prove much safer than sleeping pills. CBD oil is taken directly on the tongue at bedtime and it gently eases us into sleep.

A wide range of new studies offer supporting evidence of other benefits of CBD oil, one exciting new area even relates to children with uncontrollable epilepsy. In this area, CBD oil appears to be working where conventional medications have previously failed. In today's homework assignment you will find a short TED talk that will change your perception far beyond anything I can write. *I'd really like for you to see it.*

CBD oil currently has scientists all over the world keenly researching its many benefits, CBD oil has *zero* funky effects and it's quite an ignorant statement to suggest that it has. For your peace of mind and my amusement, I would encourage you to research this in more detail but try not to be too freaked out by one word. *That word is cannabis, I know, right? We've reached that point.* However, you should know CBD oil cannot in any shape or form get you high (sorry if that disappoints some of you).

CBD oil is a legal derivative of cannabis; however, CBD oil can **only** be sold with the TCH component extracted. TCH is the part of cannabis that's sought after by people who are looking for a high. To be absolutely clear, CBD is a world apart from this. Again let me stress you **cannot** get high from CBD oil.

BETA-1, 3D GLUCAN

If CBD oil still sounds a little too rock and roll for you then I can totally respect that and perhaps I haven't explained it well enough. If this is you, then maybe we could try something a little more traditional that's backed by research from prestigious universities around the world.

With more than fifty years of research behind it, Beta-Glucans are arguably one of the most studied naturally derived supplements on the planet. Like so many other effective compounds, Beta-Glucans isn't a one trick pony.

Beta-Glucans have a wide range of other benefits. According to research carried out by Dr. Vaclav Vetvicka Ph.D., Beta-Glucan 1, 3D even has some exciting cancer fighting benefits. However, in this chapter we are looking only at its effectiveness as a sleep aid.

It's worth mentioning that Beta-Glucans work as immunomodulators. This simply means it helps restore balance to the immune system. Think Th1 and Th2 imbalance from the previous chapter. Again, don't be in a rush to overload the body with too many things at once and be sure check with your own doctor before trying anything new.

With Beta-Glucans you tend to get what you pay for and the brand of Beta-Glucans I like best is sold by Transfer-Point. It's a little more expensive than other brands but you may find it helpful. I have no affiliation with this company (or any other). If price is an issue, first try some of the less expensive brands. If you see a positive result from the less expensive brands then more power to you.

Sometimes it can be helpful to switch things around from week to week but *it's important not to try too many things at the same time* because doing so has the potential to make sleep deprivation worse. But a little trial and error should put you on the right track.

Tip – There are lots of herbs to help you sleep and my personal favorite is chamomile tea. *If you have one, make the tea in a small hot flask and let it sit overnight, I find that steeping the tea for this length of time seems to increase its potency and you have the tea already made.*

Another sleep idea to try is a grounding pillowcase. You can find these online. The pillow connects to the earth supply in your home and it can help to calm the mind. For it to work *your home needs to properly earthed,* you should test this *before* buying the pillow.
This can be done with an inexpensive tester from any DIY store; it's a light-up device and costs around five bucks. This concept of grounding is covered in more detail later.
There are plenty more sleep tricks to try, but rather than overwhelm you, remember that using too many sleep aids at the same time is counterproductive. We covered a lot of ground in this chapter so let's quickly recap. Keep your sleeping quarters cool, quiet, and above all else

dark. Limit all blue light in the evening and perhaps even try eating some rice for supper. You could also try CBD oil or Beta-Glucan but try them on separate nights. Chamomile tea is best steeped and a salt and soda bath works well for some people.

Lastly, the mattress you sleep on plays a huge role in your sleep. I recently purchased a new mattress from Purple.com, so far I've been pleased with it. If you are in the market for a new bed be sure to check them out.

What did we learn from this chapter?

Without sleep life quickly becomes dull and stressful. Sleep is an essential part of living which is why we typically spend a third of our lives doing it. Blue light at night is a huge problem as it throws our whole system out of whack.

Homework: here's a real moving TED Talk by a dad with a pot-taking eleven year old daughter. *I know right, but this talk will totally challenge your perspective.* This is a great one so please check it out.

This TED Talk is called *"Why I changed my mind about medicinal cannabis"* by Hugh Hempel. E-book readers can simply click on the link below.

https://www.youtube.com/watch?v=3N8QMeIsX2c

Chapter 25

WHY BUY LOCAL?

Back in the day, my grandparents used to own a fruit and vegetable shop in the heart of England. With the exception of a few *non GMO* bananas, everything they sold had been grown within a ten-mile radius. Out of pure economic necessity, what came and went through the front door was either local, sustainable, or in season. At the time, this was just the way food was traded. No doubt, if the shop were around today it would be viewed as trendy or even upmarket. If my grandad were still alive, I'm sure he would be left scratching his head knowing that the organic business model he used out of pure necessity would today be seen as hipster!

After both of my grandparents passed away, the shop quickly changed hands. Today it sells bargain priced booze and the only place to buy fresh produce is at the giant supermarket down the road. Perhaps as a reflection of our changing times, all the supermarket vegetables come tightly wrapped in plastic. Quite remarkably, it is estimated that those same vegetables will have traveled an average of 1500 miles to get to the supermarket. *I know, right? It kinda makes a mockery of the whole cutting carbon emissions thing.*

To those *within* the food chain, the words "local and organic" have suddenly become lucrative buzzwords. This is where we pick up the next part of our story.

Bugs eat profits. I know this and so do large-scale organic farmers. Make no mistake, farming is hard work and you can bet anyone getting up at 5 a.m. is in it to make money like everyone else. And to be clear, there is nothing wrong with making money at 5 a.m. or any other time of day. However, if you think all your organic produce arrives on your table pesticide free **you are wrong.** Large scale organic farmers aren't about to risk crop failure and certain financial ruin just to bring you a fresh head of kale.

Ever wondered why your organic kale comes to the table *without* hundreds of tiny bug holes in it? It's been sprayed with an "organic" pesticide. What you need to quickly wrap your head around is that ALL pesticides, organic or not, share a common goal: to repel living things.

According to the USDA, the organic label only restricts the use of *synthetic* pesticides. Pesticides like copper sulfate and rotenone are permitted to be sprayed directly onto your organic produce. Am I saying *don't* buy organic? *Nope, that's not what I am saying at all,* but some of us have become so desperate to believe in the benefits of organic food *that we only see what we want to see.* The aim of this chapter isn't to tickle your ears with sweet words, it's to help you understand the value of clean, local food and show you *where* to find it.

Not all organic food is as squeaky clean as we would like it to be. With that in mind, perhaps some of the smaller local farmers without an organic seal are being harshly overlooked.

BIG PHARMA - LITTLE FARMER

Let's take this a step further by looking at that pristine organic USDA seal of approval. Would it surprise you to know that it can be handed out to products that use only 95% organic ingredients during processing? For this reason, anything carrying the organic label may not be strictly 100% organic.

Look, I'm not shooting organic food down – I'm simply saying that in today's busy world of commerce it pays to be aware that the only **truly organic** food is home grown. Your next best option is to know the name of the farmer who grows it.

The controversy over organic food can begin even before the first seed is planted. Whether or not the seeds are organic means only one thing: that the original seed-producing plant was grown according to organic standards. If a hybrid seed is planted, the resulting plant will still be organic so long as synthetic pesticides and fertilizers aren't used.

To be clear, organic food that's been grown specifically for supermarkets has its place in your recovery. It's a huge step in the right direction and an absolute upgrade of what they usually try to sell us. The point I am trying to make is this: don't be too quick to discount your small local farmer just because he/she doesn't carry that holy grail of organic seals.

Try looking at it this way: there *was* a time when our ancestors' food was truly organic. Today farmers who choose to grow "organic" food are often shackled in regulation. The irony is those nonorganic farmers who drown our foods with synthetic pesticides are less regulated.

Surely we have this all twisted. Shouldn't the *regular* farmers who are spraying copious amounts of carcinogenic pesticides on our food be the ones held accountable and buried in paperwork?

Either way, there are times when small independent farmers can't get the organic certification simply because of the added paperwork and costs involved. Fees typically include paying the government for site inspections, application fees, and annual certification fees.

If an organic farmer wishes to conform to *all* the regulations he/she must find the time to stop work whenever a government bureaucrat visits the farm. If the small local farmer wants the organic seal, he/she is inevitably forced to jump through hoops to get it and in the process loses valuable time and resources. With the small local farmer now squeezed out, I sometimes feel we are a quick to trust the large-scale organic label and slow to ask questions.

As evolutionary biologist Christie Wilcox explained in a 2012 *Scientific American* article, even "organic" pesticides can be toxic. Copper sulfate, when digested in large amounts, can lead to damage in the tissues, blood cells, liver, and kidneys. While I'm not suggesting toxic levels are being applied, we should be aware of **any** pesticide that has the potential to cause us harm.

Rotenone is another pesticide sprayed onto organic crops and is notorious for its lack of degradation. Studies show that copper sulfate, pyrethrins, and rotenone can all be detected on plants after harvest. *Hmm, I see, perhaps we need ask more questions of large scale farmers, not fewer.*

With (or without) the government organic seal of approval, enthusiastic young farmers are the lifeblood of the local food movement. They often bring clean food to farmers' markets and shouldn't be discredited for lack of paperwork.

Diversity in farming is a good thing and relying too heavily on a small number of people for our food should be obvious cause for concern. Many small farmers are the backbone of independent farming and they deserve your support just as much as any large scale organic farmer does.

The goal of this chapter isn't just to get you to buy clean food, *I'm asking you to go a step further and know the name of the farmer who grew it!* Make a connection with the person growing your food. Small farmers need you to survive and you need them to *thrive*. Ask yourself, how many of your friends on Facebook are farmers?
Still not convinced, huh?

DESERT ISLAND

Imagine we find ourselves stranded on a desert island with 150 other people and one bag of seeds. Everyone agrees that three things are needed our survival: food, water, and shelter. Fortunately, this island currently has enough coconuts to get us through the first few weeks while the (non-GMO) seeds grow. *Unfortunately,* nobody seems to have a plan beyond this so the group decides to put YOU in charge of its survival. *I know, right? Now we are* all *up the creek without a paddle.*

You quickly realize that you need to make some pretty big decisions. What percentage of this group will you send out to find water? How many do you put in charge of growing those seeds? How many do you put to work building a shelter? If you split the group evenly into 50-50-50, I think you'll eventually be okay.

Even if you split the group 20-70-60 I still think you will make it. However, if you choose to have 149 people sitting around looking at computer screens all day while just one person grows the food, I'll think you are certifiably insane.

How is this relevant?

Well, think about it. Doesn't it make you feel a little uneasy to know that, statistically speaking, the U.S. has just one farmer responsible for feeding 155 people seven days a week. This situation becomes a little more unnerving when you understand that most supermarkets have an inventory strategy called JIT (Just-in-Time).

Supermarkets employ JIT to increase efficiency and decrease waste *by receiving goods only as they are needed.* Even a small disruption in the JIT supply would see our supermarket shelves quickly stripped bare.

Are we there yet?

No?

Okay, try this. With or without an organic seal, small local farmers have a passionate connection to their land – it's in their blood. Local produce is always fresher from the local farmer and often less expensive. Superstores are now growing at an expediential rate with some of them now opening around the clock seven days a week, taking with them a huge slice of *independent* pie.

When the purchasing power of superstores is allowed to become disproportionately influential, income is taken away from the surrounding local businesses. **When all the small businesses are gone, giant superstores will be free to dictate what you eat so long as it remains profitable for them to do so.**

Fortunately, superstores are not the only game in town and you can still find *clean* food locally in small mom and pop shops or at your local farmers' market *so long as we get out there and support them.* Buying

291

food locally also gives you the added benefit of buying what's in season and fresh.

Compared to the huge superstores (which never seem to close) small farmers' markets are usually held just once a week, obviously reducing their competitiveness with the bigger players. Unless we get out and support them more, this way of trading food will soon vanish.

What's in it for you?

I know you've been paying attention, so you already know *the key to your recovery is your gut.* It takes whatever nutrients you give it and then loops it back into the cells. Rather than buying your "organic" broccoli from a superstore, when you buy local you actually get to meet the person growing it. Where there is a connection there is also accountability.

Am I saying you have to cut the giant superstores completely out of your food loop? Nope, but it's important we try to adjust the balance by sourcing as much locally grown produce as possible. *I get it,* waiting once a week for a farmers' market can increase your chances of going without, so rather than complain about it don't be afraid to take a shopping list with you on farmers' market days. *But why stop there?*

Once you have made a connection with your local growers it's totally okay to ask them if you can buy from them directly on *non*-market days. Often small local farmers will have additional eggs, vegetables, and meat for sale and they may even be pleased that you asked.

This is how food *used* to be bought and sold. Sometimes you just have to open your mind and be on the lookout for nutritional opportunities rather than following what everyone else does.

NO FARMERS
NO FOOD

Having a thriving farmers' market in every town used to be the norm, but what can you do if your town or city *doesn't* have one? The most obvious choice is to move. *Yup, finding clean food obviously needs to become a bigger priority in your life.* Failing that, I encourage you to travel to the next town or to the one after that. You could also think outside the box and approach your local supermarket produce manager and ask if he or she would consider carrying more local produce. This idea supports your local farmer and it may be a good fit for all concerned.

> *Growing your own food is like printing your own money.*
> – Rod Finley

If you *still* can't find a local farmer, then you could try hooking up with a local gardener. Anyone who grows food for a hobby usually grows more than they need. Generally speaking, gardeners are a pretty friendly bunch and they enjoy doing what they do – it's why they do it. Who doesn't like to have their hobby appreciated?

If your budget is ultra-tight, keep a lookout for garden allotments. This untapped idea can be a nutritional goldmine. This leads me nicely into the suggestion that even if you only have a small window box, you can begin to grow something yourself. This won't sustain you, but it does serve as an *important* psychological step to get you thinking differently about local food.

People often complain about the price of clean produce, which is why our ancestors played a much bigger role in growing their own. Today you can still buy a pack of 250 organic lettuce seeds for a few bucks. A single fully-grown store-bought lettuce will cost you more. Lettuce seeds are super easy to grow and even when left unattended they grow like weeds.

The same applies to tomatoes. You really don't need much skill or more than a couple of feet of soil to grow them in. I agree it all takes time, *but so does checking your email. Just sayin'.*

Once you see how easy it is to grow a few lettuces and tomatoes you may even become bold enough to grow even more things for yourself.

We spend millions of dollars keeping our lawns green, yet you can't eat the stuff and you certainly can't smoke it. Growing something, *anything*, gets you thinking beyond the scope of the supermarket.

These superstores have become masters of distraction and even with the best intentions we keep finding ourselves going back into them for organic food and leaving with a pair of socks. Think about it, these distractions put your food bill up every time you go to the store.

THOSE DAMNED SWEDISH PEOPLE

Perhaps we need to look at this problem from a different perspective. In Sweden, a small group of city folks took it upon themselves to grow just a few basic vegetables. At the end of the growing season they traded with each other for more variety. It worked out well for everyone involved. So why does this feel so unnatural to us?

A little more food for thought (author knuckle bumps reader for unintended pun): imagine if one day visitors from another galaxy dropped in to visit and began observing those crazy Swedes growing their own food.

They then observed that *other* group, yup, you know who I mean, the ones being slowly poisoned to death by pesticides. Which group would the aliens regard as crazy? The group of humans working together to grow what keeps them alive, or the group of humans eating out of cardboard boxes while sitting on their excessively manicured lawns?

So, while we are waiting for our home-grown lettuce to come to fruition let's ponder our options. They say the road to hell is paved with good intentions. Promises and plans must be put into action, otherwise they are useless. The way to make this work is to make the small local stores your first port of call and then fill in any gaps at the supermarket. Doing it the other way around rarely happens.

In all sectors, diversity is the lifeblood of healthy commerce; whether you are buying a cabbage or a carpet, small family business owners need our support.

Without economic diversity the world would become a very scary place. I'm reminded of how the Cadbury company once managed to successfully run their chocolate empire with exemplary values. Today? *Meh, not so much.*

CHOCOLATE

From humble beginnings, Cadbury's chocolate began in 1824 by a family of practicing Quakers. As they grew so did their workforce. As a way of giving back to the local community, workers were taken out of dirty slums and moved into houses built expressly for Cadbury employees in a beautiful village environment.

At a time when many workers were uneducated, Cadbury also built a school for its employees children, and a doctor's office where Cadbury workers could receive free medical care. Mr. Cadbury regularly walked the factory floor and not only knew the names of his workers, he knew the names of their family members. The Cadbury workforce had value and working conditions steadily improved year after year.

Throughout Victorian times, the Cadbury name continued to grow, in part thanks to a loyal workforce. The Cadbury brand prided itself on selling only quality products. As the business expanded, it was suggested that growth could only be sustained if the Cadbury family began to advertise. A meeting was set up and several ideas were pitched to the Cadbury owners.

After several hours, all the ideas were rejected on the grounds that it was dishonest to suggest their chocolate product was better than it was.

Fast forward and today the Cadbury chocolate company is no longer in the hands of the Cadbury family. Instead it was broken up and sold off to shareholders from around the world. I suspect many of those shareholders have never set foot on the factory floor.

While the stock price may have increased in value, the value of a Cadbury worker has never been more undermined. When American food giant

Kraft moved in to buy up the Cadbury brand, workers were seen protesting with banners that read, "Please don't sell us out." The value of those workers is now secondary to the profit line.

Try not to become a man of success,
but rather try to become a man of value.
— Albert Einstein

What did we learn from this chapter?

On average, just one farmer is responsible for growing the food of approximately 155 people. Buying local produce in season will enhance your nutritional intake as well as help the local community grow. Small independent shops often have greater ties with local growers which helps keep the local cycle going.

Homework: see if there's a farmers' market in your area and start going. Challenge yourself to know the name of your local farmer. Grow one thing from seed and see where it leads.
Also, here's an interesting short video by Dr. Axe – e-book readers simply click on this link:

https://www.youtube.com/watch?v=TUMNYkdxc9s

Paperback homies can Google "11 steps to losing belly fat by Dr. Axe."

Chapter 26

THOSE TRICKY TRIGGERS

Some foods have the potential to heal; others can cause negative reactions in some people. The latter are sometimes known as "trigger foods." The time between consuming a trigger food and having a reaction can vary quite a bit and sometimes take so long that there is a mental disconnect (or, there is no immediate obvious connection) between the food and the reaction. The aim of this chapter isn't to give you a list of what not to eat – it's to make you aware of what those potential trigger foods are.

This doesn't mean all the foods mentioned here are going to be a problem for you, it simply means as you read through this chapter you will be better informed and able to recognize patterns if and when they arise. Don't lose heart – all these problems have solutions. When we learn to recognize the connection between food and the way it makes us feel, it quickly becomes an empowering tool.

From the get-go let's kick off with the most obvious. The Big Four to be on the lookout for are always going to be gluten, dairy, eggs, and nuts. Having this vital piece of information at the very **beginning** of this chapter will serve us well as we move forward. It also pays to be on the lookout for bad fats, which we'll cover in more detail later. Better buckle up, some of this information gets a little bumpy. *Okay, here we go.*

Before illness came to pay me a visit, my diet was at best average. I guess I'd always been one of the lucky ones, I had an immune system that worked just fine, which meant I could make dietary mistakes and get away with it. However once my health was sent over a cliff, that was no longer true. I quickly went from *never* having any type of seasonal allergy or food sensitivity to being confronted with an absolute tsunami of them. *I know, right? What's up with that?*

To my horror, suddenly many of the foods I had eaten with impunity my entire life were now acting as springboards for new symptoms. Once the immune system becomes spooked, one man's food can quickly become another man's poison.

One of the frustrations I faced was trying to find accurate nutritional information. So often it felt as if the target I was desperately trying to hit was frequently moving. It really doesn't take much to find that you are wading knee-deep through a sea of conflicting misinformation. One day carbs are good, the next they are bad, yada, yada, yada.

It's not that the majority of dietary information out there is incomplete, contradictory, or wrong – the problem is we are all so different. With so many human variables it's impossible for one diet to fit every person. Unfortunately, this fundamental concept is something even the standard food pyramid fails to take into account.

Once you see the problem from this perspective the subject of nutrition begins to make more sense. Obviously there are some BASIC rules that apply to all of us. But the clean fuel *your* body was designed to run on is likely not going to be identical to that of your neighbors. The world has successfully evolved by utilizing the skill sets of uniquely different people. Perhaps Mother Nature intended food to be used as diverse fuel. *How so?*

During our early history, the nutritional needs of a hammer-swinging shelter builder would have been very different from those of person who spent most of his or her time trying to solve more complex problems, like inventing a wheel. Today we still have a *need* for that diversity; we need farmers to grow food, carpenters to build things, engineers to design things, and academics to teach us stuff. Here we begin to see the bones of the problem. Throughout history, **no single diet has ever suited everyone.**

ORGANIC TRIGGERS

As surprising as this may sound, many of the known trigger foods are *perceived* to be healthy. Some of them might even be growing in your very own vegetable garden! For that reason, it's important to note early on that even **organic** food can act as a *trigger* and with the same intensity as its nonorganic version. I'm not intentionally trying to rain on your vegetable parade here, but unless we are aware of this going forward, then everything else will be built on sand.

Once you have a basic understanding of what these *potential* food triggers are, the exploding minefield of nutrition becomes a little easier to navigate. I know what you are thinking because I've thought about it too - *why would a super smart immune system react like this to healthy food.*

Right?

In short, a spooked immune system can label something you just ate as a foreign invader. Sometimes this reaction is serious, immediate, and obvious, and sometimes it's *less* obvious. To describe this reaction, the health industry often uses terms like *food intolerance, food allergy, and food hypersensitivity* interchangeably. This is not just deeply confusing, it's incorrect.

Food intolerances are relatively common and are said to affect one in five of us. Although reactions can vary, the immune system is *not* involved in food intolerance. Trying to replicate a reaction to a *known* food intolerance can be inconclusive because there can be any number of factors contributing to the intolerance. Food intolerances are known as non-immunological reactions.

By comparison, food allergies or hypersensitivity to a particular food are both reactions to a protein found in certain foods. This *does* involve the immune system. This type of reaction is less common and is believed to affect one in fifty of us.

Once the offending protein has been identified, a predictable reaction can be replicated. With some degree of certainty, even a small amount of food will cause a reaction by the immune system. These types of reactions are known as immunological reactions.

Once the body has labeled a particular food as problematic, antigens are made that ignite the immune response. Antibodies that bind to those antigens are then formed. With so much ground to cover, what-say we avoid turning this into a stuffy old science lesson and instead think of this whole process as the body tacking a bunch of yellow sticky notes onto any foreign invader it deems suspect? The body does this as a way to help guide an attack by the immune system. That being the case, and since we know immune system is far from dumb, *why would it suddenly begin doing this in relation to food?*

> *Thinking is difficult, that's why most people judge.*
> – C.G. Jung

Due to the complexity of the immune system, that's a pretty big question to grapple with. To briefly recap, the immune system is highly intelligent and very much alive; it's arguably the most complex, impressive, and effective system of all. Its primary function *isn't* to find ways to annoy you. Its intent is to protect and yet humans insist on provoking it, perhaps to the point where it becomes totally confused.

Once the immune system is spooked, food sensitivities may be the tip of the iceberg. A confused immune system that has trouble distinguishing parts of itself from foreign invaders is better known as an autoimmune condition. A reaction could manifest itself in a wide range of problems from general fatigue to an outright attack on organs or joints. *I know, right? Always a bummer.*

To add to the problem, the word "food" has become a loosely a defined term. A spooked immune system then has the unenviable task of trying to figure out which of the 3000+ food additives are friends or foes.

The scope of the problem obviously magnifies when eating out because you really have no control over someone else's cooking. Remaining blissfully unaware or choosing to ignore food allergies, food intolerances, and hypersensitivities can potentially ratchet up the immune response and, over time, provoke a stronger reaction.

For now, let's for a moment step back from the complexities of the immune system and simply agree that the human body is an absolute wonder, and in order to function optimally it requires fewer toxins and more clean nutrients to burn as fuel.

As a rule, anything you can't pronounce on a food label should be an instant red flag. When addressing the issue of food sensitivity, food triggers, allergies, etc., it's vital to cease consuming products that come to you in a box, can, or packet. *Yup, we keep coming back to it, food that's packaged gets complicated.*

The more complicated the food, the more potential there is for an adverse reaction. Be aware that today many food additives, preservatives, and antibiotics are finding their way into the meat supply. For that reason, it's important to steer clear of the deli counter (or anything else that's been through a meat grinder) because these meats can be loaded with things that are known to trigger a reaction.

On the surface, a simplified diet may appear more basic and for sure this is how our ancestors used to eat long before supermarkets helped make us all lazy and sick. Simplifying the diet is particularly helpful in the early days when flare-ups from trigger foods are more noticeable. Again, not all food reactions are instant; and relief of symptoms doesn't happen overnight.

This disconnect in time can make it harder to find the original source of the problem – not every reaction to food has us rolling around on the floor in anaphylactic shock. *Fortunately, solutions are forthcoming* when we learn to pay close attention to those subtle signals all around us. Changes in the skin such as excessive dryness, eczema, or itching can be noticed. When a food is the cause of eczema, topical creams are often ineffective.

While these types of symptoms may be viewed as annoying to the host, they also help bring awareness to a wider problem that maybe you *can't* see. It's as if the body is trying to grab your attention by saying, *"Hey, pay attention to me, what you see on the outside is also happening inside."* If you suspect something isn't right, try seeking out a *good* doctor for allergy testing.

Tip - When the eczema creams fail, you could try cutting a thin slice of raw ginger and rubbing the clean side directly onto the area. Obviously, for a longer term solution, try *switching to a simple diet.*

Any food that causes a reaction will send out a few clues along the way. Skin issues and other symptoms may rear their ugly heads as well as bloating, long-term flatulence, chronic fatigue, and inflammation. Prolonged inflammation is believed to play a role in cardiovascular diseases, autoimmune conditions, numerous cancers, and even diabetes – just to name a few.

Some food excitotoxins like glutamate and aspartate can give the brain a source of excitatory neurotransmitters adding to the cycle of anxiety and depression. Given that psychiatrists receive little or no nutrition training, this important connection can easily be overlooked.

According to Felice Jacka, the president of the International Society for Nutritional Psychiatry Research, "A very large body of evidence now exists that suggests diet is as important to mental health as it is to physical health, a healthy diet is protective and an unhealthy diet is a risk factor for depression and anxiety."

TRIGGERS SIMPLIFIED

To help us better understand this concept we can separate trigger foods into easy to understand groups. All the following food groups mentioned here are heavily steeped in well-documented scientific data. I'm not bringing this information to your attention to intentionally piss you off; it's simply to make you more aware of potential problems.

Finding those elusive solutions becomes easier once we see the fuller picture. With that in mind, try to use this chapter as a guide. If you suspect you are reacting to any type of food then you are encouraged to research each of these subjects in more detail. *Here we go, ready?*

First off, let's establish a few ground rules. *Any* food known to trigger a reaction can also have a foot in more than one food group. I know, right? *What does that mean?* A simple example of this would be the potato. It's a vegetable, it's a starch, and it's a carbohydrate. At this stage it's not important to know what these different groups mean because they are covered in more detail later. What is important to understand is that the potato (like so many other foods) is capable of belonging to multiple groups.

To help simplify this concept, picture yourself as being a member of a tennis club and a garden club. Even though you are a member of two different clubs, you obviously remain the same person. To take this a step further, we could also say that in addition to being a vegetable, a starch, *and* a carbohydrate, this active fellow we know as the potato is also a member of yet another club called the *nightshades.* This is an important group of foods to be aware of because they can be particularly problematic. Here's why.

NIGHTSHADES

In certain individuals, foods belonging to the **nightshade family** are thought to weaken the tight joints in the small intestine which causes tiny food particles and excrement to spill into the bloodstream and trigger an adverse reaction and increased inflammation. Symptoms may include (but are not limited to) joint pain such as arthritis, fatigue, and muscle pain and tightness. *Are you catching this joint pain sufferers?*

So why would nightshades foods do this? To better understand this, know that you aren't the only one who likes to eat – so do bugs. Nightshade plants already know this, but they can't exactly pick themselves up and run away to keep from being eaten alive. So they evolved, and to protect themselves from bugs they have developed the ability to produce small amounts of reactive chemicals. Some people will react to these chemicals more than others.

So now that we know that the potato is in this group, you might be wondering what other foods are too. *Am I right?*

There are more than 2000 plants in the nightshade family. Yikes. Thankfully, the list of the ones you might want to eat is relatively short.

- Tomatoes
- Tomatillos
- Eggplant
- White Potatoes (but not sweet)
- Goji Berries
- Peppers (bell peppers, chili peppers, paprika, tamales, tomatillos, pimentos, cayenne etc.)
- Tobacco (some people chew it)

If you want to see positive results, eliminating foods in the nightshade group isn't something you can do halfheartedly. *Why?*

Once the immune system has been spooked, it's automatically on red alert. This means you can't *cheat* even a little bit. Everywhere *you* go, so does your immune system. An easy self-test is to stop eating all nightshade fruits and vegetables for 30 days and monitor how you feel.

The good news is if you fully commit to cutting out these trigger foods don't be surprised to find that after just thirty days, even those joint pain symptoms quickly subside. While some people have no problems eating foods in the nightshade family they *can* present problems for anyone with any type of autoimmune condition. This is something to keep in mind particularly if you don't feel well after eating. Unfortunately, foods that are capable of triggering an adverse reaction aren't confined to the nightshade family. As we have some ground to cover let's leave nightshades for the moment and take a closer look at food mold.

MOLD

Most of us are exposed to low levels of food mold at every meal. This type of mold isn't as obvious to the naked eye as is the mold we are used to seeing grow on bread. In sensitive individuals, repeated exposure to an undisclosed food mold can make the diagnostic process all the more challenging, hence awareness once again becomes your key.

In certain individuals, low level exposure to food mold can present itself as headaches or brain fog, higher levels can result in more serious problems. All foods can be susceptible to these molds and there is currently a school of thought that suggests that a peanut allergy may in part be due to the mold found on peanuts. While the nut debate remains speculative, I thought it an interesting addition to the subject.

With so many everyday foods prone to mold, even coffee can become a culprit. It might surprise you to know that EU countries, South Korea, and Japan have strict regulations regarding levels of mold found in coffee; the U.S. and Canada have no such limits. If you are a coffee drinker, where your coffee comes from is important and it's obviously something we are going to look at in more detail later.

LECTINS

Although you may not have heard of lectins, scientists have known about them since 1884. Lectins are found in abundance in certain fruits, vegetables, beans, nuts, legumes, milk, and members of the nightshade family (hello again).

Lectins (not leptins) are a type of protein that can bind to cell membranes. They are sugar-binding and become the "glyco" portion of glycol-conjugates on the membranes. *Lectins can be extremely problematic for anyone with a suspected autoimmune condition.* There are literally thousands of versions of lectins and not all of them are truly problematic, but some *are* capable of causing irritation to the gut lining. The worst offenders, deemed to have vastly higher lectin contents, are listed below.

Obviously try to keep in mind that *some people* are more likely to have sensitive reactions than others. With lectins, these reactions can be widespread and far reaching. Mother Nature devised lectins as a way to allow certain fruits and vegetables to defend themselves against the microorganisms and insects intent on eating them. Lectins help the seed part of the plant survive.

In most cases, seeds can be notoriously hard to digest. They are constructed that way to ensure that when an animal eats the fruit or other plant its seed will later be pooped out intact, thus allowing a new plant to grow. For that reason, if you are going to eat any type of edible seeds it's probably best to soak them until they sprout a tail, which will help with digestion. All seeds aside, some fruits and vegetables have a much higher lectin content than others, and the genetic engineering of some plants may cause some fluctuations. *Gee thanks.*

In susceptible people, lectins are thought to wreak havoc in the gut by causing spikes in inflammation and a general degeneration of the lining of the gut. *A confused digestive system runs parallel with a confused immune system.* Dr. Gundy, the director of the International Heart and Lung Institute in California, believes autoimmune conditions such as rheumatoid arthritis and lupus are greatly helped by restricting the overall amount of lectins we eat. For sure, Dr. Gundy is one smart cookie. He has also written several books on the subject. And he has plenty of interesting YouTube clips. If you find yourself leaning toward the autoimmune camp it might be worth taking a look.

Foods with lower levels of lectins include mushrooms, broccoli, onions, bok choy, cauliflower, leafy greens, pumpkin, squash, sweet potato, carrots, and asparagus, as well as berries, citrus fruits, pineapple, cherries, and apples. You can also add to this list animal protein from fish, seafood, eggs, meat, and poultry, as well as fats from olive oil, avocado, and butter – all of which have low levels of lectins.

FOODS HIGH IN LECTINS

- All grains and cereals

- Nightshades, including tomatoes, peppers, potatoes and eggplant
- Gluten from wheat, rye, barley, malt and maybe oat because it can cross contaminate during processing
- Beans and legumes, including soy and peanut. Cashews are considered part of the bean family
- All dairy, including milk, cheese, cottage cheese, yogurt, and kefir
- Yeast (except brewer's yeast and nutritional)
- Fruits should be restricted during the first 30-day trial period and then gradually reintroduced

The good news is you can reduce your *overall* lectin intake by cooking with a pressure cooker. This method of cooking will help lower the overall the number of lectins in your foods. Moving along nicely, let's take a look at our next trigger – grains.

GRAINS

Grains are found in everything from pasta to spice mixes, cakes to processed meats, and even salad dressing. The list is impossibly long so it's important to note that grains can be found in just about any subset of food. *Because of the way grains are stored when harvested, they can also be susceptible to hidden molds.* In certain individuals, any grain can become a problem but the one most talked about is the one I'm sure you have already heard of and that is gluten.

While some people may believe that going gluten-free is some kind of new fad, the discovery of this problem grain was actually first made in Holland by professor Willem-Karel Dicke back in the early 1950s. As many already know, gluten is the seed of wheat and an insoluble protein composite. In plain English, this simply means it's difficult for the digestive system to break down. If I were a betting man (and I'm not), I'd be tempted to bet that grains are, at least in part, contributing to your symptoms.

As set out earlier, intolerance to gluten isn't the same thing as an allergy. An intolerance is the lesser of the two evils and it can certainly rear its head in any number of ways. But comparing a gluten intolerance or sensitivity to an allergy is the equivalent of comparing a very bad sunburn to a third degree burn. Obviously, you wouldn't want either, and to the person dealing with it on a daily basis neither illness is desirable. My point is that they are as different as Donald-T and Malcolm-X ... *just sayin'*.

A true allergy to gluten becomes a more serious autoimmune condition known as celiac disease. This results in damage to the small intestine whenever gluten is ingested. For some, the problem with grains goes beyond gluten.

The most common mistake people make when they are told they have an issue with gluten is they wander around the supermarket loading up on bags of gluten-free breads, gluten-free cookies, and other gluten-free snacks. *But, wait, that's good, right? Meh, not so fast.*

Once you have a problem with gluten you have a spectacularly higher probability of reacting negatively to other grains. Simply switching to a different grain that doesn't contain gluten is no different than switching to a different pack of cigarettes – they are equally bad.

Some people have an immediate and noticeable reaction to gluten; others have a delayed reaction that can occur gradually over several days. This type of disconnect is obviously more challenging to deal with.

If you suspect you have a problem with gluten, the easiest way to test it is to go totally grain free for thirty days. After thirty days, carefully watch what happens as you reintroduce grains into your diet. Yup, you could also get tested by your doctor, but any treatment is going to involve a strategy of total avoidance.

You might wonder why gluten is suddenly getting so much heat when bread clearly dates back to biblical times. That's a nicely thought of question and I'm going to award you five points for effort, but if you are thinking of wheat as being three feet tall and blowing gently in the wind think again.

Sadly, those types of romantic golden wheat fields are long gone and have been replaced by a much smaller, genetically modified version. This type of wheat is often soaked with a broad-spectrum systemic herbicide known as glyphosate (Roundup) and is designed to produce higher yields rather than higher quality. *Is it me, or is Roundup beginning to cause more problems than it was intended to solve?*

We could easily fill up the rest of this book talking about problems relating to glyphosate and gluten, but for simplicity's sake, let's agree that for some, gluten avoidance has the potential to bring huge health benefits and its worth trying for thirty days. Try to keep in mind that gluten can hide in anything that comes to you in a box, a can, or a packet. It can even be in salad dressing!

To do this right, you need to stop looking at this as being gluten-free and go completely *grain free.* This is the single biggest reason people with a gluten problem fail to see progress. Until then, you may find it beneficial to avoid *all types of grains*, especially wheat, corn, barley, oats, rye, and rice.

Tip –
To help you on your way, check out a book called *Against all Grain* by Danielle Walker. It's packed with good ideas and healthy recipes.

MILK

As discussed earlier, there are many reasons why milk can cause problems, even milk from grass-fed cows. In part it may be because the protein component of milk (casein or BCM-7) or the milk sugar (lactose), are not well-tolerated. And remember, cheese and "healthy" organic yogurts form part of the same problem.
However, casein and BCM-7 are largely absent in butter made from cows raised in open pastures and generally doesn't seem to pose as much of a problem to those who are sensitive to milk.

CHECK IT

Below is a list of foods believed to cause approximately *90% of all food allergies*. Take a look and ask yourself which of these foods you consume on a regular basis?

Wheat and other grains with gluten, including barley, rye, and oats

- Milk and milk related products, yogurt, and cheese
- Eggs
- Peanuts (prone to molds)
- Tree nuts, like walnuts, almonds, pine nuts, brazil nuts and pecans
- Soy
- Fish (mostly in adults)
- Shellfish (mostly in adults)
- Food additives

Just about everything leading up to this point has looked to remove stressors from your body. Bacterial, viral, and parasitic infections are all known to induce or **worsen** symptoms of food sensitivities, mainly through the mechanism of molecular mimicry. Hence, previous chapters in this book have looked to eradicate them.

Finally, I'd like to invite you take a moment to hear the story of a one woman's recovery which was helped in part by avoiding certain trigger foods and replacing them with key nutrients.

Terry Wahl was a patient with a chronic, progressive disease and found herself confined to a wheelchair. As a qualified doctor, she used all her medical connections to the fullest. Even so, her condition got steadily worse. *Hmm, I see.*

In desperation, she tried a new path that included nutrition and – can you believe it? – today she walks freely. Coming from a doctor I found her particular TED Talk fascinating and it's in today's homework.

What did we learn from this chapter?

Our individual needs cannot be measured with a single diet or blanket approach. Once you have a spooked immune system, the funky world of food can become an exploding minefield. To complicate matters, some of these trigger foods are often perceived as being *healthy organic foods*.

Homework: listen to Dr. Terry Wahl's TED Talk. If you are reading the paperback version of this book, a simple Google search will take you there, for all others here's the direct link. Enjoy.

https://www.youtube.com/watch?v=KLjgBLwH3Wc

Chapter 27

SIMPLY SIMPLIFY

In the last chapter we learned about some of the foods you may need to avoid. *Solutions to those problems are coming,* but for now let's keep things interesting by switching gears and looking at something new. Of all the recommendations offered in this book, the ones in this chapter are probably the *easiest* to implement and I hope they will make the *biggest* difference to you and those around you.

Our perception of success is often judged by the number of dollars we are prepared to exchange for each measured unit of toil. We then exchange a percentage of those dollars for material things. More than ever before, the retail industry is keen to help you do this. Gone are the days where we needed to physically stand inside a store. Today, online shopping brings the store to us at any and every hour of the day or night. We can literally *shop till we drop* while still in our PJs. Left unchecked, this has the potential to become a huge problem. *How so?*

As it turns out, your financial health, your mental health, your shopping health, and your physical health are all closely connected. The mind tells money what to buy and the body gets to tag along for the ride. So where has the mind been going and how does that affect your health?

$

Well, in this day and age that's actually pretty easy to find out and you need only click one button. Take a quick look at your browsing history over the last twenty-one days and see what it says about you. Tracking your browsing history is sometimes described as a tool "to enhance user experience," others call it "data-combining." Either way, it also doubles as a way to constantly monitor *everything* you view, and does so with astounding efficiency. Somebody, somewhere obviously wants that information.

Why?

In a word: *money* – and lots of it. It's a scary thought, but you already *agreed* to this intrusive monitoring the moment you clicked that "I accept" button without reading that long list of terms and conditions. *Don't panic, nobody ever reads that stuff because we all need our internet access at any cost, right?* This is *not* just an attack by those annoying pop-ups ads. Once your computer has you all figured out it works on learning what you are going to buy, *perhaps even before you do.* When it learns to cater to your spending habits, money (yours) usually flows in one direction, *out.*

No?

Okay, if you feel that your spending habits are *not* being directly influenced by the internet then take a look at your credit card statement over the past two months. Hmm, notice it forms an alarming correlation with your browsing history? *Sheer chance? I think not.*

You are being gently encouraged to buy more things whether you care to admit it or not. *Okay, so even if this is true how does owning more stuff fit in with my health?* Well, stuff is just stuff until money changes hands and then it turns into pollution. *We all like to drink clean water, breathe fresh air, and look at the big blue sky, right?* But there's another problem and it goes by the name of stress.

It's an illusion to think more money automatically equals more happiness. Once self-value comes from owning more stuff it can quickly lead to a never-ending cycle of want. The more we have the more we want. Left unchecked, this line can easily become unhealthy and blurred. If we aren't careful, the things we own **begin to own us!**

Think of it this way: if a news flash suddenly came on the radio and said you had just fifteen minutes to evacuate your house, what items would you throw in your suitcase? Now ask yourself, what could you gladly leave behind? Perhaps we don't need as much stuff as we think we do.

Over the years I've met with some incredibly wealthy and interesting people, some of whom are used to seeing more money in a day than many of us will in earn in our lifetimes, and yet many of those people were unhappy beyond description.

There's nothing wrong with being wealthy or wanting a better quality of life, but we have to be careful that wanting it (or having it) doesn't take on a life of its own. Many of us have been led to believe that luxury is a standard worth chasing after, yet it also has the potential to bring the most stress.

A preoccupation with accumulating more luxury "stuff" can become a trap that tends to lead into a downward spiral of self-inflicted stress. Somebody somewhere will *always* seem to have more, and yet this thirst for material things steals the one thing we need more than anything else – our *inner peace*.

Give a man a million-dollar house and it isn't too long before he's peeking over the garden fence at the sixty-foot boat his neighbor owns. The problem with this concept is twofold. First, you should know the definition of a boat is a hole in the water that must *constantly* be filled with money. Second, *nobody cares.*

Throughout this book I have strived to be upfront with you. To be honest, there was a time in my own life when I too was a dollar-chasing victim. I followed the herd and drove my overpriced pretentious car and even bought the gold Rolex to match, but no matter how hard I worked it never seemed enough. Some twenty years later, wealth no longer impresses me. I find genuine contentment looking at a full woodshed knowing that I have enough fuel to see me through the coldest of winters. To me this has a real and tangible value beyond money sitting in a bank. Today, I really don't care what car I drive, but I do pay close attention to what food goes on the end of my fork.

A man who views the world the same at fifty,
as he did at twenty has wasted thirty years of his life.
– Muhammad Ali

I once sat on a plane next to an elderly Irishman who had a twinkle in his eye. At some point he and I could hear the couple behind us arguing about money. This elderly fellow turned to me and in the softest of Irish accents said, "Son, in this life you can be sure of this, if a man has a wife or a set of wheels, he's heading for problems." In a crude sort of way, he was right, stress does indeed come from two things, the people we surround ourselves with and the *things* we own.

It's estimated that in a lifetime, the average American will purchase his or her way through a cool 2.7 million dollars' worth of stuff. If owning more stuff enhances your life, more power to you. But take a look around, how much of that "stuff" is *really* making you happy or has it become like a ball and chain around your neck?

Ever notice how some of the brightest smiles seem to come from people who live in remote parts of the world and who have the fewest possessions. *What's really going on here? Why are they so happy and how does this affect our health?*

It seems odd that many of us drive around with more spare change in our cars than some people live on per day, and yet somehow we still manage to go into debt to buy more things. According to American credit card statistics, in 2015 the average US household carried $15,675 in credit card debt and $132,158 in total debt.

That's a lot of stuff, and potentially a whole lot of stress. People now own so much stuff they can no longer fit it all inside their houses. It has to be stored out in a shed, over in the barn, crammed into the attic, stuffed in the basement, or taking up all the room in their garage. And when all those places are full, the trend now is to rent a storage unit! How much stuff do we *really* need?

YOU DON'T NEED MORE SPACE
YOU NEED LESS STUFF!

As I write this, Black-Friday has just come around and I happened to see on YouTube some of the scuffles that break out when greed sweeps the mind and flat screen TVs go on sale. Even though I don't own a TV myself, I fully appreciate that some people like to watch TV. But still, it's hard to imagine what TV show warrants such acts of aggression. Maybe Black-Friday should be renamed Black-Eye-Friday. Although I offer no proof, I suspect it could even be the Jerry Springer show those folks are in such a desperate rush to watch... Jerry! Jerry! Jerry! .. *just sayin'*.

I get it, people want to save a buck or two on Christmas presents, but greed can soon become a bottomless pit with a deeply *repulsive* element to it. Wait a second, didn't Gordon Gekko, the lead character in the classic movie *Wall Street*, once tell us that greed is good?

Huh ... really?

With rising sea levels and darker environmental skies, maybe that classic line from *Wall Street* should have been replaced with the following quote from Seneca: "The highest wealth is the absence of greed."

This planet that feeds you, your children, and your grandchildren can sustain all of us – it just cannot sustain the current level of consumerism. It's estimated that a truckload of plastic is dumped into the sea *every minute of every day.* If we continue buying cheap imported plastic at the current rate, some estimates suggest that by 2050 there will be more plastic in the sea than fish!

They say a picture is worth a thousand words. At the end of this chapter stop what you are doing and Google "Plastic -Midway Island." It's shocking to see where all our garbage ends up. The key to solving this problem isn't recycling. *If we all just bought less stuff we could automatically recycle less stuff.*

If you really do have disposable income, think about buying an experience rather than a thing. My wife likes Chris Stapleton (a musician, I think) and has just ordered a ticket to see him perform live. The ticket was more than she wanted to pay, but we justified it because she isn't a typical consumer. Had she paid that much for a new hat we might not have seen eye to eye. My point is this: enjoyable experiences are what tightly bond people together, these lasting memories will be around long after material things hit the garbage can.

It's really clear that the most precious resource we all have is time.
— Steve Jobs

Given half the chance, kids seem to get this concept too. It's funny how they always remember the days when we stopped to color with them on the rug, but quickly forget all the money we spend on plastic toys.

Sometimes we are *forced* to buy things: roofs leak, cars break, kitchens cupboards wear out. *I get it.* Reducing stress by reducing clutter is one thing, but the day an *unexpected* repair bill comes our way the whole stress cycle starts all over again. **Don't underestimate stress, it can be a killer,** anything you can do to reduce it should be tried. If you are faced with a bill that's over $500 it makes good sense to always get three estimates.

IMPULSE BUYS

Impulse buys on the other hand are a totally different animal. An impulse buy is anything that winds up on your credit card that *wasn't* a burning desire to buy twelve hours earlier. I'm not sure who wakes up in the middle of the night and says, "Hey, I must buy another windmill for my garden." It's an impulse buy packaged as a bargain along with a gazillion other bits of plastic that we don't need.

For those who need it, the definition of a bargain is something you don't need at a price you find hard to resist.

It's estimated that a single plastic bottle can take *450 years* to completely degrade. Perhaps when man has exhausted the world's oil supply it will no longer be economically viable to sail a boat full of plastic goods from China all the way to the U.S. with the intention of then selling those goods on the open market for one dollar each. Given the amount of pollution we are now creating for our children's children, is it me or is it a tad selfish to keep buying more stuff?

318

Simplicity is the ultimate sophistication.
– Leonardo da Vinci

Buying less $1 clutter inevitably means less plastic heading for the oceans and landfills. If you aren't sure whether something is clutter or not, try to think of it this way: if you don't *love it or use it* then technically it's become clutter. The two exceptions to this rule are dangly wind chimes and dreamcatchers, even if you love them they are still clutter.

Tip –
for no-nonsense practical advice on how to quit the rat race and live frugally check out a book by the name of *Possum Living, How to Live Well Without a Job and with (Almost) No Money*, by Dolly Freed.

Sadly, the ones who sometimes seem to get sucked into buying those *strategically* placed "point-of-sale" items are the ones who can least afford to buy them. Bad spending habits are really just that, *a habit* that stifles cash flow and increases acidic stress.

One way to break free is to make a list of all the essential things you need BEFORE you go to the store *and then stick to it.*

THREE STEPS TO FREEDOM

If you need help to peel out of a repetitive cycle of buy, buy, and bust here's an easy three-step way to do it. Step 1: Streamline. Step 2: Use the N-word. Step 3: Repeat.

Step-1: Streamline.

Look around your house and work out which things you absolutely need and what is clutter. How do you know what's clutter and what's not? Simple, *if you don't use it, or absolutely love it then technically it's not serving a purpose and it's become clutter.* (Yup, worth repeating.)
If at any point you feel motivated to liberate yourself of clutter –don't wait to sell it. Simply drop it off at your favorite charity shop *today.* Procrastination is the thief of all time.

Step-2 Use the N-word.

This is a little trickier because it takes a certain level of practice to say the N-word right. Stay with me on this, it's a great technique and I guarantee it works. Okay, make an nnnn sound with your tongue (you may need to practice this several times until you feel comfortable.) Only when you have the nnnn sound down can you move onto the next step which is the ohhh sound. Keep alternating between the two sounds and then speeding up until finally a whole new sound evolves.

If you keep practicing the nnnn-ohhh sound over and over it will eventually become shorter. If you are unfamiliar with this sound, it's the opposite of the Yes word. Whenever you go on a shopping field trip make this new sound whenever you see the words 50% discount, final reduction, or half off. Instead of saying Yes, just say Nnnnohhh.

STEP 3: Repeat.

From today on, continue using the N-word (NO) rather than hitting the Sales or the Buy Now button. This new sound can help save your sanity, the planet, and your wallet!
Finally, I once heard of woman who was so addicted to shopping that she chose to marry for money rather than love as a way to fund her habit.

At some point in the marriage her purse, containing all her credit cards, was stolen. For two months, her wealthy husband did not to report the theft to the police. When his wife demanded to know the reason for the delay, he calmly explained that the thief was spending less than she was!

What did we learn from this chapter?

Ownership is an illusion; we might think we own something, but if that purchase requires any form of maintenance then it can just as easily own us. Clutter can create self-inflicted stress; the wider implication becomes industrialized pollution.

Homework: please check out "Plastic -Midway Island" a simple Google search should take you there, or click link below

https://www.youtube.com/watch?v=yCb8UKuTzZ0

Chapter 28

SIX TYPES OF DIETS

Over the course of this book dietary information has been slowly bleeding its way through and already we know about toxic food ingredients, excessive sugars, processed foods, deceptive sales tactics, where to buy food, food types, and trigger foods. We've also learned that it can be an incredibly ignorant assumption to think we can lump all our nutritional needs into one single diet.

So the aim of *this* chapter is to guide you toward six diets with a proven track record for success. Some of them you may already know, some you may not. If you are drawn to any one of these diets, great, run with it *for a month* to see how you feel. If not, no pressure, just continue reading, your answer is in here somewhere – we just have to find it. This isn't a rule book, it's a book to help you find your best fit. And, rest assured, by the time we finish very few stones will be left unturned. So *here we go, ready?*

It often seems that diet is easily the most divided and confusing topic of all, at times experts will line up to disagree with each other, and finding that single *perfect* diet can be an elusive dream to chase. A good rule of thumb is don't worry what everyone else is doing, if you find a diet that makes you feel good *then keep doing it,* if not, consider trying something new. It's safe to say whatever works for the gut flora of one person will not work for everybody. The idea here is to give you several effective options to choose from rather giving you a *rigid* diet to follow. In the long run, having an open mind will serve you better than becoming entrenched in dietary battle grounds.

Identifying with diets such as raw, vegan, vegetarian, ketogenic, paleo, etc. are great if they are working for you, but don't shoot yourself in the foot over it. The only thing we can say with some degree of certainty is if something comes in a box, a can, or a packet then it needs to be viewed with an element of caution. (I might have mentioned this before.) Before we get too far into this chapter, let's quickly recap.

Often a food product label can be part of a slick marketing campaign and not an accurate reflection of how the food was produced. That cozy "all natural" farm design logo on the label is purely meant to entice you into a making a purchase. Once we become drawn in, food manufactures are keen for us to count units of energy rather than looking deeper at their nutritional content. While calorie counting sounds good in theory, this is a classic bait-and-switch routine that *rarely works in practice*.

Either way, whatever types of food we *perceive* to be healthy we then pay for, bring home, and begin spoon-feeding into our bodies. At this point it's important to realize that every time we eat, we are taking something from the *outside* world and forcing it deep *inside* our delicate digestive system. *I know, right? It all starts with putting the right foods inside our shopping carts.*

Avoiding processed foods should be a given, but in today's world, unless a diet has a name to it then it's not really a thing. We could call this the BCP avoidance diet (**B**ox-**C**an-**P**acket), some people call it the paleo diet, others lean more toward a ketogenic diet. However, the more mainstream diets become, the more we see it backsliding into foods that are once again trapped inside a box, a can, or a packet. Wherever there is a fast buck to be made, problems inevitably follow.

I've touched on the paleo diet in previous chapters. If you are unfamiliar with the paleo diet then the good news is you can eat as much as you like, *you just can't eat everything that you like.* For that reason, the paleo diet is a good stepping stone for anyone trying to escape a poor diet because there are no calories to count.

While paleo has obvious benefits, it's worth noting that the standard version doesn't take into account many of the food triggers we mentioned earlier. Fortunately, this time around we are now delving a little deeper and looking to offer you practical solutions. For anyone with a steadfast desire to overcome illness, one of these six classic diets will prove helpful.

1.   THE CAVEMAN DIET

Looking at the image below, it seems we are now beginning to evolve into a less than healthy species. Some people refer to the paleo diet as the caveman diet because this is how our ancestors were thought to have fed themselves long before supermarkets came along and made us lazy. Historically speaking, eating fruit when it's out of season or eating carbs out of a box would have been impossible back then, so there are times when claiming to be truly "paleo" can be a bit of a stretch.

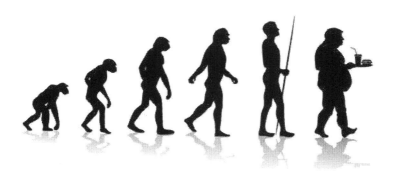

Compared to eating heavily processed foods, a strict paleo diet has obvious benefits – clean, whole foods beat anything you can get out of a can. That being said, we should also exercise a degree of common sense because there are some modern day paleo meals that may have an unnaturally high sugar content. As with any growing trend, everything you could ever need to know is *already* in print, which is why I'm surface skimming through these diets as opposed to writing a whole book on any one subject. This is good news because finding paleo cooking ideas is now the easy part.

If you are looking for more in-depth answers you can't go too far wrong with the book *The Paleo Approach* by Sarah D. Ballantyne Ph.D. It's pretty detailed and has a lot of solid scientific background information that's well presented. The author also links to lots of recipes that can be found on her website (PaleoMom) which helps give a clear idea of what the paleo diet is *and is not*. Again, my role isn't to copy what someone else is already doing right, it's to guide you to good people. For anyone with a suspected autoimmune condition *The Paleo Approach* is an important book to have on your shelf.

2.   THE ELIMINATION DIET

Let's assume that you are already onboard with the idea that the road to health is to eat only whole foods – problem over, right? Meh, not so fast, *remember, once you have a spooked immune system all bets are off and you could potentially react to any food, even those found in an organic vegetable grower's garden!*

As the name suggests, the elimination diet looks to eliminate problem foods. For anyone just starting off, it is again worth noting that the foods most likely to cause a reaction are gluten, dairy, eggs, and nuts, closely followed by corn. Today, it's not uncommon to find all of these foods on one plate – think of a BLT with mayo. If you can get away with it, great, if not once we simplify the diet anything that causes a reaction is going to be easier to spot.

Ever wonder why you can't eat one cookie or cheese chip? Both gluten and dairy have an addictive quality to them, *no seriously,* they contain "opioid peptides." Yup, that's the same family as opium. Peptides from both gluten and casein (a protein molecule found in dairy) react with opiate receptors in the brain. Yup, that's right, it has the same effect as if you were taking opiate-like drugs such as heroin or morphine.

When a person comes off gluten and casein they can expect to experience withdrawal symptoms. This is why the cardboard diet described in Chapter 14 is so important – it removes all temptation. (In case you've forgotten, that's the one where you stand before your pantry and refrigerator and toss everything you *now* know you should not eat into cardboard boxes.) I can't imagine there are too many people who quit smoking or drinking by having cigarettes and booze within easy reach – the same applies to gluten and dairy.

The trick here is to stack the odds in your favor by eliminating suspect foods for a minimum of one month and then slowly reintroduce them into your diet, one at a time. If your symptoms spring back, then bingo, you nailed your kryptonite. To help you do this I recommend picking up a day planner and making a note of everything that passes your lips while making a side note of how you feel throughout the day.

If you (or someone in your family) are reacting to food then keeping a detailed food journal is invaluable because so many foods today have random "things" added to them, things you wouldn't expect unless you were keeping a record. Again keep in mind that in some people reactions can happen much later, hence keeping a written account is very helpful to glance back at. Once food has become a trigger, simplifying your diet will help highlight problems. If this is a new concept to you, then the elimination diet should be something to consider. This isn't a diet to lose weight, it's a diet to lose symptoms.

As the name suggests, this involves cutting out certain foods. *I get it, changing old habits isn't always easy,* but if you are grounded in illness then it's possible that your current diet is either making you sick or keeping you sick. Whenever food enters the digestive system it's scanned for foreign invaders by the immune system. Once a problem is spotted, a code-red is sent out and a reaction occurs, this could result in a food sensitivity or even full blown allergy.

The elimination diet works, yes, and it takes effort, *but the rewards for doing it are real.* Before we look at the list of foods you may need to break from, let's first take a look at the looong list of symptoms you could be leaving behind. *Sometimes we have to give up what we have to get what we want.* When you commit to doing the elimination diet you could potentially be saying goodbye to:

- Chronic fatigue
- Arthritis
- Asthma
- Mood disorders, including depression and anxiety

- Skin flare-ups like eczema, hives, and acne
- Autoimmune disorders
- Atherosclerosis (hardening of the arteries, a precursor to heart disease)
- Cognitive decline and neurodegenerative diseases, including Parkinson's and dementia
- Learning disabilities like ADHD
- Trouble sleeping or insomnia
- Muscle and joint pain, such as from arthritis
- Weight gain and obesity
- Migraine headaches
- Nutrient deficiencies
- Kidney and gallbladder problems

The whole point of doing this diet is to pinpoint exactly which foods you are reactive to. You can't always exercise or medicate your way out of a reactive diet. The elimination diet needs to be followed for a minimum of thirty days. When you look at the list of symptoms above, thirty days really isn't that long. This isn't a diet you can throw yourself into half-heartedly, and if you aren't mentally prepared to give it 100% then there is no point in doing it.

Why?

As discussed previously, when the body reacts negatively to trigger foods the immune system makes antibodies to fight the perceived threat. It takes a while for these antibodies to calm down and some believe this process can take three weeks or more. For every cheating nibble you sneak, a new bunch of antibodies are launched and the whole cycle starts over again. Yup, you can hide under the stairs eating trigger foods if you like, but once your immune system is on red alert it *never* stops watching what you do. For that reason, keep in mind if you cheat you won't feel *any* benefit of doing the elimination diet and sneaking trigger foods will *undermine* the whole process.

Before looking at the list of foods you need to eliminate, you might want to make a mental note about why you are doing this. *This is a good time to ask yourself WHY you want to be free of your symptoms.* For encouragement, take a look at the list above again. And, as you read the list below, note that it is a much shorter list than the list of symptoms you stand to lose. Okay, here we go, take a deep breath, it's time to rip the band aid off and remember that *quitting these foods could set you free from a lot of those symptoms in that much longer list.*

- No gluten (or any type of other grain)
- No diary
- No soy
- No refined/added sugar
- No peanuts
- No corn
- No alcohol
- No eggs

That wasn't too bad was it? It should come as no surprise that gluten tops the list and, as previously mentioned, you simply can't use this as an excuse to munch your way through the gluten-free section of the supermarket. *I never said this was easy but I am telling you it's going to be worth it.*

To help you pull this off, check out Tom Malterre. Tom comes to this subject first as a dedicated father of five and, just for good measure, he holds a bachelor's and master's degree in nutrition. His book, *The Elimination Diet,* is essential reading and is full of tips to set you on the right road, you can also find his talks on YouTube.

3. THE AIP DIET

AIP diet stands for Autoimmune-Paleo and it's a leaner version of the basic paleo diet. It also involves the elimination of all the usual suspects such as grains, dairy, eggs, seeds, legumes, as well as some foods found in the nightshade family which would obviously include tomatoes, tomatillos, eggplant, potatoes, goji berries, tobacco, and all types of peppers. The AIP diet is not without merit as it goes a step further and also removes certain trigger foods such as lectins.

To better understand this diet, your lifeline comes in the form of a well-written blog by the name of autoimmune-paleo.com. The blog is run by two extremely knowledgeable ladies, Angie and Mickey. Both have a well-balanced common sense approach. Their blog is packed with reliable information that is also easy to follow. For anyone struggling with trigger foods, the importance of this information cannot be overstated.

4. THE KETOGENIC DIET

The ketogenic diet is rapidly gaining mainstream momentum. The problem is there is a right way and a wrong way to tap into this highly effective diet. It's fair to say that the ketogenic diet requires an element of self-discipline, but once you get there, food becomes a matter of choice rather a carbohydrate eating emergency. I've been in true ketosis and I liked how it felt. Ketosis also helps clear the mind. But what is this diet and how do we get there?

Think of the body as dual fuel burner, pretty much in the same way a hybrid car is capable of running on either gas or electricity. The body can run on either glucose or fat. At times when glucose is low, the body is perfectly capable of switching fuels. It was once thought that the body *only* burned glucose for fuel, but we now know that's not strictly true. This is good to know for reasons we will go into later.

Regardless of whether we find ourselves in times of feast or famine, the brain requires an enormous amount of energy to function. When glucose supplies are exhausted, the body begins to convert fat in the liver into energy cells known as ketones. Any time the body burns fat, the metabolic state is described as ketosis. This simply means your body has switched from burning glucose for energy to burning fat. The body has a two-day supply of glucose in the form of glycogen, so the effects of ketosis aren't always immediate. Most people go into a state of ketosis after several days of consuming no more than 20 grams of carbohydrates per day. While this might sound daunting to some, it's worth noting that this is a totally natural process that helped your early ancestors evolve. Back then, food wasn't guaranteed three times a day or any day. Chugging down a quart of orange juice and eating a box full of carbohydrates would have been enough to get you stoned as a witch. *Hmm, I see.*

The full name of what we are describing here is lipolysis/ketosis. Lipolysis simply means that your fat stores are being burned as the primary source of fuel. The by-products of burning fat are ketones, so ketosis is a secondary process of lipolysis.

Some people refer to this as Ketogenic or Keto diet which is really a just shortening of the term. The ketogenic diet has been around since in the 1920s and was originally started at the John Hopkins Center Medical Center. A ketogenic diet is similar to the paleo diet – however it's typically lower in carbohydrates and high in healthy fats. As always, the devil is in the details because not all fats are the same; some trans-fats can be darn right dangerous! Don't panic, trans-fat (and good fat) is explained in more detail later.

Once the body enters a state of ketosis it becomes more efficient at burning stored fat. For some people, ketosis reduces blood sugar and insulin levels. Some studies also report a marked improvement in diseases such as Alzheimer's, epilepsy, and diabetes.

There are always going to be exceptions, but for me personally, I've found that when I'm periodically in a state of ketosis my thoughts are clearer and I have noticeably fewer food cravings. Essentially what's happening here is we are switching from being a sugar burning mammal into a fat burning one – and some would say this was once our preferred state.

There are a couple of variations on the ketogenic diet which include:

- A **standard ketogenic diet** which is typically a very low-carb, moderate-protein, and high-fat diet that contains 75% fat, 20% protein, and only 5% carbs.
- A **cyclical ketogenic diet** which involves periods of higher-carb intake, such as 5 ketogenic days followed by 2 high-carb days.
- A **high-protein ketogenic diet** which is similar to a standard ketogenic diet, but includes more protein with a ratio of 60% fat, 35% protein, and 5% carbs.

If all that sounds too confusing, then I have the perfect guru for you. Her name is Leanne Vogel and she has a free blog that I urge you to take a look at. Her blog is called "Healthful Pursuit" and Leanne also has a new book, *The Keto Diet,* that I've just started reading.

As we have already mentioned, ketosis is a normal metabolic process. Unfortunately, its name is sometimes confused with a life threatening illness known as keto**acid**osis, an illness driven by a lack of insulin in the body typically seen in diabetics. Although ketosis and keto**acid**osis sound alike, they are as similar as chalk and cheese.

It could be argued that keto**acid**osis is aggravated as a result of consuming excessive amounts of sugar-spiking carbohydrates. As I'm sure many of you already know, diabetics produce either too little insulin, or the body doesn't respond to insulin at all. When that happens, blood sugar levels can rise and the blood can become dangerously acidic.

Given that the ketogenic diet strives to lower blood sugar levels, it may be something that some type 2 diabetics find useful. As always, *before* attempting anything new it's best to work it out with an informed healthcare provider.

Although the brain is made mostly of fat, it cannot use fat directly for energy. It can, however, use ketones which the body makes when there is not enough insulin in the blood. From time to time you may hear the argument that the brain needs glucose to run – and while this may be true, it's actually a very small amount. Interestingly, this small requirement can be achieved without resorting to eating donuts. How so? Your body can make small amounts of glucose through a process called gluconeogenesis.

As a final note of caution, keep in mind that although most people do absolutely fine with the ketogenic diet, a sudden switch to consuming 70% fats may, for some people, stress the gallbladder. As always, listen to your body for clues that might include pain in the mid- to upper-right section of your abdomen.

5. THE GAPS DIET

Okay, almost there. Four diets down and just two to go. Again, keep in mind that I'm not trying to bust your balls here, I'm simply saying that statistically speaking, there is a pretty good chance one of these diets may benefit to you, especially if your health problems have been difficult to figure out.

At the beginning of this chapter I emphasized that you need to be patient and find the *right* diet for your *unique* circumstances. The GAPS diet is another well thought-out diet and some people claim to have success treating autism, ADHD, dyslexia, dyspraxia, depression, and even schizophrenia with this diet.

The *only* reason the GAPS diet is being mentioned here is because of the dedication of Dr. Natasha Campbell-McBride. I have listened to this lady at length and she has a proven track record for bringing solid results to the table. It also helps that Dr. Natasha Campbell-McBride is incredibly smart and has not one but two postgraduate degrees: a master of medical sciences in neurology and a master of medical sciences in human nutrition.

The GAPS diet has too many benefits to list here, so the list below is just a **small** cross section of the many advantages people often report.

• Psychological improvements

- Boost immunity
- Reduce food sensitivity
- Improve neurological function
- Heal inflammatory bowel disease
- Improve type II diabetes
- Improve lactose digestion
- Kill candida
- Support detoxification

Dr. Natasha Campbell-McBride is well known for developing a concept known as GAPS (Gut and Psychology Syndrome), which is described in her deeply informative book, *Gut and Psychology Syndrome*.

6. FODMAPS DIET

Our final diet in this chapter is the FODMAP diet. **If you have tried cutting out gluten and failed to see positive results, then FODMAPs are something to be aware of.** These are yet another collection of misunderstood foods that can have a foot in more than one category. Just as some people are sensitive to gluten, a person with a FODMAP sensitivity will react in much the same way. For some, FODMAPs are the cause of a wide range of digestive upsets that are particularly prevalent in IBS (Irritable Bowel Syndrome), Crohn's disease, Celiac disease, and just about any other type of digestive disorder you can think of.

What foods are FODMAPs found in?

Many of these foods can be thought of as healthy in their own right which makes **awareness** all the more important. FODMAPs can be found in a wide range of foods with some foods having a higher count than others. While the list below of FODMAPs is extensive, don't lose heart because there *is* some good news. This condition is *unlike* a true food allergy and may even be reversible. A reaction to FODMAPs can be greatly reduced by restricting all FODMAPs for a given period of time to allow the gut to calm down. *Are you catching this? I'm saying with a bit of luck; you may be able*

334

to slowly reintroduce many of these foods into the diet without too much problem.

Again the idea here is to give you something to grab onto when all else has failed, this time your go-to-gurus are Doctor Sue Shepherd and Doctor Peter Gibson. They recently coauthored a nicely presented book that is actually sitting here at my elbow as I write.

Again as with anyone I choose to recommend, I have no direct link with them other than I admire the good work they do. Doctors Shepherd and Gibson take all the guesswork out of what to eat and what *not* to eat and it's all neatly covered in their easy to follow book aptly named, *The Complete Low FODMAP Diet: A Revolutionary Plan for Managing IBS and Other Digestive Disorders.*

In case you were wondering, FODMAPs stands for: fermentable oligosaccharides, disaccharides, monosaccharides, and polyols. If it's easier, we can simply think of them as fermentable carbohydrates. FODMAPS are poorly absorbed by the small intestine and as a result can enter the colon where they are fermented by bacteria, and as they do so, they draw on water and expand causing excessive bloating and diarrhea.

TEST

There is a standard test that your doctor can carry out that doesn't even require blood to be drawn. It's called the Hydrogen Breath Test and it could save you an awful lot of guesswork. Again, rather than let this section overwhelm you, if you have been dealing with stomach issues this is all good information to know. Try to hold onto the positives. You now have a whole list of good people and some new ideas to try and you probably also know a lot more than you did just a few hours ago.

Below is a list of vegetables that are low in FODMAPs, again, let's not forget that some of these foods may have a foot on more than one camp.

Low in FODMAPS = bell peppers, bok choy, carrots, eggplant, common cabbage, endive, fennel, green beans, kale, lettuce, spinach, potatoes, and zucchinis. Fruit low in FODMAPs include bananas, grapes, kiwi, cranberries, lemons, mandarin oranges, blueberries, cantaloupe, honeydew melon, oranges, pineapples, raspberries, strawberries, and tomatoes.

Examples of vegetables **high** in FODMAPs are garlic, onions, celery, broccoli, all kinds of potatoes including sweet, turnips, sugar snap peas, seaweed, artichokes, asparagus, bean sprouts, Brussels sprouts, and cauliflower. Fruits high in FODMAPs include apple, apricot, avocado, blackberry, canned fruit, cherries, cranberry, dates, grapefruit, mango, nectarine, papaya, peach, pear, persimmon, plantain, plum, prunes, and watermelon.

I get it, some parts of this chapter may have seemed a little heavy, but don't let any of this overwhelm you. The idea is to find what works for you, in order to do this, you have to be aware of your options. Only then can you find the best fit for *you.* I know you can do this or you wouldn't still be reading. The good news is that more solutions are coming, just hang in there for me.

> *Life's battles don't always go to the stronger or faster man.*
> *But sooner or later, the man who wins is the man who thinks he can.*
> – Vince Lombardi Jr

Before we leave this chapter here's a few more foods that are high in FODMAPs.

Grains – wheat and all gluten-containing grains, amaranth, barley, buckwheat, corn, millet, oats, quinoa, rice, rye, spelt, teff, and wild rice

Legumes – cannellini beans, chickpeas/garbanzos, fava beans, kidney beans, navy/white beans, pinto beans, soybeans, peas

Dairy Products – all dairy (except *pure* butter without additives)
Proteins/Meats – bacon with sugar or maple syrup, broth made with onions or garlic, deli/processed meats

Nuts – cashews, chia seeds, flaxseed, hazelnuts, pistachios

Fats – margarine, soybean oil

Sweeteners – honey, maple syrup, molasses, sugar alcohols, stevia, sucralose, sugar/sucrose

OK, if you made it to this point and you still aren't sure what to do then simply start by cutting out *all* gluten and dairy for one month. Done right this alone can have a dramatic effect on your overall health, but remember, no cheating. Once you have gluten and dairy out of your diet then be sure to try any one of the diets mentioned in this chapter.

What did we learn from this chapter?

Because there are so many variables, some people may have better success with one diet over another. This does *not* mean the diets recommended here can't work for you, it simply means your individual dietary needs are uniquely different from those of others. A little trial and error should set you on the right track.

Homework: for anyone who appreciates independent values, you might find a TED Talk by Sharyl Attkisson interesting – it's called *"AstroTurf and Manipulation of Media Messages."*

https://www.youtube.com/watch?v=-bYAQ-ZZtEU

Chapter 29

FAKE-BOOK

According to a new report from Oxfam international, Bill Gates, Warren Buffett, Carlos Slim, Jeff Bezos, Mark Zuckerberg, Amancio Ortega, Larry Ellison, and Michael Bloomberg are collectively worth an eye-watering $426 billion. Those eight men now control as much wealth as the world's poorest 3.6 billion people. Every year, *one million* of those billion people die from drinking contaminated water. *When you stop and think about it, that's a lot of people with a very* basic *need that is not being met!*

As for the rest of us, stress often comes from having too little money and trying to own too many things. Stress is the body's way of flooding the system with hormones to heighten response to any perceived or real threat. Great if there is a Bengal tiger loose in your back bedroom, but it's *not* so helpful if you are delayed in traffic and your boss is a jerk.

Stress hormones include adrenaline and cortisol which pump through the body in preparation for emergency action. The good news is short term exposure to stress has no lasting effects. However, a *constant* level of stress can take a more serious toll on our mental and physical wellbeing.

Many of us already know this, but it's worth reiterating that medium term stress can manifest itself as headaches, muscle tension, fatigue, stomach upsets, loss of libido, sleep problems, increased levels of anxiety, restlessness, irritability, and sadness. A feeling of being overwhelmed by stress can even change a person's mental state and can manifest in emotional outbursts. If stress is left unchecked, a person can easily become withdrawn and depressed.

Have I got your attention yet?

No?

Okay, let's keep going. In addition to the many mental and physical health problems stress can create or exacerbate, it also speeds up the aging process and makes your body more acidic (hello again pH). A constant high level of stress has the potential to disrupt nearly every system in the body. As stress levels increase, *immune function decreases,* blood pressure rises, and the digestive, reproductive, and nervous systems all get out of balance. *Are you getting this? Stress is a killer!*

Any sharp increase in blood pressure can result in chest pains, a hardening of the arteries, heart disease, and even stroke. Rather than try to resolve this mountain of health issues, maybe our time would be better spent *reducing* the main causes of our stress. In part, this can be accomplished when we take a different view of our spending habits and make more efficient use of our time. It may also help to reexamine our reasons for doing what we do.

MAN-STRESS

Science has shown that men and women react differently to stress. Men have the capability to overreact to overwhelming stress in more *extreme* ways. I am statistically drawn to the fact that men are three times more likely to commit suicide than women. When stress gets to this heartbreaking level, I suspect it's not one thing that pushes good men over the edge, but a relentless chain of smaller things that have been allowed to build up over time. I suspect that people who commit suicide aren't always looking to end their lives; they are simply looking for a way to end their suffering. If this is you, *please find someone to talk to.* Suicide is an irreversible and permanent solution to a temporary problem. Some men find it harder to talk openly to their peers about financial difficulties for fear of being judged. Men may also have a tendency to *internalize* things far more than women who (generally speaking) often have a better support network of friends in place. Outside of the complications of interpersonal relationships *(yup, that would be a whole 'nother book)* men generally blame their stress levels on two things: a need for *more* time or a need for *more* money – and it's not uncommon for both to be spent unwisely.

Maybe what men are really saying is they would like to be shown more respect. Men are constantly bombarded with idiotic statements from

340

luxury car manufacturers like Porsche who claim that "there is no substitute" for owning a $250,000 car. *Really? I've driven a Porsche and it really didn't bring me any peace.* All too often we are encouraged to relate success with owning objects.

Men are frequently dangled a *karat* from expensive diamond retailers who are keen to tell you, "Diamonds are a girl's best friend." If men only knew, ownership is an expensive illusion and inner peace doesn't come from what we buy; it comes from the things we can live without. If you can't freely give away what you own, then you don't own it, *it owns you.*

While we all have different income streams, each and every one of us gets the same amount of allotted time every day. What we spend our time and money on is a choice. Some men may spend it on a new car, a new suit, a bigger desk, all of which are rewards for having too much money. But these are short term rewards that cannot compete with having the freedom to do what you want *when you want.*

> *A man is a success if he gets up in the morning and gets to bed at night, and in between he does what he wants to do.*
> – Bob Dylan

So what's the solution for a chronically stressed man who has fallen into the shallow trap of equating success with ownership of more stuff? That's easy – remember 102-year-old Edie Simms from chapter 8? Turns out she was right; you *can* liberate your soul by humbling it. *I know, right? WTF? (What's the Formula?)*

Edie does something on a regular basis that not only keeps her going, it's been scientifically proven that her life is enriched every time she helps another person. *No really, there is enough scientific data about that to fill the rest of this book.* The term "Helper's-High" is based on national research done by Allan Luks (feel free to Google) which revealed the powerful physical feelings people experience when directly helping others— results were measurable and showed improvement in both physical and emotional health.

Friend, it's not your money I'm after; it's your time. *Time* has a value; the love of money gets people into this mess. The fastest way to alleviate any type of self-inflicted stress is to *find a problem that's bigger than you are.* People are hurting all around you, and yet there is something uniquely valuable about looking another human in the eye and saying, "Hey, are you okay in there, Bud?"

To someone who's going through hell, the simplest of human interactions can be more valuable than the shiniest of gold. Find someone who needs help in your local community *and be part of the solution.* I'm offering you a way out of this shitty cycle, take it!

Stepping out of our comfort zone to help another person is the fastest way to finding your own sanity. The trick here is to do a little but do it often. This doesn't have to be a huge drain on your time. Maybe offer to help a sick or elderly neighbor, at the same time try to be respectful of the fact that the transition into vulnerability isn't easy for anyone. In today's fast-paced world we have become quick to measure ourselves by the quality of the car we drive, the size of our houses, or the number of electronic digits we have that represent our net worth. Perhaps a man would be better judged not by economic wealth but by the way he treats the most vulnerable members of a society.

Committing huge portions of your time can lead to frustration. The idea here is to do what *you* are comfortable with rather than turning it into a form of resentment. *For this tip to work it doesn't matter how little you do, so long as you do something.* What do you have to lose? If I'm right, you will begin to get back something your money cannot buy – *a quiet sense of inner peace.* Have you ever wondered why volunteers don't ask for money? It's not because they have no value, it's because they are priceless.

Man is not made for defeat.
– Ernest Hemingway

Do this quietly and for the right reasons. *Work for a cause, not applause.* There's no point if this morphs into a boasting opportunity and no, you don't need to tell the world via a Facebook post what you just did for someone. You may find your inner peace helping out at a local soup kitchen, others find it rewarding to volunteer at a local hospital; you know your personality better than I do, find something you are comfortable with. Do this and a month from now you will be happier and less stressed, you'll also care less about your neighbor's stuff. If anything, your neighbor will be looking over YOUR fence thinking, hey, what's with *this* guy and his new inner peace?

WOMAN-STRESS

If you think men have it bad, then women have an *added* stress. Almost every woman who engages with any type of media is immediately faced with images of younger women with increasingly bigger eyes, bigger lips, bigger boobs, and even bigger butts. Sheesh, way to make a person feel uncomfortable in her own skin. If *that* isn't stressful, I'm not sure what is.

Today, one of the primary causes of stress for women is the constant pressure to conform to a certain physical type in order to be accepted. Social media has become quick to present us with a carefully staged digital image of perfection, but scratch below the surface and you sometimes find the deep roots of insecurity. Perhaps the world doesn't need more skinny women taking selfies in bathroom mirrors. It needs more normal, content looking people. I sometimes wonder if it's called a "selfie" because narcissistic is too difficult a word to spell? *I digress.*

More than ever, people are desperate to show you an updated *snapshot* of their happiness, often this is nothing more than an elaborate hoax in need of debunking. When your Facebook feed is constantly bombarded with photos of people having 24/7 fun, it's important to understand that not everything is how it seems.

I once watched a young mom take at least ten grinning selfies next to a shimmering hotel swimming pool, and yet standing off to one side was her small child in a damp polka dot bikini complaining that she was cold and hungry. Given the time it took the woman to get the perfect selfie I have probable cause to believe the kid with the tears in her eyes failed to make it to the final cut. Maybe a better name for Facebook would be to call it Fake-book. I guess one advantage of *not* having a Facebook page myself is that *I wouldn't have to worry about whether people **"like"** me or not.*

At times, social media can be a warped distortion of reality where nothing much is the way it seems. It can even make us feel as if *we* aren't enough. Recently I read an article about how some women in the U.S. are so desperate to fit in they turned to an illegal underground practice where bigger butts are offered on the cheap. Sadly, this is done by injecting dangerous chemicals under the skin. These butt-boosting shots include injecting mineral oil and a can of roadside tire inflator directly into the muscle. *Nope, not joking.*

If you haven't seen this product before, it's sold in car accessory shops and its intended use is to inflate a blown tire with rapid set expanding foam. I know, right? What kind of message is social media sending out to impressionable young minds when it makes them feel as if they need to pump it up with fix-a-flat tire weld?

Perhaps our wives, sisters, and daughters are constantly being told that in order to fit in they need to have a totally different body shape. Might I remind those who are caught in this trap to look at any old photo of a family member to see how quickly ridiculous fashions come and go. Once it might have been a curly perm, ridiculously tall platform shoes, or a pair of flared jeans. Bad fashion is one thing, but can you imagine ten years from now how a body that has been surgically altered to meet a current fashion trend might look?

It would seem that even the clothing industry is geared to keep young women hooked on buying more clothes. Fashions now change before you can say the word *overdraft,* often leaving some women feeling compelled to buy a new outfit every day of the week.

Trying to extract value from ever-changing fashion is just another form of negative stress and, left to ferment, it simply becomes unhealthy. Is it any wonder, that the global apparel market is currently valued at an eye-watering three trillion dollars!

Buy less, choose well.
— Vivienne Westwood

I get it, we all long to be accepted, but it seems that our minds have become polluted with an unsustainable lust for material things and the mundane gossip of people we will rarely meet. Take comfort from the fact that your uniqueness has value — it sets you apart from the crowd, so FCUK the fashion industry.

Just as men are striving for more respect from their peers, it seems women, above all else, just want to be valued, but that value needs to come from within. Regrettably, wants and *needs* are often two very different things.

For sure, we all *need* clean food and water, a warm safe place to sleep, and clean clothes to wear. Maybe even a friend to turn to in our time of need — but beyond that, it rarely bodes well to have an emotional attachment to material *things.*

HAPPY HOMESTEAD

Sometimes it can be a challenge to let go of material things. I was recently reminded of this in my own life when I gave up my home in the U.S. It wasn't a big or a fancy place but over the years we were truly happy there. This little gem was the absolute epitome of sustainable, simplistic living and minimalism. I'd worked hard to transform this property into a super-efficient homestead.

Set in the mountains, this house had become an *integral* part of our lives, it gave us clean food and safe shelter from the outside world; it had been our school, office, church, and hospital. Flanked on all sides by organic gardens and fruit trees, it's fair to say I'd worked every inch of the land and it had just begun to give back more than it took. With a small barn for chickens and a workbench for a collection of hand tools all neatly lined up like a surgeon's operating table, we bothered no one and no one bothered us.

Living off the land had been my end goal and to help me achieve this I built a small high tunnel to extend the growing season. This final addition was the last piece of the puzzle because it allowed me to grow year-round. Little did I know at the time, but this "improvement" was going to be my downfall.

Unfortunately, I must have built it a little too well because it quickly provoked a visit from the town tax inspector. I guess he liked what he saw because over the next twenty-four months our property taxes steadily increased until they had almost doubled! In Northern New Hampshire this rapid increase amounted to several thousand dollars. When you are trying to live a simple life, this rate of increase was not just unwelcome it was, sadly, unsustainable.

Ultimately we were priced out of the small town we had come to love. If I'm honest I'm still a little irritated by this. We enjoyed being part of the local community and had friends there. But with no sign of the man letting up, this became a matter of principle as well as economic hardship.

We had no choice but to put the place up for sale. Perhaps with hindsight we'll see this as a mistake. Either way, a lady from Florida saw the photos online and was *immediately* smitten. She flew up the very next day and said it was the sharpest looking house she had viewed to date.

She particularly liked the friendly feeling of the house and commented on how clean and well-organized everything was. Her husband was suitably impressed with the efficiency of this house which could be heated year-round with just four cords of wood.

This was really important to him (just as it had been to us) because he wanted a small place with affordable utility bills. It seemed to tick all the right boxes, but after several days of deliberating, the wife finally decided *not* to buy. *The reason?*

She had once travelled to Japan and while there had bought a large collection of china vases that she then imported to the U.S. For the past fifteen years, wherever she lived, *they* lived. No matter how hard she tried

346

in her mind, she simply couldn't find a place in our house to put them all. As her husband rolled his eyes for the third time it made me realize this was a classic case of something they no longer owned. These vases truly owned them!

The love of possessions is a weakness to be overcome.
– Alexander Eastman

Someone else soon came along and snapped it up. This actually brought heaviness to my soul, but it also made me thankful that for the last seven years of owning this house and its things, none of them owned me.

For now, this American dream had come to an end and as I write this we have decided to sell up and try our luck back in the motherland. As liberating as this may sound, it's probably the first time I've packed a suitcase and not wanted to be somewhere else.

For now, I'm really not sure where the wind will take me, and although we all miss the stability of our homes, my message to you is clear: *things* shouldn't define who we are. When all else fails we must dust ourselves off and keep going.

Finally, I'd like to ask you for just four minutes of your time and direct you to an unusually short but inspiring four-minute TED Talk. Mark Bezos is a volunteer firefighter and he quickly retells a short story of heroism that didn't quite go as expected — it taught him a BIG lesson which was *don't wait.*

What did we learn from this chapter?

Stress can make us even *more* acidic, a subject we seem to keep coming back to. We can reduce our own stress quickly by finding a problem that's bigger than we are. Stress can come from owning too much stuff, the media, and yes, even social media.

Homework: find someone today who needs help and do something about it. Please find time to watch the four-minute TED talk by Mark Bezos, this guy is my kind of hero!

https://www.ted.com/talks/mark_bezos_a_life_lesson_from_a_volunteer_firefighter

Chapter 30

THE WEAKEST LINK

Take a sneaky look behind any website and you will see long lines of computer code. Take a peek behind the dashboard of your car and you will find lots of wires. Take a hard look at the underlying cause of illness and you will almost certainly find that its roots are deeply intertwined with chronic inflammation. *Wait a second are you catching this? There is a link between serious illness and inflammation!*

Inflammation is associated with just about every health condition; even PubMed is awash with strong scientific data connecting inflammation to a list of diseases ranging from cancer to obesity. Given the importance of this, perhaps we have things a little twisted. In every hospital we have swarms of oncologists, cardiologists, and neurologists, but not a single *inflammation-ologist!*

We have a medical system that's rich in cash and yet fails to address the underlying cause of chronic inflammation. During a routine doctor's visit it's not unusual to hear your doctor talk about preventative medicine and yet the root causes of inflammation are rarely mentioned.

What's interesting is that developing countries that spend statistically far *less* on healthcare consistently outperform the West on everything from infant mortality to longevity. *I know, right? What's up with that?*

Allow me to repeat myself with emphasis: inflammation and illness go hand in hand. Given the importance of this subject, let's take a look at what inflammation is and then see how all this fits in with what we have learned so far. Inflammation is an essential part of the repair process within the body; it can be acute or chronic. Many of us will have already experienced acute inflammation which is an early-stage response to obvious physical trauma (think of a twisted ankle or bruise). Acute inflammation is obvious and rapid. It will include an onset of pain, heat, redness, and swelling. This is also a sign of a body that's healing. Think of acute inflammation as being similar to a small campfire that's *under control.*

Chronic inflammation, on the other hand, is less obvious and has more of an insidious quality to it that can span weeks, months, or even years. As the diagram below suggests, chronic inflammation is the common denominator that's weaving its way throughout so much serious illness. The good news is that chronic inflammation is totally reversible. *If this is true, it suggests that many illnesses are also reversible* – but you already know this because of course you watched the suggested homework video in Chapter 5.

Think of chronic inflammation as a smoldering, lingering type of fire always on the lookout for a puff of wind. Once chronic inflammation ignites, it can be likened to a raging forest fire.

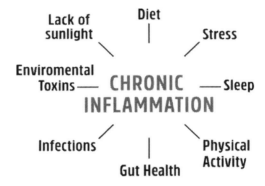

Looking at the diagram above, can you see how all this is beginning to fit neatly together? If illness has you in its grip, there is a pretty good chance that something in this image led to your downfall. And by the same token, something here also holds the key to your recovery!

These eight categories can be thought of as our pillars of good health. The good news is once we get these bad boys in line, good health is yours for the taking!

We seem to have covered a lot of ground together and I fully appreciate it can be a lot to take in. The idea of this chapter is to take stock of what we have learned so far. Just to keep things interesting I'll be mixing in a few new things that I hope you will find interesting. If repetition is the mother of all learning, let's quickly begin our short recap with stress and continue working our way around the diagram in a clockwise fashion.

STRESS

In this life there is no shortage for the causes of stress, some of these we have already taken a look at. Stress has become an omnipresent part of life and even with the best intentions it can follow us around like a bad smell. The people we surround ourselves with can bring us stress and certainly our jobs can.

Everything of true value either has a heartbeat or it is free. With that in mind, the one category *we do* have full control over is the things we buy. As discussed previously, our value should not come from material things nor can it be found in the approval of others.

I will not let anyone walk through my mind with their dirty feet.
– Mahatma Gandhi

Magnesium plays an important role in stress reduction. Long- to medium-term stress will quickly deplete magnesium levels. Certain foods such as dark leafy greens, avocados, and almonds have a high magnesium content. Do a little homework and you will find there are others.

Stress can also lower the function of the immune system making us more susceptible to infections. One way to combat stress is to increase the things in your life that bring you pleasure. It's very hard to remain stressed when you are doing something that gives you joy. If eating junk food gives you pleasure, then sorry, you can't include that. *Nice try though.*

SLEEP

Although we should aim for a *minimum* of six hours, some people will absolutely need more. The *quality* of our sleep is just as important as the quantity. Sleep is where our body gets to work cleaning the brain and accomplishing all those internal repairs; sleep is like the maintenance crew that comes in to do essential shop cleaning at night. For this reason, it's important to protect your sleep. Keep your bedroom cool, dark, and quiet. Avoid all forms of blue light in the evening because it will disrupt melatonin production.

Around bedtime be mindful of what you eat. Sugar and protein will almost certainly keep you awake; instead, go for clean carbs at supper such as a bowl of rice. We aren't trying to win culinary awards here; we are looking for a better night's sleep. Medications and certain health supplements can also disrupt our sleep. If you are having trouble sleeping, try not to take anything after 6 p.m. You can find more sleep tips in Chapter 24.

PHYSICAL ACTIVITY

Cells like movement and all motion is lotion for the joints. As discussed earlier, even something as simple as bouncing on a small yoga trampoline can have a big impact on our health. These types of trampolines are relatively inexpensive and allow the user to ease into exercise at their own pace. Personally, I like the trampolines sold with springs and the one I have is called "ANCHEER." For some people, joining a gym is never going to happen – that's okay. If committing to an exercise program is a step too far, look for cheats like parking your car farther away from the store. This becomes a subtle way of forcing us to walk. A brisk walking is less traumatic on the body than running long marathons. Whenever we exercise, our lungs begin pumping more oxygen and this helps with the pH of the body. **Remember, sitting is the new smoking!**

Incorporating a hobby makes exercise less of a chore which means you are more likely to do it.

Prior to selling my tiny homestead, I managed to get my daily workout from gardening. This usually involved a lot of bending and lifting. Providing you don't overdo it, lifting is an important part of any exercise routine because it helps maintain testosterone levels. Contrary to what you may think, women also produce testosterone, albeit in much smaller quantities. Low testosterone can cause symptoms ranging from low sex drive to depression.

GUT HEALTH

This is huge in more ways than one. We might think of the skin as being the largest surface area to come into contact with the outside world, but some estimates suggest that if the GI tract were laid out on the floor it would fill a tennis court! The gut is the cornerstone of your physical and mental wellness. Repairing the diet doesn't happen overnight, foods loaded with excessive sugars are intended to be addictive and it takes effort to change. Gluten and dairy also have an addictive quality to them which is why it's so difficult to "just have one." Poor diet and medication can fuel the destruction of those delicate gut bacteria.
Sometimes we have to make a leap of faith so I need you to just trust me when I say your mental state is often a reflection of your gut bacteria. Feeling grouchy all the time has more to do with your gut than your brain. The good news is this is fixable.

Some medications prescribed to alleviate symptoms can have an adverse reaction on gut bacteria. As we've discussed, antibiotics can be lifesaving but indiscriminate overuse of antibiotics has become a huge problem coupled with the fact that antibiotics are now regularly used in the food supply. Restoring gut flora takes time; treat it as a steady marathon and not a sprint. Fermented foods and probiotics can help, but it's best to do this slowly. Keep in mind we don't want to cause the bad bacteria to die off too quickly or we *will* feel worse. Some people are drawn to yogurt for their probiotic content. Be aware that store-bought yogurt is often pasteurized and is more likely to be filled with sugar than any useful probiotics.

Food plays a key role in both gut health and inflammation. Years of eating the wrong foods cannot be overturned in a day. Be patient, the road to recovery takes time. Foods that heal rarely come from a tin, nor do they have a high sugar content. Bone broths are covered in more detail later and they are a valuable tool for anyone looking to repair the gut.

INFECTIONS

Infections can be caused by living organisms such as fungi and bacteria. Some of these organisms cause disease while others can be quite harmless and some even help our bodies work properly, including those found in the gut. Trillions of these bacteria and other microbes are *already* living inside your body and it's often said the number of microbes inside us outnumber our cells by about ten to one! Essentially we are a collection of bacteria with a human host. *I know, right? Who are we, really?*

Bacterial, viral, fungal, and even parasitic infections all receive their nourishment from you. Often in illness we alternate between hot and cold sweats. In the short term this can be a positive sign of healing. A fever is a common sign of illness, but that's not necessarily a bad thing. In fact, fevers seem to play a key role in fighting infections as some illness-reducing pathogens are killed off at higher temperatures.

Understanding that fevers play a key role in fighting infections means you will need to exercise a degree of common sense when deciding whether to let a fever run or call the doctor. As a rule of thumb, if you are an otherwise healthy adult, not immunocompromised or taking chemotherapy drugs, and haven't recently had surgery, then up to 102 F (38.9 C) it can be beneficial to let a fever run – but, obviously, drink plenty of fluids to stay hydrated. Ultimately this is dependent on your circumstances. It's not a hard and fast rule and it's not intended to replace medical advice.

Most common infections are no match for an immune system that's supported by good nutrition. The problem is we don't always realize this until *after* we become sick. Antibiotics are sometimes used to treat certain infections. While they obviously have a place in medicine, overuse brings its own problems and antibiotics won't do anything to treat any type of viral infection.

Natural alternatives worthy of further investigation are tea tree oil, colloidal silver, cistus-incanus tea, *food-grade*-hydrogen peroxide, and MMS 1. The latter two being the most controversial, but they are both treatments I have used in the past to good effect. Am I saying they are right for you?

No, I'm saying here are five **separate** things that are worth more research. In the right *diluted* dose, some things are helpful and others can be darn right dangerous! Dose is the key to EVERYTHING, even common table salt when eaten in too great a quantity is deadly. Heed the warning: moderation will always serve you better than excess.

ENVIRONMENTAL TOXINS

Industry is fueled *not* by oil, but by consumer demand. It's estimated that by 2050 there will be more plastic in the sea than fish. These tiny plastic partials are now entering the food chain and *nobody* knows the long-term effects of this. The most effective way to recycle is not to buy it in the first place. Buying plastic goods in ignorance is no longer sustainable or acceptable. THE MOST EFFECTIVE WAY TO DEAL WITH PLASTIC ISN'T TO PUT IT IN THE RECYCLE BIN, IT'S TO STOP BUYING IT!

SUNLIGHT

The positive effects of broad spectrum light on the body are wide reaching and profound. Think of a summer evening around 7 p.m. – most main streets are a hive of activity as people walk around feeling alert and awake. Natural sunlight plays a key role in how we feel. Natural light also affects mitochondrial function – these are the tiny energy cells of the body. Now think of a dark winter's night around the same time. By 7 p.m. on a winter's night some of us are probably already in our PJs, right? Light is energy, embrace it!

Sensible daily exposure to sunlight also helps our bodies produce vitamin D which is essential for healthy immune function. Sunlight also increases dopamine release in your body. Even plants grow measurably stronger when exposed to sunlight.

DIET

Food has a profound effect on our health and yet today food is such a loosely defined term. Clean, locally grown food often has a higher nutritional content than large scale commercially farmed crops. When you buy local it's a WIN-WIN – your community thrives and you get to eat food that's in season and at the peak of nutritional value. As a commodity, food is often exploited; as a medicine, food is often misunderstood.

Typically, fast food also has excessive amounts of manmade sugars. This will drag the immune system down and deplete the body of key minerals. All food turns to sugar anyway, and dumping more into the system only adds to the problem. Fruit is naturally high in sugar. In nature we wouldn't find everything ripe at the same time or in the same place. Fruit was meant to be eaten in moderation and in season. Until you get your health issues under control, consider giving fruit the boot. You can slowly reintroduce it into your diet later. When the body can no longer cope with the amount of sugar circulating in the bloodstream, the problem goes well beyond diabetes. One illness loves sugar above all others and its name is cancer.

Today most fast foods are cooked in vegetable oils which have been shown to cause oxidative stress; this simply means the oils create free radicals in the body which in turn **causes inflammation**. Oils high in omega-6 will promote inflammation, as will dairy products and grains. If this is all new to you, don't panic.

If you are new to the subject of nutrition and feeling overwhelmed by it all, a good rule of thumb is to simply fill half of every plate you serve yourself with organic leafy vegetables. Do this one thing and your portion sizes will naturally become more balanced and tackling the remaining 50% of your plate will be less daunting.

Treating symptoms is as easy as popping a pill but unless the underlying cause is addressed, progress will *always* be slow. When we become ill our delicate filtering organs such as the kidneys, lungs, skin, and liver are already working under pressure. Everything we swallow has to be processed, so let's be aware of the things we ingest whether they be food, liquid, or pills. In effect, the things we swallow can tax the body; this is even true of vitamins and herbal supplements (as previously discussed).

A healthy liver is essential to good health because it does far more than just detoxify toxins. If one organ above all others deserves the title of being a true *multitasker,* then it's the liver. It performs over 500 different functions, including fighting off infection, neutralizing toxins, manufacturing proteins and hormones, controlling blood sugar, and helping clot the blood which is probably the reason for it being the largest and heaviest of all the internal organs.

The liver is the most metabolically complex organ in the human body. It plays such an important role that it's the only visceral organ to possess the remarkable capacity to regenerate itself. Get this: if part of the liver is surgically removed or chemically damaged it can actually regrow itself. *I know, right?* It has to be the coolest tool in the toolbox and any time you are ill you can bet the liver is either being overused or abused.

A liver that's been overworked can sometimes outwardly manifest as frustration or increased emotional instability. If you find yourself easily crying, becoming easily irritated, or acting out in anger, look to the liver. To help improve liver detoxification naturally, a **castor oil pack** is sometimes used. The idea is to apply a liberal amount of high *quality* castor oil to a piece of cloth, then place it over the liver and hold in place with a hot water bottle to help stimulate lymph and liver function. A simple Google search will give you the exact details for this effective protocol. Another way to assist the liver is to drink fresh lemon juice first thing in the morning (see Chapter 15).

It seems highly probable that if we have a problem with the liver we can also expect underperforming kidneys because the two are so closely intertwined. Once the liver and kidneys are struggling to cope with the demands put on them, you may also notice an increase in body odor. When the kidneys are underperforming, itchy skin conditions such as eczema may also flare up and odor is prominently noticed in the feet.

Another reason for increased body odor (and there are many others) could be a low-grade biofilm infection. Cistus-incanus tea is something worthy of further investigation. When used over a two-week period, most infections give up and the body odor disappears. As always, moderation will serve you better than excess, and small amounts of tea taken regularly is more helpful than excess.

Gentle herbs such as milk thistle can be helpful to detoxify the liver. Herbs have been used safely for thousands of years, but as with anything that detoxifies – *go slow* or risk dumping toxins into the bloodstream faster than they can be removed. Using herbs that support the liver and kidneys may help bring an improvement to overall health.

Enlisting the help of a knowledgeable, local herbalist can bring faster, safer results. Be mindful that the effects of other drugs/supplements can be magnified as they are dragged through the liver or kidneys. Where possible, it's best not to mix/take them at the same time.

Sodium bicarbonate has been shown to be helpful with certain kidney issues. You can find this in most regular supermarkets and it's often called baking soda. The preferred brand is sold by Arm and Hammer because it doesn't have any other ingredient apart from sodium bicarbonate. It's important that it has NO aluminum added as with some other brands.

Before you rush to shoot me down for suggesting you drink baking soda, let me first tell you that this research comes direct from the Royal London Hospital and findings can also be found published in the Journal of the American Society of Nephrology.

As always, do your own research and before trying anything new always speak to your doctor. I sometimes find it helpful to add a quarter of a teaspoon of sodium bicarbonate to a glass of water and drink it on an empty stomach.

Another firm indicator that the kidneys are running out of sync is a change in urinary frequency, either too few trips to the bathroom or too many. These are often reflected in the color of the urine, i.e., too dark or too light. This was already covered in some detail at the end of Chapter 7.

Let's not forget that the skin *and* lungs form part of the detoxification process. Problems with the lungs are obviously easier to notice because anything that affects breathing is instantly going to be on your radar. Here, the herb mullein can be an effective ally along with staying hydrated.
Mullein helps lubricate the lungs and throat membranes while reducing swelling, which can help alleviate irritation. Mullein has traditionally been used to remedy bronchitis, asthma, croup, whooping cough, pneumonia, asthma, and tuberculosis. It can be made from loose tea and sipped, or in tincture form added to water. As always, *my* goal is only to guide you to these things and *your* role is to research them to the point where you make your own judgment calls. Keep in mind these are delicate filtering organs; less will always serve you better than more.

HAVE A PURPOSE

I've long suspected that people with a passion for a project usually hang around long enough to see it completed. In my honest opinion, this is one of the more powerful tips offered in this book which is why I'll be covering it again in another chapter. Having a purpose (in spite of an illness) can get us through the toughest of mental days.

Look, I know it sucks being ill and, trust me, you can go back to being ill for the rest of the day, so for now just humor me. Find something – *anything* – that is important to you, even if it's only for five minutes a day. Make no mistake, a passion, when combined with a determined spirit, is a *powerful* tool to have in the box. People who are passionate about finishing a project rarely seem to die while in the process.

There is no right or wrong answer here. You can commit to painting a landscape or a bedroom at your own pace. Fly a kite or fly a plane, make a video or write a book, start a club or join one, plant a tree or cut one down – it's all good.

Even if I knew that tomorrow the world would go to pieces; I would still plant my apple tree. – Martin Luther

What did we learn from this chapter?

Illness is always going to go after your weakest link. It's well documented that chronic inflammation is behind a wide range of diseases. The good news is it is reversible. This means that something in this chapter could be your silver bullet.

Homework: for a better understanding of how things link together in the body, check out "How the Body Works," by Dr. John Bergman. You can find this video on YouTube. Over the years I've gotten a lot of solid information from this person. Or click the link below:

https://www.youtube.com/watch?v=mActHjsX5pc

Chapter 31

MY DIET IS BIGGER THAN YOUR DIET

Ask ten foodies what constitutes a healthy diet and you are in for a polarized debate. It seems no topic is more divided than what should go on the end of your fork. Making a claim to be vegan, paleo, vegetarian, a raw foodist, or ketogenic has almost become like pledging an allegiance to a particular religion. And once the rigid battle lines are drawn, people are quick to become defensive.

Vegans and vegetarians – know that I feel your pain and much of the advice, information, and suggestions in this book should guide people *away* from barbaric farming practices. But at this stage, encouraging someone who is just now seriously thinking about nutrition to go 100% vegan is simply a bridge too far. Raw foodies – know that I have no beef with you either (yup, intended pun) and we could endlessly debate the pros and cons of yours and other diets, but the most important and first thing I want to stress is that *any* dietary choices that take us away from the heavily processed and very sad SAD (Standard American Diet) are important steps in the right direction.

Rather than divide ourselves into opposing groups, can we at least all agree that if your diet makes you feel great then it's the right one for you. By contrast, we can say with equal conviction that if you are experiencing a number of health issues perhaps your diet has room for improvement. When our thinking is rigid it's easy to prove ourselves right, but in the process we run the risk of shooting ourselves in the foot.

Let's also remind ourselves that so much of this is open to interpretation. A person eating pizza, fries, and cake could technically claim to be vegetarian, just as a person eating deep fried chicken and fries could claim to be paleo, and someone on the ketogenic diet could certainly be eating greater than normal quantities of cheese. Are these healthy, balanced ways to eat? I would say not. However, the idea behind *this* chapter isn't to tell you what foods to eat, it's to look at your *current* diet with a view to plugging any nutritional gaps it might have.

Everything I have learned (and continue to learn) has come as a direct result of trying to keep an open mind. Periodically, I find it helps to write down everything I know about nutrition on a blackboard **and then wipe the blackboard clean.** Looking at problems from different perspectives allows us to see things we might have missed. Who knows, perhaps nutrition started to go wrong as far back as Columbus when he decided to inflict his discovery of potatoes, corn, and tobacco on the rest of the world ... *just sayin'.*

MITOCHONDRIA WTF? *(Where's-the-Fat?)*

Mitochondria are a fascinating subject and what you are about to read is an oversimplification of probably the most amazing and powerful sequence of events your body performs every second of every day. While simplification helps us cover more ground together, I have to say that the subject of mitochondria warrants a book solely devoted to it. This, clearly, is not that book.

But fortunately, there are two new books on this very subject. The first is Dave Asprey's book *Headstrong*. Dave did a real nice job on this and for sure it's worth checking out. Not to be outdone, Dr. Joseph Mercola has just released a new book titled *Fat for Fuel*. As with anything Dr. Mercola puts out, it's a wealth of cutting-edge information.

Mitochondria are tiny cigar-shaped batteries found inside almost every cell in the body. They can be thought like the battery in your car. When that battery is fully charged, the engine bursts into life on demand, but when the life of that battery is almost drained your car's engine is slow to turn over.

When mitochondria perform well we feel energized and healthy. Mitochondria really don't care what particular diet group you belong to; they simply demand raw materials to make energy. You can take it to the bank that when the mitochondria are undernourished, illness, fatigue, and brain fog are all present. Let's take a closer look at nutrition from the mitochondria point of view.

Mitochondria are perfectly formed powerhouses that produce energy by utilizing oxygen and breaking down food and then releasing that energy in the form of ATP (adenosine triphosphate), along with some byproducts such as carbon dioxide, water, and free radicals. ATP is the fuel of the cell and it's used for everything from blinking to sprinting. *Why is this important?*

Think of it this way: we can go months without food, we can go days without water, we can go minutes without air, but when it comes to going without ATP? *Meh, you have about fifteen seconds before it's game over.* ATP is the energy currency of life and it's mostly produced *inside* the mitochondria. We could think of ATP as gasoline used by a car, but as we all know, gasoline doesn't come straight from the ground ready to use, it has to be refined from oil.

Making ATP is a process similar to refining oil and it happens mostly inside the mitochondria. Given that we cannot go fifteen seconds without making ATP, we could argue that this process is more important than the air we breathe. *Can you see where I am going with this?*

We know that the highest numbers of mitochondria can be found in the brain, eyes, and heart, and in women there are also high concentrations of mitochondria in the ovaries. Rather than asking which set of dietary rules we must defend and obey, let's flip the question around and ask, *hey, what do my mitochondria need to function optimally?*

When we look at nutrition from this perspective we will do well to remember that the greatest number of mitochondria live in the brain – and as we already know, the brain has an extremely high fat content so it makes sense that we need to consume foods that are high in fat. *Duh.* This doesn't mean we have to throw all other diets under the bus, it simply means we should increase the fat content of the foods we choose to consume.

This also highlights the *problem* of following a strictly low fat diet which, as it turns out, makes absolutely no sense whatsoever. *I know, right? WTF? (Where's-the-Fat?)*

Fat goes by lots of different names, including saturated, unsaturated, polyunsaturated, healthy, unhealthy, trans-fats, omega-3 fats, omega-6 fats, etc. This is a topic fraught with confusion and, depending on who you ask, everyone seems to have a different opinion.

GOOD FATS

While it might not be politically correct, I'd like to simplify this mess by splitting it into only two groups: good fat and bad fat. Be warned, in some circles even these can be viewed as the same thing – remember, mitochondria really don't care what advice others have for you, they just need the raw materials to function optimally. One of those raw materials is good fat. Not all fats, however, are equal.

Let's first look at fats found in animal products like grass-fed butter, whole raw milk, and fatty meats. I don't expect everyone to agree, but in my opinion these are all good fats. Butter sometimes gets a bad rap, but the devil is always in the details. Cows that graze on open pastures make the best butter and it's nothing like the margarine humans make. *You know that, right? Manmade = bad.*

Other sources of good fats can be found in avocados, pasture-raised eggs, coconut MCT oil, raw cacao butter, and raw nuts such as pecans and macadamias. These types of fats are friends to your brain.

Animal fats contain beneficial levels of (good) omega-3s. Omega-3s can be found in healthy fish such as Alaskan salmon, sardines, and anchovies because these fish are lower in toxins. Krill oil supplements can also help boost omega-3 and they generally have fewer problems than regular fish oil supplements because they have a lower mercury content.

Omega-3 fatty acids are a class of essential fatty acids. The two principal omega-3 fatty acids are EPA (eicosapentaenoic acid) and DHA (docosahexaenoic acid). For all ages, DHA is critical for optimal brain function. If you want your kiddo to be smart, best you pay attention.

Omega-3 is essential for optimal brain health and, in a perfect world, omega-3s should be balanced with omega-6s. A balanced ratio would be in the approximate range of 1:1.

Unfortunately, the standard western diet has this balance massively out of whack in favor of omega-6s. Some estimates put this imbalance as high as 25:1 in favor of omega-6! When the ratio of omega-3 and omega-6 is out of balance, the stage is set for inflammatory health problems. As mentioned earlier, inflammation is heavily implicated in all forms of illness.

High concentrations of omega-6 fatty acids can be found in vegetable oils – for example, per tablespoon grape seed oil has as much as 9744 mg; sunflower oil, 9198 mg; corn oil, 7452 mg; wheat germ oil, 7672 mg; soybean oil, 7059 mg; shortening, 4771 mg; and margarine, 3323 mg. With so much of fast food being fried in these types of oils, it's easy to see why the balance is so far off.

BAD

The real kicker is that foods high in good fats are sometimes shunned by the medical profession. For this we can thank a flawed study by the late Dr. Ancel Keys. His work linked higher saturated fat intake to higher rates of heart disease and ever since it has stuck in the minds of some doctors. But the problem isn't healthy fats – it's another group of fats known as *trans* fats. Trans fats can really mess with your insulin receptors. Some research suggests that trans fats can even increase your risk for chronic diseases such as cancer, heart disease, and diabetes.

Personally, I try to steer well clear of *all* commercially fried foods because they tend to be fried in trans fats. Trans fats are found in margarine, vegetable shortening, and partially hydrogenated vegetable oils. Trans fats are just unhealthy and you should avoid them entirely – they are typically used in low-quality products and your mitochondria can't use them (so neither can you). **Trans fat = bad.**

Bad fats aren't helpful to you or to your mitochondria; it's the equivalent of trying to build a house with substandard materials. As we seem to have come full circle back to talking about the nutritional needs of your mitochondria, let's also kick out all those excess sugars, processed flours, gluten, and dairy. *Ahh, that feels better already.*

Avoiding trans fats, as well as taking gluten and dairy off the table, is a good starting point. Do you remember why? The correct answer is gluten and dairy (closely followed by eggs and nuts) have the **highest** probability of triggering an unwanted food reaction. As a gentle reminder, let's keep in mind that gluten isn't only found in bread, it's in pastas, pastries, crackers, cakes, cereal, granola, pancakes, waffles, croutons, sauces and gravies, flour tortillas, brewer's yeast, and just about anything else that has wheat flour as an ingredient.

To keep things interesting, it gets even trickier when eating out because it's in soooo many other foods. When you have an immune system that's watching *everything* you do, you can't cheat even a little.

Mitochondria also enjoy fresh fruit, *albeit in moderation.* And they also like an abundance of fresh vegetables with a wide variety of colorful greens. Ideally aim for six to nine cups a day. Sulfur rich foods can help the body produce glutathione which you can find these in cruciferous veggies: bok choy, broccoli, cabbage, cauliflower, horseradish, kale, kohlrabi, mustard leaves, radish, turnips, and watercress.

There is some debate surrounding the goitrogenic effect of some of these foods which are thought to affect thyroid function by inhibiting synthesis of thyroid hormones. While this may be true in extremely large doses, cooking and steaming reduces this effect. So, too, does supplementation with selenium, vitamin E, and iodine – but let's not get ahead of ourselves when there are still plenty of food options on the table.
If it's not clear by now then it's worth repeating that taking either selenium or iodine in isolation has the potential to causes more problems than it solves. This synergistic gang of three should be taken in direct relationship to each other. Other supplements that can be thought of as mitochondria-protectives include acetyl-l-carnitine, alpha-lipoic acid,

coenzyme Q10, N-acetylcysteine, NADH, D-ribose, resveratrol, and magnesium aspartate. But for now, let's stick with food.

Fiber is important for good digestion and can be found in fruits, vegetables, and grains. But because we are trying to avoid grains, here's a list of foods that are high in fiber but do not contain any grains: avocados, Asian pears, berries, coconuts, figs, artichokes, peas, okra, acorn squash, Brussels sprouts, turnips, black beans, chickpeas, lima beans, split peas, lentils, nuts, flaxseeds, and chia seeds. Seeds and beans are best soaked overnight to aid digestion. Men and women have slightly different fiber needs. It's recommended that women get approximately 25 grams of fiber a day and men between 35 and 40 grams.

Autoimmune conditions can wreak havoc on the mitochondria. If you aren't sure whether or not you have an unrecognized autoimmune condition remember that a good indicator that you do is if you've seen multiple doctors and are still *without* a firm diagnosis. The joy of autoimmunity keeps on coming and anyone with this condition should also consider the possibility of a leaky gut. If this is you, then bone broth can be a useful food staple because it is rich in glutamine and other amino acids known to be beneficial for the lining of the gut.

CRUISING FOR OYSTERS

There can't be too many controversial neurosurgeons out there smart enough to make your head hurt and abrupt enough to cause offense. If you are blissfully unaware of Dr. Jack Kruse, be warned – his critics call him an undiplomatic quack and his supporters label him a revolutionary genius.

Personally, I find his style refreshing *although his stance on mercury fillings is at odds with my own experience.* Perhaps it's the mercury in his own teeth that makes his style somewhat abrasive. Either way, the magnetic pull of Dr. Jack Kruse is something I find strangely fascinating.

You are probably wondering why we are suddenly talking about a controversial neurosurgeon, right? I'm glad you asked. It's fair to say the average brain surgeon knows more about the brain than the rest of us. Whether you love or loathe him, there is no getting away from the fact that Dr. Kruse is smart.

Dr. Kruse sometimes catches flack for being too far out there, but he's basically a proponent of eating paleo, keeping seasons in mind, eating more ketogenic in the winter and more carbs in the other seasons – something I think most people can get their heads around.

In his professional capacity, Dr. Kruse is quick to tell us that DHA is an important brain nutrient. He also believes that of any food, oysters are the most nutrient dense for optimal functioning of the human brain. *Is he right?* Who knows? But whenever I come across fresh oysters I now eat them and so far I've lived to tell the tale.

Oysters have no central nervous system, so the theory is they do not feel pain. Perhaps this might sit well with vegetarians looking for an alternative protein? Oysters are considered a powerful aphrodisiac and a good source of essential minerals including phosphorus, calcium, potassium, and zinc. Some people eat oysters raw and do just fine with them. For my money I prefer to have them cooked because there is a risk of raw oysters carrying the hepatitis A virus. It's really not the oysters' fault; Hep-A is sometimes found in water that has been contaminated by humans.

Cooking oysters is super easy. Simply place the oysters in a flat bottomed pan and add a little water. Slowly apply medium heat until the oyster shell opens and, bingo, you are good to go. The whole process usually takes between five to ten minutes.

The US Food and Drug Administration also warns that oysters should be cooked to avoid contamination with pathogens. And of course, a good rule of thumb is if something doesn't look or smell right, throw it out.

To balance things out I also listen to another board-certified neurologist by the name of Dr. Perlmutter. He's on the absolute cutting edge of innovative medicine and when he talks, I like to listen. Check him out in today's homework.

What did we learn from this chapter?

While it's true that not everybody is going to have the same dietary needs, we can with absolute certainty say that *everybody* has mitochondria. When the mitochondria are fired up they go hand in hand with good health. The eyes, heart, and brain all have a high density of mitochondria.

The brain needs fat in the diet to function optimally. The ideal ratio of omega-6 to omega-3 fats is 1:1. You can help maintain this balance by regularly taking krill oil supplements and eating fish such as Alaskan salmon, sardines, and anchovies because these fish are lower in toxins.

Homework: check out these two interesting sites, drperlmutter.com and Jack Kruse.com.

http://www.drperlmutter.com/

https://www.jackkruse.com/

Chapter 32

SEVEN BIG GUNS, NO CARROTS

In this chapter we will look at six things that have nothing to do with food but can have a profound effect on your overall health. The good news is each one is easy to do and totally free! Every day I try to incorporate some aspect of these things into my daily routine.

#1 SET THE CLOCK

With the precision of a Swiss clock, birds migrate, flowers open, roosters crow, and at 5:15 p.m. every evening it was common for two deer to walk through the back of my property. I suspect neither of them owns a wristwatch, and yet they must absolutely have body clocks. Animals, plants, and humans all respond to changes in darkness and light. These changes follow the approximate 24-hour cycle and have a profound effect on physical and mental health. This cycle is better known as the circadian rhythm.

Like the deer, we also have a body clock and there's a price to pay when it's out of whack. Fortunately, resetting it is pretty easy to do. For best results, this should be done each morning *within five minutes of waking* by simply exposing yourself and your eyes to as much natural sunlight as possible.

If you find yourself stuck indoors on a dull, overcast day, be sure to open the blinds and turn on lots of bright lights. Setting your clock is a two-part trick. To keep your circadian rhythm in check, it's also essential to keep to a regular bedtime schedule. *I get it,* establishing consistency takes discipline, but I promise you, the rewards for doing this are rapid and real.

Science recognizes that a "master clock" in the brain coordinates all the other body clocks so that they are in synch. Circadian rhythms influence hormone release, body temperature, sleep-wake cycles, and hundreds of other important bodily functions. Abnormal circadian rhythms have also been associated with diabetes, depression, obesity, bipolar disorder, seasonal affective disorder, etc. Sleeping in on weekends can throw your whole body clock off; if you need extra sleep on the weekend, try going to bed earlier. For those of us who are now too old to rock but too young to die, this is easy advice to follow.

The importance of keeping the circadian rhythm in sync cannot be overestimated; a brisk walk in the morning sunlight is an incredibly powerful way to give you an immediate energy boost as well as help you reset your circadian rhythm. When your eyes sense morning light, your body responds by being more awake and alert. For that reason, be sure not to obscure the sunlight with sunglasses. Did I just say you need to stare at the sun until your retinas bleed out? *No, of course I did not. That would be idiocy.*

As the evening sun sets we want the *opposite* of bright light. The electric light has been an invaluable asset to mankind, but as the evening rolls in we risk sabotaging not only our circadian rhythm but our melatonin production. Keep in mind that before the invention of the electric light bulb humans relied heavily on the soft glow of candlelight. Today we are bombarded with harsh blue light almost around the clock.

In most houses, electric lights throw off a harsh blue light. This is also true of LED lights and compact fluorescent bulbs. You may recall from an earlier chapter that some of those compact fluorescent bulbs (the curly looking ones) have mercury in them! The best solution is to use a small evening lamp, preferably with one of those older incandescent light bulbs – something with an amber glow will suffice.

> *Humans are the only species bright enough to make*
> *artificial light and stupid enough to live under it.*
> – Jack Kruse

Bottom line: after dark it is important not to confuse our brain into thinking it's still daytime. Some of the worst culprits for artificial blue light are laptops, tablets, and cell phones. Be sure to power down tech devices at least three hours before bed. You can also apply a filter to them such as F-lux. This is available as a free download and it works really well.

Check this out: in 1994 the *Journal of the American Medical Association* (JAMA) published a study showing that surgeons performed measurably better while listening to music. The best results happened when music was selected by the participants. *Hmm, I see.*

Music can reach into parts of the brain faster than a shot of tequila. A recent study showed that music improved cognitive performance and recall abilities in patients suffering from dementia. Music has also been shown to reach Alzheimer's patients where medications fail. I recently put this to the test when my wife and I went to visit an elderly relative. Serious illness has been ravaging her ailing body for quite some time. She can no longer speak, is bedridden, and spends her days staring at the ceiling. Familiar voices mean nothing to her and are often met with a blank stare. But the day my wife played her favorite hymn, "Amazing Grace," I swear, her eyes opened wide and she turned her head and smiled.

Music has the ability to lift the soul. Sometimes we just have to be reminded to use it as part of our daily health routine. Whenever I find myself in a funk, the fastest way I know of to turn my day around is to jump on a small trampoline while listening to a short music video via YouTube.

They say you can tell a lot about a person from the music they listen to. Personally, I can find something to bob my head along to in just about any music genre. *I know, right? Square peg, round hole.*

When my body dies, my wife knows to play Louis Armstrong's, *"What a Wonderful World"* going into the church and, just to keep the energy up on the way out, I've requested "I'm a Firestarter" by the Prodigy (true story). Like me, it seems my musical taste is a little difficult to put into a box.

For just a moment I'd like to challenge you to imagine living in a world with zero music. (I know – *bummer.*) Now write down three of your favorite songs. At the end of this chapter I'm going to ask you to play them. See how quickly music has the power to stir up your emotions. Obviously you want to *steer away* from sad songs; the idea here is to *lift* your spirits.

#3 EARTHING

If I had to choose only one tool to tackle illness, that tool would be an open mind. Opening ourselves up to new ideas allows us to see problems from a different perspective. You might want to hold onto that thought as we now look at grounding, also referred to as earthing.

For consistency, I'll use the latter term from here forward. We like to think we are biological beings but really that's only part of the story. Your brain, heartbeat, and neurotransmitter activity all rely on *electrical* signals. Without these electrical signals there would be no life. Fundamentally, you and I are *electrical* beings.
To be clear, there are plenty of credible, published scientific studies surrounding earthing. More important, earthing is something you can put to the test for yourself right now and monitor your own results. If the weather outside allows, try reading the rest of this chapter outside with your bare feet touching grass, stone, or concrete. This experiment will **not** work on asphalt (that's tarmac for my European homies).

I know what you are thinking because I thought it too – *what's with this hippy shit, right?* Do yourself a huge favor; postpone your judgment until you have all the facts. Better still, ask yourself when the last time you placed your feet on bare earth was. For many of us, this probably happens once a year on vacation. *Walking barefoot on the beach felt good, right?*

Apart from that beach vacation, the rest of the year we keep our feet wrapped in plastic boxes, walk on nylon carpets, drive our cars on rubber tires, and expose ourselves to ridiculously large amounts of electromagnetic pollution. If I were a gambling man, I'd bet the farm that these events play a huge part in systemic inflammation. *Why?*

When you look at blood samples under the microscope the differences between earthed and non-earthed blood is quite remarkable. It's sometimes said, *what can't speak can't lie.* When the two samples are set side by side it's almost like looking at red wine and tomato ketchup. Make no mistake, earthing improves blood viscosity.

It seems the smarter we become, the dumber we become. Maybe future historians will look back on *this* period the same way we look back on the Roman Empire. Those Romans became so smart they began moving water around in lead pipes which we now know is a toxic heavy metal. It wasn't long after they began doing this that the empire crumbled from within. Perhaps over time Wi-Fi will be the equivalent of lead pipes.

Studies reveal that earthing has an effect on heart rate variability, cortisol dynamics, sleep, autonomic nervous system (ANS) balance, and reduces the effects of stress. In short, earthing helps put out the fire of inflammation! If you take only one thing from this chapter let it be this: earthing is missing in our modern day busy lives, *illness is not!*

Earthing appears to minimize the consequences of exposure to "dirty electricity." *How often should you practice earthing?* If you are exposed to Wi-Fi daily, then it pays to make this a daily habit. I try to do this every morning, ideally for twenty minutes a day – longer is better, and less is better than nothing.

Tip - Anytime you find yourself unable to think straight, find a quiet spot outside, slip off your socks, and let your feet touch the negative charge of the earth. This allows the transfer of electrons to your body which in turn helps neutralize damaging free radicals. In a relatively short space of time, the world and all its problems begins to look like a very different place.

Earthing can be done any time simply by making contact with the earth or walking barefoot outside. In parts of the world where walking barefoot isn't possible, there are now special shoes that incorporate copper contacts into the soles. Long before manufactured rubber soles became the norm, leather-soled shoes acted as an effective semiconductor. These types of shoes were sometimes worn by our Victorian ancestors.

Earthing devices are not restricted to shoes. Today it's possible to purchase an earthing mattress, mattress covers, and even pillow cases that work by using the ground plug of a house. Although you tend to get what you pay for, some people report deeper sleep with less mind chatter and fewer aches and pains in the morning. In one study, participants who slept on a special earthing mat showed significant changes in key biomarkers including serum sodium, potassium, magnesium, and iron.

The key to effective grounding indoors is to ensure your outlets are properly grounded because all grounding mats use the ground wire in your home. If you are in any doubt, ask an electrician to check them for you.

Sleeping while earthing makes good sense because you don't have to do anything other than sleep to reap the benefits. For those who are more technically minded, you can see the difference this makes when you hold a simple voltage meter. To better understand what's happening, think of earth as being abundant in negative ions. Another ideal place to have a grounding mat might be at your feet as you work on your computer. If you find yourself on a limited budget, you can make an earthing mat with a few basic supplies from a hardware store. YouTube has lots videos to show you how to do this. Ideally, whenever you use a laptop put it on a desk. If you don't have a desk, try placing a thick book beneath it along with some kind of pillow. This will help reduce the EMF felt in the body to some degree.

If you really want to be blown away by earthing, invest in Clinton Ober's book *Earthing: The Most Important Health Discovery Ever?* Just reading the reviews on Amazon will make your head spin!

#4 COLD THERMOGENESIS

WARNING: cold thermogenesis may not be suitable for those with a serious health condition, please consult a medical doctor before trying it.

Compared to wandering around shoeless with a flower in your hair, cold thermogenesis is a little more hardcore. While it's not for everyone, if you can pull this off the rewards are plentiful which is why it's a favorite with top sports people to aid in recovery. There's also a couple of easy cheats to help you do this.

Cold thermogenesis helps alleviate pain, improves mood, and increases production of norepinephrine in the brain (which is connected to focus and attention.) It's also known to be helpful in reducing inflammation and can even help with migraines. *But wait, there's more.* Cold thermogenesis is said to lower body fat, increase sexual performance, and improve adrenal/thyroid function. If it feels like I am giving you all the benefits before revealing exactly what cold thermogenesis is, you are correct. *Why?*

Cold thermogenesis involves cold water, a bath of sorts, and you. *I know, right? Had I opened with that you would have probably stopped reading by now.* Fear not, cold thermogenesis was something I stumbled upon even before I knew it had a name. Back in 2011 my body intuitively knew the value of cold thermogenesis and given how ill I was I just went with it. Years later I was surprised to learn there is actually a lot of published scientific data to support this concept.

At the time, my sitting in ice cold water must have made it seem as if I'd lost my marbles. No doubt my wife (bless her) had me pegged as bat-shit crazy, but it's one of the many things I've done that helped in my own recovery. The part that left my wife scratching her head was when I started doing it outside in the dark. *Why?*

With inflammation raging through my body, the outside temperature had dropped to where I needed it, and doing it in the dark spared the neighbors having to see a sickly looking, semi-naked Englishman sitting outside in a tub of ice cold water. WAIT! Before you turn the page on me, remember I have some cheats to help get you through this. You don't have to do what I did to get a benefit. The good news is you can tap into cold thermogenesis gradually by starting small. There are a couple of ways to do this.

Method #1: for this you need to find a pan the size of your face. Fill a third of it with water and then place the pan in the freezer. Once frozen, take it out and top off the bowl as needed with cold water. Next, place your face in the ice water for as long as you can stand it. The first couple of times you probably won't be able to do it for more than a few seconds but over the week you should be able to withstand it for longer periods. Congrats – you are experiencing the benefits of cold thermogenesis with all your clothes on.

Method #2: you could try incorporating the James Bond shower from an earlier chapter, *yup, that old chestnut's back.* The easy way to do this is to start by taking a hot shower and then **gradually** turn the water to warm and then in the last thirty seconds of your shower, on cold. Aiming the cold water on your face and chest may also help you breathe easier throughout the day. The cold water also stimulates the lymphatic system. Gradually, easing into this rather than jumping into a cold shower makes the whole process less daunting, and believe me, once you get used to it, it's actually quite invigorating – no, *seriously.*

Method #3: over time you may feel ready to take the plunge and try an ice cold bath (obviously assuming that your doc says it is okay for you to try). It's easier to do cold baths if you focus on the **benefits** of doing it and it may help to start off with lukewarm water and gradually add in more cold.

You might not be able to do this for very long to begin with and that's okay. Over time I managed to do it for half an hour at a time without even shivering, although I suspect if I tried it today I'd be lucky to do a few minutes. If you try this, it's helpful to keep your head, fingers, and toes out of the water because these extremities are particularly susceptible to cold. A final word of caution to men: when you get out of a cold bath it's probably not the best time to take that naked selfie ... *just sayin'.*

#5 LET THERE BE LIGHT

Recently, while passing an antique shop, I happened to notice in the window an old light box for sale. The box measured approximately 4ft x 4ft with a hole in the top for a person to poke their head through. Inside, the light box was lined with mirrors and lights. Back in the day, a person would pay to sit inside the box and have their body blasted with light.

What's cool about this box is the company that made it also installed the exact same model on the *Titanic*. This made me think, light therapy really isn't anything new, but it's incredibly powerful. Here's why.

The skin acts almost like a solar panel charging up the body with ultraviolet B waves and a cholesterol derivative found in the skin. Once the skin comes into contact with natural sunshine (or light that mimics sunshine) vitamin D (which is actually a hormone) is synthesized.

Make no mistake, light has a profound effect on the body and the aim of artificial light therapy is to mimic elements of natural sunlight. Light therapy is known to affect brain chemicals linked to mood and sleep. But wait, there's more.
In 1903 the Nobel Prize for medicine was awarded to Niels Ryberg Finsen for his outstanding contribution to the treatment of diseases, particularly Lupus vulgaris which is a form of tuberculosis (TB). This was treated with concentrated light radiation. Finsen believed that tissues that had been attacked by bacteria might respond well to treatment with light.

In 1895 he used concentrated beams of ultraviolet light to successfully treat patients with lupus vulgaris. For a time, light therapy was widespread but was eventually replaced in medicine with antibiotics.

Today, some smaller light therapy boxes can fit on a desktop and are designed to help those with seasonal affective disorder (SAD). This is a particular type of major depression that occurs at specific times of year when sunshine is least available.

Exposure to a light box for as little as thirty minutes a day can help stimulate a change in the hormones that affect mood. If you live in a part of the world where the sun doesn't shine, then you really should have a light box (otherwise called a SAD lamp) somewhere in your house. You can find light boxes for sale at Amazon.

The benefits of natural sunlight cannot be understated. Any morning when the sun is shining I immediately make a beeline outdoors to get a skin-full, preferably *before* the geoengineering-gods see fit to block out the blue sky. *I know, right? Humans controlling the weather, what could possibly go wrong?*

RED LIGHT THERAPY

Red light therapy differs from the light therapy just described. Again, it's light that you can see but, as the name suggests, it's light that comes in the form of a red glow. There are a couple of different types of red light and they each play a different role. In this section you need to pay attention to those differences because understanding them will impact your health in different ways.

Red light therapy falls into the visible light spectrum between 630-700 nm on the electromagnetic scale. Red light therapy is often used to treat the surface of the skin. Red light therapy can be thought of as healing and regenerative; it accelerates wound healing and can be applied to muscles or joints to reduce swelling or pain.

Last year I pulled something in my shoulder while working and I used red light therapy to help fix it. I liked using this option because it's noninvasive and drug free. There are lots of options out there, some offer good value for the money and others can be quite expensive.

The one I've been using lately is made by a company called Tendlite. It's the size of a flashlight but don't let the size fool you. It's really well made and a powerful tool to have in the toolbox for relief of joint pain. Relief doesn't always happen overnight, but if you stick with it results do come.

As with any of the following therapies, it's important to *keep the light away from your eyes.* Ideally you should invest in a set of inexpensive goggles similar to those used on some tanning beds. The light sold by Tendlite comes with dark glasses.

Tip – If you are on a shoestring budget, simply purchase a red heat bulb found in most pet shops. They are often used to keep young chicks warm and come with an inexpensive lamp holder. Bingo – you have a red light therapy for less than twenty bucks!

Red light therapy also soothes inflamed tissues, is good for headaches, sinus pain, nasal congestion, sore throats, earaches, and coughing. Red light therapy can help you get a deeper, more restful night's sleep, promotes relaxation, and is known to reduce anxiety and irritability.

Okay, now here's where we switch to a totally *different* type of light so it's important to make the distinction. Before you dismiss this idea you should know that the folks at NASA were early proponents of the following types of light.

INFRARED (AND NEAR INFRARED) THERAPY

Here we are talking about two different lights, the main distinction relates to the wavelengths. Infrared light typically falls into the invisible part of the light spectrum with wavelengths between 700 and 1200 nm, while near-infrared light falls into the spectrum of 700 nm to 2500 nm. Of the two, near-infrared can be thought of as *deeper* penetrating,

Near-infrared frequency can have a healing effect on our individual cells. Inside the mitochondria of every cell there are receptors that respond to near-infrared wavelengths. This light triggers an increase in cell metabolism, protein synthesis, and antioxidant activity which helps the cells detoxify. Near-infrared light reduces inflammation and pain while simultaneously triggering growth and regeneration in the cells.

Near-Infrared light comes to us in the form of halogen, laser, and LED. The preferred technology is LED because the surface temperature can be controlled. It also disperses over a greater surface area giving a faster treatment time. Near-infrared LED also has a gentler delivery, will not damage tissue, and carries less risk of accidental eye injury.

Benefits of near-infrared therapy are

- Boosts metabolism
- Recharges mitochondria
- Stimulates white blood production
- Reduces body fat
- Promotes cell regeneration
- Increases energy
- Reduces inflammation
- Improves circulation
- Heals wounds faster
- Provides pain relief
- Rejuvenates the skin
- Lessens joint and muscle pain

If you have the means, you can look into investing in your own infrared sauna. For the rest of us, we can tap into this technology by joining a local gym that has an infrared sauna as part of its membership. If you spend enough time researching the health benefits of light, it isn't long before you come across the name of Dr. Joseph Mercola (whom I've mentioned before). Dr. Mercola was talking about light therapy *long* before it became mainstream.

Dr. Mercola is a highly reliable source for cutting edge medical news and I use his site often. If you are looking to expand your knowledge, I urge you to check out his vast library of videos at mercola.com.

#6 PROJECT PASSION (IKIGAI)

Make no mistake – having a project you are passionate about can help keep you out of the doctor's office. The Japanese have a word for it: *ikigai* (pronounced ee-kee-guy). Roughly translated, it means having something to get out of bed for in the morning. Ever notice how a Monday morning feels different than a Saturday morning? Both days have the same number of hours, so what's changed? As kids, many of us remember that Christmas morning feeling when we bounced out of bed at 5 a.m. Yet trying to get out of bed on a school day even an hour later always felt like a challenge. Obviously not every day can be Christmas, but it serves to make a poignant point: having a meaning to the day adds purpose to a person's life.

Every one of us has something we enjoy doing even if there is no money involved. It's as if the human soul is hardwired to have a purpose. Take my advice, if you want better health, go find your ikigai. When you learn to tap into what motivates you, something freaky happens at the biological level. Ever notice how motivated people rarely get sick?

#7 LAUGHTER IS MEDICINE

Finally, it's sometimes said that laughter is the best medicine, unless of course you are laughing out loud for no apparent reason, in which case I suspect you *need* some medicine. Learning to laugh in the face of adversity is a powerful cure for all known stress. At some point during the day, give yourself permission to smile, even if it's only for a minute. Sometimes when my wife and I were waiting at the hospital, I'd see a worried look come over her face. The challenge was always to find something to make her laugh so hard that no sound would come out and she would be forced to clap like a demented seal. It really was a beautiful sight.

> *A wonderful thing about true laughter is that it*
> *just destroys any kind of system of dividing people.*
> – John Cleese.

What did we learn from this chapter?

Each of the light therapies in this chapter offers a wide range of health benefits. Light therapy can affect mood, circadian rhythm, and many other body processes. Red light therapy is helpful with joint and muscle pain and near-infrared therapy can act as a cell rejuvenator, among other things.

Homework: check out Dr. Mercola at mercola.com, or click on this short video. Then go play your favorite three songs as **loud** as you possibly can!

https://www.youtube.com/watch?v=2bo_lqFG_20

Chapter 33

LIQUID LIFE

Water is water right? *Meh, not so fast.* Science tells us that water can occur in three phases: liquid, solid, or gas. Liquid water is wet and fluid. Water as a solid is water that freezes. And water as a gas is the vapor present in the air all around us. But what if I told you there was a 4th phase to water that's rarely talked about and yet has a profound effect on your health?

This is not H20 but rather H302 – it's more alkaline, dense, and thicker than regular water, and it's actually alive and even holds a negative charge much in the same way that a battery does. In terms of benefits to you and your health, this living water is capable of tackling a wide range of health problems with astounding results.

When you have this piece of the puzzle in your toolbox it changes everything and, nope, *it's not holy water.* This 4th phase water is already inside you and by the time this chapter ends you will know how to give it a boost and where to get even more of it. Most medical students learn that water is just a background carrier to more important chemicals and bacteria, but according to Dr. Gerald Pollack, a PhD in biomedical engineering, water is central to everything the body does, and in relation, everything the cell does.

As early as Chapter 5 we first began exploring the idea that a healthy body requires healthy cells and now that concept comes full circle. An average adult is thought to be made up of 50-65% water, with the percentage of water in infants being much higher, typically around 75%. This type of water isn't the same as the water we drink from a plastic bottle. This water becomes highly-organized and appears in abundance inside most of your cells, even our extracellular tissues are filled with it.
Dr. Pollack has published numerous peer-reviewed scientific papers and his understanding of the physics of water is uniquely valuable to anyone in search of better health. Dr. Pollack carried out extensive experiments at the University of Washington on this 4th phase of water which uncovered

some remarkable findings. One experiment showed that the water molecules acted like telephones to carry messages throughout the body. Dr. Pollack's team also discovered that this type of water has the ability to exclude things it doesn't like, even small molecules. Given this unique property, it's sometimes referred to as "exclusion zone water" or EZ water for short.

The negative charge found in EZ water helps form cellular energy. *Are you getting this? Your body is made up mostly of water and that water is alive and it takes what it needs and excludes what it doesn't. It then sends signals around your body creating enough energy to keep you moving throughout the day!*

Light is a key ingredient for creating EZ water, whether in the form of visible light, ultraviolet (UV) wavelengths or infrared wavelengths that we are surrounded by all the time. If the goal is to maintain wellness or recover from a serious illness, it's important to understand that energy comes from the light we absorb which in turn affects the cells.

Laser therapy can help increase EZ water by penetrating the cells. In doing so, some laser therapy treatments have also been shown to reduce pain and inflammation which can help shorten healing time in muscles, ligaments, and bones.

Infrared light is the most powerful, particularly at wavelengths of approximately three micrometers. Hence the reason infrared sauna may prove helpful because the cells in the body are deeply penetrated by infrared energy which in turn helps build EZ water. The same can be said for spending time in the sun, although to get the full benefits of natural sunlight you need to step outside rather than sit behind a glass window. Glass will filter out much of the natural light spectrum. For the same reason, if you are a wearer of glasses you may find it helpful to periodically remove them and let the natural light gently and indirectly filter through to your eyes.

The fear surrounding natural sunshine and skin cancers is not without justification, but it might surprise some to know that *statistically speaking* skin cancer rates failed to go down when the use of sunblock became more widespread. Equally confusing is the fact that many skin cancers appear on parts of the body the sun doesn't reach.

Sunshine also plays an important role in the way your mitochondria communicate. Increased vitamin D levels play an important role in creating EZ water. Am I saying you should stay in the sun until your eyeballs burn out? *Nope, that would be foolish.* But keep in mind some of those sun blocking creams contain toxic chemicals, and anything that goes onto the skin goes into the bloodstream. Who knows, perhaps over time some of those toxic chemicals may prove to be equally problematic ... *just sayin'.*

Sun in moderation appears to be the preferable key. Personally, I try to get a skin full of sun in the morning *before midday.* If the afternoon sun is strong I either stay shaded or cover up with a brimmed hat and long sleeved shirt to give my arms some protection. Let's be clear, full spectrum light from natural sunlight is important to your health, manmade light by comparison can be more of a problem.

Spend enough time under fluorescent tube lighting and some people begin to experience fatigue and even migraine headaches. If you are particularly sensitive, even LED lighting can have a negative effect. Given the number of hours we spend indoors, as mentioned earlier it may be a better option to switch back to the older incandescent type light bulbs (obviously not those curly ones that contain mercury).

Light aside, EZ water can also be found in glacial melt, but unless you have a spare iceberg in the back garden you might want to consider locating a natural deep spring, the deeper the better because EZ water increases when under pressure. There are actually some products on the market that attempt to emulate this natural process by creating something known as vortexed water. Personally I haven't used any of them so I can only speculate about their effectiveness.

Vibration also plays a role in increasing EZ water and, to a lesser degree, so does rebounding on a trampoline. Movement is important to your health. If for some reason you find yourself immobilized with ill health there are products on the market to help achieve the sensation of intense movement. Whole body vibration plates come in all shapes and sizes and can be a useful tool to anyone standing or sitting at a desk for long periods of time.

If you don't have access to a vibration plate, an underground natural spring, an iceberg, natural sunlight, or infrared light, then fear not, all is not lost. EZ water can also be extracted from living foods, which brings us neatly to the subject of juicing. Juicing is simply a way of squeezing the juice out of vegetables and fruits and then drinking the liquid. *I know, right?* But just trust me on this one. *There are few things capable of turbo charging your health faster or better than juicing!*

If you are unfamiliar with this term you are in for a pleasant surprise. Juicing can form part of *any* diet which simply means you can dip your big toe in the water without too much disruption. Done right, this process doesn't just boost your nutrient intake, juicing also helps clean out the GI tract which can over time become clogged with mucus, rancid fats, undigested proteins, and parasites. *I know, right? It's nasty, but a cleaner GI tract will result in better absorption of nutrients into the cells.*

The idea that *you are what you eat* isn't strictly true. A more accurate description would be you are what you *absorb.* By now, we should all know the benefits of eating more vegetables – but let's be realistic, not many of us can eat two heads of broccoli, a bag of carrots, and five lettuces every day. Even if eating large amounts of vegetables were sustainable day in and day out, your poor digestive system would be working overtime to break it all down. Fortunately, juicing allows us to bypass this whole process and those nutrients are easier to absorb when juiced than they are if you try to eat your way through the same amount in solid form.

In solid food, fiber is important to aid digestion, but because juicing is a liquid, it's okay that most of the fiber is removed by the juicing machine. Keep in mind that this is a balance. I appreciate that if the juice doesn't taste good, some people will be reluctant to drink it. But we don't want to fall into the trap of adding too much fruit, either. Once the fiber is removed from fruit you should really think of it as liquid sugar. This is really important to remember. Moderation is always key, more so if you are dealing with a particular low grade fungal or bacterial infection.

There are lots of juicers on the market, some big, some small, some are affordable and some can be darn right expensive. Some are quality built and some are junk. Some juicers will outperform others and the tradeoff for doing so can be more time spent cleaning up. So before you rush out and buy one, know that the best juicer to buy *is the one you will use.* Even a top of the line juicer is useless if it sits in the cupboard because it takes too long to clean.

In my humble opinion, owning a juicer is better than having money in the bank. For sure, buying a juicer can be an investment, but there are few things in this life worth investing in more than your health – and let's be clear, *illness ain't cheap!*

Finding the right juicer for your needs is important. I urge you to check out a guy by the name of John who runs the YouTube channel DiscountJuicers.com. John has an unbiased passion for putting juicers through their paces. If anyone can tell you which juicer will fill your needs, it's John. Personally, I like the Omega VSJ843. As a first juicer, it's got a decent warranty and it's pretty simple to use. Ideally I would have liked the excess pulp to be a little dryer, but hey, the tradeoff is that compared to some other juicers it's relatively easy to clean.

By adding selective fruits (in moderation) juicing can be a pleasurable experience. *No seriously, get this right and you can even get the kids to drink their greens!* Think apples, with a hint of ginger, mixed with blueberries, celery, and lime, perhaps add a hint of fresh mint, parsley, or even kale. *Huh?* Just relax, kale is nothing more than angry lettuce, *when the amount of kale in the juice is right you won't even taste it.*

Before you diss the kale, know that it's loaded with thiamin, riboflavin, folate, iron, magnesium, and phosphorus. It's also a good source of vitamins A, C, K, B6, as well as calcium, potassium, copper, and manganese. Compared to popping a pill can you see why the health benefits surrounding juicing are unique? Juicing drives nutrients into the digestive system while at the same time packing a nutritional EZ punch. Some people run juicing alongside their current diet, and some use it as a standalone way of intermittent fasting, the benefits of which were covered in Chapter 15 (Hit the Reset Button). The trick to juicing is to make your green juice taste good and the good news is there are now hundreds of free juicing blogs to help give you additional support.

It's kinda difficult to narrow it down because there are soooo many good ones out there. I guess Kimberly Snyder would be one of the better known ones. Kimberly not only radiates with health; she also has a genuine passion for helping people. Her website has all kinds of wonderful information. There is a link to her in another chapter, or if you are rolling as a paperback homie, check out KimberlySnyder.com

Over the years I've always tried to get my information from a diverse pool of people. I find this helps give my research a healthy balance. So when it comes to juicing blogs, I'd also like to give a big shout out to Dan McDonald.

Of all the admirable qualities a man can possess, overcoming adversity is the one I admire most. Lord knows, Dan's life hasn't always been easy and on the surface he might seem like an unlikely health guru. A former drug addict whose mom died when he was just three years old, Dan was then raised by an extremely abusive father.

With over 1500 unscripted YouTube videos under his belt, Dan turned that adversity into something uniquely positive. For me, Dan's honesty is deeply refreshing. There is no slick editing and in some of Dan's early videos he makes mistakes, sometimes says weird shit, and simply carries on. What you see is what you get, which is often a man wearing no shirt but looking great! His show, *The Life Regenerator,* can be found on YouTube. Check it out.

WHEATGRASS

When talking about juicing I'd be doing you a great disservice if I didn't tip my hat to the subject of wheatgrass. Wheatgrass juice packs a real nutritional punch, and it's something I used to grow. The vitamins and minerals found in just two ounces of freshly squeezed juice equal three pounds of organic vegetables!

Wheatgrass juice is approximately 70% crude chlorophyll which is nearly identical to the hemoglobin found in red blood cells. Chlorophyll in wheatgrass juice has been shown to increase the function of the heart, help the vascular system, the intestines, and the lungs. It's also said to speed up blood circulation, cleanse the blood of waste, lower high blood pressure, and stimulate healthy tissue cell. Wheatgrass is rich in vitamin K, which is essential in bone formation.

Wheatgrass juice also contains 90 out of 102 vitamins, minerals, and nutrients, including vitamins A, B (niacin, riboflavin, thiamine), C, E, and K, as well as choline, calcium, chlorine, iron, magnesium, phosphorus, potassium, sodium, sulfur, cobalt, and zinc, not to mention twenty amino acids and about thirty enzymes. I know, right? It beats taking that harsh multi-vitamin.

If you can keep a houseplant alive then growing wheatgrass is totally doable. The grass grows quickly and in seven to ten days will be approximately 8" tall. Then you cut the grass and turn it into juice via a hand cranked juicer.

Although wheatgrass takes a little more effort, it is another good tool to have under your belt.

Wheatgrass juice can also be bought in some juice bars but it should ALWAYS be consumed fresh. There are lots of books out there on wheatgrass and the one I like best is *The Wheatgrass Book* by Ann Wigmore. It's a small, well-written and easy to understand book.

Finally, for anyone looking to overcome serious illness the Gerson Therapy is a natural treatment that activates the body's extraordinary ability to heal itself through an organic, plant-based diet, raw juices, coffee enemas (yup you heard me right), and natural supplements.

With its whole-body approach to healing, the Gerson Therapy is a *powerful* treatment to have in the toolbox. If you find yourself in a tight medical spot there is also a movie on YouTube called *The Beautiful Truth* that covers the Gerson Therapy in more detail.
Dr. Max Gerson first developed this therapy in the 1930s, initially as a treatment for his own debilitating migraines and eventually as a treatment for a *wide range* of degenerative diseases. Over the years many people have claimed to have used this therapy in the fight against cancer. Dr. Gerson's work was later carried on by his now 95-year-old daughter Charlotte.

What did we learn from this chapter?

Keeping an open mind allows you to explore practices that may have a significant impact on your life, for example seeing liquids in a different way. Juicing is truly transformative. Health is an investment, not an expense.

Homework: check out the Gerson Therapy documentary, *The Beautiful Truth* on YouTube. Here's the link:
https://www.youtube.com/watch?v=jEvQLNg3OJM

Chapter 34

YOU HAVE A GIFT

Growing up in government housing as I did wasn't always perfect but it *was* always interesting. At times people were perhaps a little too quick to settle their differences the old fashioned way, standing toe to toe with clenched fists, thus ensuring the ointment of life always had an element of grit to it. In the middle of this madness I was extremely fortunate to have someone in my life who was respected by all.

Dad was one of those unusual people who could turn his hand to anything *and do it well*. He could fix the toaster and the car; he was a meticulous maker of intricate things, he knew his way around a boxing ring, and he could play the guitar. With his magical tricks and witty jokes, he could entertain a room full of people with ease.

They say you can't teach an old dog new tricks but he once rewired a whole house to an impeccably high standard and then grew a prize vegetable garden from seed! At the age of fifty he started running in marathons and, just for good measure, he always crossed the finish line by doing a forward roll – in spite of his bad back.

Over the years he developed an uncanny knack for being right and people often came to ask his advice. He lived his life free of debt and spent money wisely. He never drank and he never swore.

And yes, he could even fix the TV set and the radio, but Dad's greatest gift was his handwritten notes which *always* carried a beautiful majestic flow.

Writing seemed to light a fire deep inside him and in his *spare* time he would leave informative notes for anybody who would read them. Before leaving for work he often left Mom a page-long letter, and when eBay first came along he spent an hour writing the most eloquent description just to sell an old coat. It's fair to say Dad's writing was not only his gift, *it was his passion.* The problem was he didn't know it, and so he settled for less.

Dad never skipped a day of work, not even when he was ill. For thirty-five years he fed his family by driving a double-decker bus that, because of his precise nature, *always* ran on time. His bus driver uniform was always neatly pressed in a certain way, and his clean, polished shoes stood out from a meter away.

No matter how late he worked, Dad remained honest and friendly with everyone he met. With an unblemished driving record that stretched more than three decades, his number one goal was to deliver people safely to their destination.

Late one night a man boarded and left his wallet behind. The wallet quickly found its way back to its owner. Another night a drunk spat in his face – *he* wasn't quite as easy to trace. If you asked my dad why he drove a big red bus he would joke, "It's an easy job, my load walks on and walks off." He found a positive in every situation.

Sometimes he wrote so much that I found myself skipping through his eloquent handwritten letters. If only I had been a bit smarter back then I would have said, *"Hey Dad, why don't you write down all those practical tips that you know?"* He often told us things like, "Never buy a house at the bottom of the hill."

Earlier this week the local news ran a story about a street that had been flooded out, except for the house that stood at the top of the hill. Dad was gifted in so many ways and I'll never know why such a meticulous mind spent eight hours a day driving a big red bus. Sadly, Dad's not here anymore so my question to *you* is this.

What's *your* passion and why aren't you doing it? In this chapter we hope to find out.

To better understand ourselves it's important to understand our psychological traits. Are you introverted or extroverted? Do you lead with your head or your heart? Are you goal oriented or people orientated?

The Swiss psychiatrist and psychoanalyst Carl Jung founded analytical psychology. He believed our distinguishing characteristics have a tendency to fit into four basic personality types. For ease of understanding, Jung color-coded these four categories using the colors yellow, red, blue, and green. See if you can recognize yourself in any of them. *Ready?*

YELLOW

Yellows like to be around people and are very much the life and soul of the party. They are sociable, expressive, imaginative, and enthusiastic. They are also informal, optimistic, and animated. Yellows have creative imaginations that can sometimes run away with them as they are *very* fast paced thinkers. Yellows don't like to be slowed down with intricate details or formalities.

RED

Reds like to take control. They are strong-willed, fast-paced thinkers, risk takers, purposeful, less patient, overtly competitive, formal, and rational. They don't like small talk and prefer people get straight to the point, which is why this description is short.

BLUE

Cool blues are deep thinkers, analytical in nature, very detail focused and formal in their thinking. They are deliberate, systematic, precise, and pay great attention to detail. They like things in their place and have excellent time management skills. They are much slower paced than the reds or yellows. Blues like to have all the facts and then logically put together a suitable answer. Blues don't like to be rushed into things or be disorganized.

GREEN

Greens are laid back, relaxed, and patient. They are easy to get along with and informal in their approach. They are social and focus more on relationships and may at times come across as emotional. They are much slower paced in their thinking and are very democratic people. They are very understanding and agreeable. Greens sometimes make the perfect go between for Reds and Yellows, who are much faster paced. They also act as the facilitator to conflicts. Greens don't like to be pushed or put on the spot.

Did you see yourself in any of these four groups? How about family members or your partner?

When we choose a partner we are *sometimes* drawn to personality types that are opposite us. We can then spend our whole lives being driven crazy by them, and they us!

Knowing what color best suits your partner can help unlock those complicated interpersonal relations. If you want to show your affection to a green, give them a hug, if you want to show affection to a red, offer to complete a task in record time. Knowing what makes a person tick is halfway to a lasting relationship.

Understanding ourselves helps us better understand our role in the workplace. When we are happy in our work we are less stressed. All too often we base our entire working lives on our academic achievements rather than taking into account our *specific* personality traits.

Knowing who and what you are may help you fit into a job you **enjoy**, although it seems quite odd that we are told to choose a career before we can even legally buy a beer. If you are currently stuck in a job that you dislike this chapter may prove particularly insightful. The good news is **it's never too late to change.**

> *The privilege of a lifetime is being who you are.*
> – Joseph Campbell

When you look at the diagram below there are no right or wrong answers, only relevant ones. It's not uncommon to find yourself 80% dominant in one color and 20% in another. Check which category best suits your personality best and then see *how* it could be put to good use in a working environment.

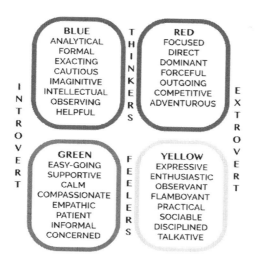

Once you have a basic understanding of these four categories life becomes less enigmatic and even teenage kids become easier to understand. Keep in mind if you are hoping to ground a *blue* teenager be sure to give them all the reasons, if you are going to ground a *red* teenager give them the fastest way to become *un*grounded. Understand that a *green* teenager needs compassion and good luck clipping the wings of a social yellow!

If we relate these colors back to the work place, can you see a blue introvert working in customer sales? *Nah, I don't think so.* How about a yellow extrovert working in sales? *Hmm, maybe.* How about a fiery red dentist? *Nah, I think I'll take my chances with the more supportive green one.*

My point is this: the only way to do great work is to love what you do. If you hate your job, *it shows*. Maybe the real reason you dislike your job is because you are not being true to yourself.

FIND YOUR GIFT

No matter which color you identify with, *you,* my friend, have a gift somewhere deep inside you. *Everyone does.* Your job is to find it. A clue might be that subject that you *love* to talk about. Once you know where to look, your gift is actually pretty easy to find. What's the one thing that you do that seems easy or obvious to you, while others may struggle or muddle their way through? Congrats, *that would be your gift.*

> *The meaning of life is to find your gift;*
> *the purpose of life is to give it away.*
> – Picasso

Once you have your gift, own it, nurture it, fight for it. It's the fastest way to a meaningful life. All too often we are told we must run with the pack, swim with the current, or follow the crowd.

Often we are conditioned to think it's too late to change; you can't do this, obey the rules, accept the limitations imposed by others. Life is good at getting us to conform the same way my dad did for most of his working life.

Do what you love and all good things will come. *This should be easy to do right? Meh, not so fast.* Let's not forget some of us were educated in decaying inner city schools and taught from an early age to think *inside* the box – such impressionable young minds all programmed to *expect and accept less.*

> *People will forget what you said, people will forget what you did,*
> *but people will never forget how you made them feel.*
> – Maya Angelou

Unfortunately, that last quote strikes a chord with my school experience. Standing in the corner facing the wall can be a deeply humiliating experience. Once used to shame those who failed to grasp basic information, it also served to suppress the human spirit. I don't ever recall my teachers every saying, "Follow your dream, do what you love, we believe in you!" Instead we were forced to learn about algebra.

BROKEN TOILETS AND BAD KNEES

As a result, I am sometimes caught up in self-doubt and conflict. Like my dad before me, I've spent much of my life doing work that perhaps I wasn't destined to do. Over the past few years I've been used to earning my money the hard way – with my hands. Give me two young guys with strong backs and I can fix your house from the ground up – although these days I find it less stressful to work quietly on my own.

Yeah, that's right, I'm the guy without an education whom you call to come clean up your yard or fix that broken gutter.

You see, I'm *still* fighting for my gift – even this minute as I write this, I'm still tormented with an internal debate about whether I should abandon this foolish idea of writing this book and just stick to being a construction worker. In the winter months when work is thin on the ground, I either read more or I write. But it might surprise you to know that over the course of the previous two chapters I've also been busy painting the side of someone's house, repairing a toilet, and hanging a new door for a customer.

Between construction gigs, I can be found with a small notebook in my pocket containing a collection of thoughts that I reshape daily until they become something interesting or new. Like my dad, I *refused* to believe old dogs are incapable of learning new things.

> *The capacity to learn is a gift;*
> *The ability to learn is a skill;*
> *The willingness to learn is a choice.*
> – Brian Herbert

While carrying out those recent home repairs, I noticed the elderly homeowner had a problem with his knee. To fix his toilet, I replaced the inlet valve, to fix his knee I suggested he apply dimethyl-sulfoxide (DMSO) directly to the area twice a day and then refrain from eating all reactive foods in the nightshade family for one month.

From the look on his face I guess he thought handymen only fixed toilets. Fortunately, he was in enough obvious pain to see past my overalls and within a week the treatment had taken most of the inflammation out of the joint. Either way, my customer was grateful even if he was a little mystified as to why he could suddenly walk unaided again.

As a rule, I generally keep my thoughts to myself for fear of being misunderstood. I was once updating a kitchen for a customer whom I overheard complaining of eye pain. When I suggested she immediately get herself checked out by a doctor, she scoffed at my advice. *I know, right? What could the handyman possibly know about optic neuritis?*

Maybe I just see things differently; I guess I've always been a bit of a square peg in a round hole. Whenever I'm asked the dreaded question *what I do for work,* I cannot claim to be a writer without a *published* word to my name, although this is how I spend my evenings. I cannot claim to be a nutritionist, although I do have an understanding of nutrition. I cannot claim to be *formally* educated, and yet I am not *un*educated. So I usually reply, "I'm just a handyman." This is generally met with a silent nod as if they already know my type. It seems that people like to pigeonhole us as a way of helping them work out who we are. I'm currently toying with the idea of telling people *I blow up bridges* just to gauge their reaction.

So by now you are probably now wondering how does a fifty-two year old, often underemployed handyman with no previous medical experience come to know all this stuff? It's called unbending persistence, although if you were paying close attention you already know this from Chapter 2.

It's true that where there is a will there is always a way. When something is important to us we either find a way or we find an excuse, *and nobody cares how good the excuses are for not doing something!* To some, I'm sure I must appear quite odd as much of this book has been written while living out of a suitcase and there are times when the only quiet place I have to type up my notes is parked in my vehicle.

With hindsight maybe this year wasn't the best time to try and write this book. In recent weeks attempting to balance work, family life, and find a new home has become a challenge. When I pick up my tool belt I can expect to get paid on Fridays, when I pick up my pen it becomes a source of friction.

I'm as human as the next guy and when something becomes stressful I also hear that uneasy loop playing over in my mind – *Give up, go back to what you know, you shouldn't be doing this.* Or my personal favorite – *This is a waste of good time.*

In my darkest hour when I was on the verge of saying, *to hell with it all, I quit,* hope came from another unpublished writer, *my daughter.* Her simple note below has been driving me to see this project through to the end.

Dad,
I want to remind you of something. You're not writing this book for you, you are writing this book for people who have little hope left, for people as ill as you were, who have no way to get out. You're writing this book for your kids and your kids' kids. You're writing this book because you said you wanted to help people. You wanted to write this book so that nobody had to go through what you went through.

You are writing this book for a reason, for a purpose. You were meant to be a writer, not a carpenter, not a mechanic, not a handyman, you were meant to mean something, to change something, to be an inspiration to people who have none left. There's a fire in you to write, a certain creativity. You were meant to be a writer and I just wanted to tell you that.

P.S. I Love you. X

It seems that regardless of my situation, this book **isn't** going to leave me alone until it's written so I have no business quitting.

What did we learn from this chapter?

Often we are *conditioned* to believe our foolish dreams are too big and we should give up on them. But the simple truth is you need only to find your gift *and then use it to do what you were put here to do.*

People generally fit into four basic groups, knowing which one you belong to will help in both your career *and* your relationships. This in turn helps reduce stress which makes you more acidic, a subject we keep coming back to. To have any chance of inner peace we should first know who and what we are.

Homework: you can see Dr. Jacobs talk about the healing power of DMSO (Dimethyl sulfoxide) for yourself by watching the short video clip below. Keep in mind there is no big money to be made from DMSO which is perhaps why some people like to jump all over it.

DMSO is sometimes used to help protect delicate donor organs while they are in on their way to transplant patients. The FDA also approved DMSO for the treatment of interstitial cystitis suggesting it has a valid place in medicine. Am I saying DMOS is right for everyone? Nope, never did say that, but for someone facing the surgeon's scalpel and a 50k bill for a knee operation, it sometimes pays to have a few options on the table (or to keep you off the table).
The video clip below is taken from 60 minutes and although it's a little dated, the information remains as valid as ever.

https://www.youtube.com/watch?v=H_szhaOS9V4

Chapter 35

WOBBLY FOOD

While I haven't always been a country boy, it's fair to say I've always been a home boy. Over several months we spent so much time wandering across Europe looking for a new home that the adventure aspect of living out of a suitcase wore thin. All the upheaval brought a new heaviness to my soul and I began to miss my orderly life, my OCD vegetable garden, and a familiar place to hang my hat.

Living in a state of limbo became too stressful and, unable to find a new place to call home, we found ourselves back in the city in a rented apartment. This has been something of an adjustment, but compared to another day of uncertainty I am, for the moment, gladly embracing my new concrete garden.

Being out of my comfort zone will no doubt come through in these final few chapters. Perhaps it's refreshing to learn that *there are days when we all struggle and* this path to clean living isn't always going to be easy. Even the best laid plans can misfire on us. As John Lennon once said, "Life is what happens while you are busy making other plans," although you never know because he also said, "I am the egg-man, I am the walrus."

Keep in mind that for much of the past decade I've been living in a small rural community, growing my own food, and heating my house with wood cut from my own land. Now I find myself living in an apartment where heat is available at the touch of a button which has the magnetic allure of a new tire in a monkey park. I've been used to preparing for cooler nights six months in advance. That usually involved dropping a tree early in the spring (to give it time to dry out) before splitting it with an axe in the fall.

Chopping down a tree may sound like work, but in many respects my life was much easier when I didn't have to worry about paying for heat. I also had access to a local freshwater stream, an organic garden, and I had gotten to know all the local farmers by name.

Although I grew up in the city, coming back has me feeling a bit like a fish out of water. The tranquility of listening to a babbling brook has been replaced with the sound of my upstairs neighbor walking across my ceiling.

As I struggle to adjust back into city life, I've taken to sucking water out of plastic bottles like everyone else and my once pristine diet has fallen. It's not that I'm being lazy. Shipping everything across the Atlantic after we'd sold our tiny homestead made no economic sense. But suddenly being disconnected from the things I had come to rely on has shown me that it is not always easy to maintain a healthy lifestyle on the fly.

Over the years I've spent enough time listening to online health gurus to form the opinion that *most are genuinely nice people* who never misplace a nutritional foot as they are carried from podcast to podcast on the shoulders of infidels. Alas, I can no longer pledge my allegiance to such high standards so I'm afraid you are going to have to tolerate a little more of my disappointing honesty. I'm a real person and sometimes I mess up.

Last night I found myself ill prepared, hungry, and staring into an open food cupboard where the only thing looking back at me was a lone box of cereal. I'm not going to pretend I'm perfect or even explain why it was there, but in a moment of weakness I ate the whole stupid box. *I know, right? What's next, Flakka?*
At the moment I seem to be backsliding faster than a speeding ticket. This morning I even caught one of my kids trying to eat *yellow Jell-O for breakfast.* The fact that yellow Jell-O has to be made ahead of time is what worries me the most. Not only did they manage to sneak yellow Jell-O-O past me, it was a premeditated attempt to eat a food group that *wobbles* and now suddenly *I'm the bad guy.*

It would seem that at any given point in this life, we are all either swimming with the current, floating on a log, or drowning. Today it feels as if I'm spluttering on a little more water than usual.

As unwelcome as this experience is, it's also inspired me to write these remaining chapters with fresh eyes. So, while I'm over here taking a hit for the team, here are a couple more home truths. You probably won't like hearing them, but I'm going to spill the beans anyways. I've recently rediscovered that unless you have access to your own year-round organic garden or limitless funds for your own private chef, there is going to come a point when you find yourself standing in a sterile supermarket feeling overwhelmed by it all, *am I right?*

For those of us struggling to find organic food grown by one armed monks or who have fallen off the no-gluten wagon, know that we are not the first nor will we be the last. There is no point in beating ourselves up over it; tomorrow is another day and we will pick ourselves up, dust ourselves off, and go again. If this is you, take a deep breath and know that it's going to be okay, okay? Let's draw a line under today and begin moving forward.

Whenever I fall from nutritional grace, I find it helpful to ask: *why the hell am I doing this, anyway?* Maybe, like me, you are just sick of being sick. Maybe you are simply tired of being tired. The only right answer is an answer that motivates *you.* Perhaps you simply want that elusive summer beach body to show off, or you need more energy to play Frisbee with the grandkids.

This whole finding what motivates you thing is pretty important – fear, pain, bikinis, accountability, family, and even recognition are all powerful motivators. Knowing which one motivates you can make the difference between success and failure.

Find the driving force behind why you do what you do – *that* has to be your reason for wanting more health and less sickness. You don't have to make this complicated; the right answer is always going to be the one that motivates you. One way to turn that thought into a powerful commitment *is to write it down.*

NOTE THE EXCUSES

Whatever it is that's motivating you, know that better health starts with what goes on the end of your fork. *You might think that's waaaay too simple, but it's actually true.* It's important to be honest with yourself here. Are there any patterns that may be creeping in – like you didn't have time to cook, or you couldn't find the right ingredients?

Then ask yourself whether these *genuine reasons* or whether you let a handful of excuses trip you up? You know the ones I'm talking about, those lame excuses like the kids made me do it, everyone else was doing it, or my personal favorite, "I thought I could have just one." *Yeah right, damn you hard licorice Scotty dogs.*

We would do well to remember there is no shame in falling down. The shame is to keep falling down in the *exact* same place! Knowing our excuses in advance helps us see the same repetitive pattern. You really want to *own* this one and sometimes writing down three reasons why we fell off the nutritional wagon forces us to acknowledge these are areas that trip us up.

So far we have our motivating reason for doing this and our excuses for not doing it, if you have your paper and pencil handy what say we go the extra mile?

Ready?

Even though we may have fallen off the wagon, starting today let's set five ground rules that we absolutely refuse to budge on *even on days when all else fails.* Setting a new baseline makes it harder to fall below the standard you deserve. For me, I'm going to say no matter how dysfunctional my current environment gets, I won't drink soda, I won't eat white bread, I won't drink milk, I won't eat any more licorice candy, and I absolutely, point blank, refuse to eat yellow Jell-O for breakfast! *I know, right? Let's hope somebody just browsing the book section didn't turn to this paragraph first.*

Once we have our shit together let's get back on the horse. To help us stay in the saddle I have some breakfast tips coming in the next chapter. They probably won't win any culinary awards, but they may help you survive meal times when all the low hanging organic fruit has been replaced with concrete. *The good news is the morning after the night before breakfast is super easy to get right.*

What did we learn from this chapter?

We all mess up – own it. Quit whining about it and try again. If you still need pizza check below.

Homework: to help you stay on track, check out this short video by Kimberly Snyder. Here Kimberly offers simple step by step advice for those looking to find a healthy pizza! If you get the opportunity, please feel free to mention where you found her information.

https://www.facebook.com/KimberlySnyderCN/videos/1510961885593465/

Chapter 36

WHAT THE HELL DO I EAT FOR BREAKFAST?

It's often said that breakfast is the most important meal of the day, this is the one piece of mainstream advice I think we can all agree on, *alas not for the reasons you may be thinking.* Breakfast is the most important meal because getting this *wrong* can set up failure for the rest of the day.

Starting the day off with a boxed cereal containing dried fruit, grains, added sugar, topped with a splash of cow's milk is sure to promote inflammation and a sugar spike even before the day has begun. *Sheesh, talk about a cereal killer.*

Even worse, many think swiping a banana off the counter as we head through the door is a "healthy" breakfast option. But ask yourself, when you eat this way, how's your hunger and energy level at about 11:30 a.m?

You may have noticed that sugar has become rampant in this world, and so too has illness. We can now walk around an0y supermarket and find fruit (another form of sugar) even when it's out of season. Let's keep in mind that not only does fruit turn to sugar, so too does protein, as do carbohydrates, as does fruit juice, so the last thing we need are more manmade sugars like sodas, cookies, and a million other additives adding to the sugar burden. As Nobel Prize winner Otto Warburg pointed out waaaaay back in 1931, cancer cells need sugar to replicate.

Now we know what breakfast *isn't,* let's be clear about what breakfast *is.* Break-fast literally means, "breaking the fast" and it's usually the first meal we eat after sleeping. For some of us, it could have been twelve plus hours since our last meal, although this isn't necessarily a bad thing. *Here's why.*

Given the average breakfast choices of cereal, toast, or fruit we might be better off eating no breakfast at all. This alone is an interesting concept. The body is smart. Ever notice how the first thing to leave us when we feel ill is our appetite? The body automatically sends us into intermittent fasting mode. This is a process that actually dates back to biblical times and even the modern day science behind fasting is pretty mind blowing.

Once again, I could easily fill up the rest of this chapter with scientific references to support this notion, but life is short and there is absolutely no time left to waste. Let's summarize by saying that intermittent fasting can (and does) help with everything from cellular repair to human growth hormone, from gene repair to improved insulin levels, yada, yada, yada. But for my money, the most interesting aspect of intermittent fasting is that it *increases* energy.

While I'm not advocating any one diet over another, many aspects of the ketogenic diet seem to fit this concept quite well because it flips the body into fat burning mode rather than using glucose as the primary fuel. And please note that I'm not saying other diets *can't* work. There are some people who obviously thrive on a vegetarian diet while others do not. The idea is to try to keep an open mind, and if your health is in a ditch don't be afraid to try new things. The only diet I can't imagine people thriving on is the Standard American Diet which, despite its name, has now been exported to many other countries around the globe. So SAD.

When we push back on the morning urge to eat sugary carbs two things happen: first, we aren't being slowed down by excess sugars and second, the body is encouraged to burn fat in the form of ketones. Ketones, as you may recall from an earlier chapter, are produced in the liver during periods of low food intake. The body then uses them as an alternative fuel source. The benefits of burning ketones for energy are many, and absent a recognized eating disorder, pushing back on carbs isn't too big an issue for most of us.

Either way, in this chapter you will find six breakfast ideas to help you break away from all those sugary carbs. These ideas are so simple even I can do them and best of all there are no calories to count. The trick is to play around with these ideas until you find one that works best for you. Ideally, in the morning we could slip into intermittent fasting mode but if that's a little too rock and roll for you, then let's kick around with the idea of increasing our intake of healthy fat while reducing our overall carb intake.

BREAKFAST IDEA #1, THE BULLET

Up until now I've been pretty good at taking things away from you and your reward for sticking with me is about to be paid. How would you like a breakfast that gently lifts brain fog and gives you more energy? Better still, it can make you feel good and, in the process, you won't even feel hungry until midafternoon. Welcome to the world of butter-coffee or "Bulletproof" coffee!

Bulletproof coffee is the brain child of Dave Asprey. Dave is one of those curious people who refuse to accept illness as an acceptable destination and while he makes no claim to have invented intermittent fasting, he certainly came up with a novel idea for a better way to do it.

First, let's address why some data suggests that drinking coffee is bad for you. It might help to know that whenever you read a study relating to coffee, the **quality of that coffee is rarely taken into account.** This is huge because the difference between regular coffee and **high quality coffee** is the same as the difference between night and day. When the two are treated as the same, results are always going to be skewed. Make no mistake, Bulletproof coffee is an upgraded version of the stuff sold in the average coffee shop.

Ever wonder why your cup of Joe makes you feel good and then a few hours later you crash? It's all to do with *where and when* the beans were harvested. Mycotoxins are a form of mold that the naked eye cannot see, once they get into the coffee harvesting process they are thought to be the reason for that crash.

So yes, finding the right bean is key, and beans grown at higher elevations in Central America are less likely to be affected by such molds. For that reason, stay well away from blends that are almost certainly going to include beans from lower down on the mountain. There are lots of options out there and Dave Asprey himself sells a brand of coffee that has been carefully screened for such molds.

Coffee sometimes gets a bad rap for stressing the adrenal glands. This is something I am well aware of, but again it's more likely to be lower grade coffee so let's not be in a rush to throw the baby out with the bathwater. If you are suffering from any type of adrenal dysfunction, supplementing with cordyceps has a wide range of health benefits. Cordyceps have adaptogenic properties which is something we will look into later.

Research shows its powerful effect to improve kidney, **adrenal,** brain, pancreatic and hormonal health. You may also find relief from a wonderfully helpful herb by the name of ashwagandha, both of these supplements have adaptogenic qualities, an important subject I'd like to try to squeeze in before this book ends.

Use Bulletproof coffee as an alternative to eating energy-zapping cereals for breakfast. I've been doing this myself for the past few months and trust me, Bulletproof butter-coffee hits the spot, it's something to try at least once and see how you do.

The science behind Bulletproof coffee is impressive, but more important, *this is a tip that works.* Bulletproof coffee is easy to make, but in order to pull it off you need three **key** ingredients.

1. A high quality coffee bean.

2. MCT oil which is short for Medium-Chain Triglycerides. MCT oil is a form of saturated fatty acid that has numerous health benefits ranging from improved cognitive function to better weight management.

3. Grass fed butter such as Kerrygold.

Please note: **Inferior substitutions simply will not work.**

Bulletproof coffee has plenty of good fats that come in the form of MCT oil and butter from grass-fed cows. If you feel good doing it, then keep going, if you feel worse, don't hesitate to stop and try something else. I hope by now the take-home message is loud and clear: *there is no one size fits all.* Don't be shy in trying out other options until you find something here that works for *you.*

A deeper reference to these key ingredients can be found in this helpful how-to video by Dave Asprey himself. To learn how to make Bulletproof coffee, click the link below.

https://www.youtube.com/watch?v=4YjLMdx3YZY

Dave can also be found on his podcast "Bulletproof radio" which is something I regularly tune into.

BREAKFAST IDEA #2, BACON SALAD

If bulletproof coffee didn't do it for you, then this next breakfast suggestion is relatively quick and easy to make, the idea here is to give you a few workable tools as opposed to being a culinary tour de force.

So our mornings look to be leaning toward the higher fat and lower carb spectrum. This leads us neatly into bacon salad.

To save time, simply pick up a box of mixed salad from the store. These types of pre-made salads aren't perfect, but they do cut down on time and waste. Bonus points if it's organic. If not, don't panic, just do the best you can. Know that this breakfast is a step up from that boxed cereal and it really doesn't take much to prepare, it's also going to help save us from a sugar crash later in the day.

I'm not going to micro-manage you on the bacon, you know how you like your bacon cooked better than I do, so long as you aren't cooking with bad fats. While the bacon is cooking grab a clean plate and throw a handful of mixed salad onto it. Add a squirt of apple cider vinegar and a pinch of salt. As soon as the bacon is done, add it to the salad and eat. The simplicity of this meal means food triggers are kept to a minimum.

If you have it, you can also pour a little MCT oil over the salad, again this ensures your breakfast starts with plenty of good fats which will keep you from feeling deprived throughout the day.

As with anything new, be aware of how this makes you feel. While most people will experience a positive health benefit from adding MCT oil, I can think of at least one person I know who seems to do better without it. If your regular breakfast is usually cereal, then you may need to give your body a chance to adjust to this cleaner, leaner way of eating breakfast. Sometimes it just takes a little time.

You may be wondering why eggs are missing from the bacon salad. While it may be true that eggs are nutritious, there are many, many people who react badly to them. For now, let's try this breakfast without the eggs and then perhaps a month down the road add them in and closely monitor how you feel. As mentioned in a previous chapter, not everyone will roll on the floor and turn blue; some reactions will be delayed and subtle, such as general fatigue.

BREAKFAST IDEA #3, GO-AVOCADO

Technically a fruit, avocados have a lot of vegetable-type qualities. Avocados are nutritionally dense and a *better* source of potassium than bananas. Do I like avocado? No, I can't stand the damned things but it's another form of good fat and if it keeps me on my feet I'll eat them.

Although the idea is to limit fruit for breakfast, adding a little lime juice and a *few* blueberries makes an avocado more palatable. You can even add a pinch of Himalayan sea salt for added kick. Avocados come loaded with heart-healthy monounsaturated fatty acids. Need more fiber? Go avocado.

BREAKFAST IDEA #4, BUDWIG

If we haven't found your thang yet, then rest assured, the Budwig breakfast is an interesting one. This idea is accredited to German biochemist Johanna Budwig who was also a highly respected pharmacist and held degrees in physics and chemistry. She lived to be ninety-five and was nominated seven times for the Nobel Peace Prize. *Why am I bothering to mention all this?* Obviously Johanna Budwig was a very smart lady and her simple Budwig diet has been suggested by some to be a powerful protocol for certain cancers. You can find more information relating to this on a website called Cancer Tutor. Am I saying this is a cure for cancer? *Nope, never did that, never would, just thought you might find the information behind the Budwig diet interesting reading.*

The reason I've included the Budwig breakfast here is because it's simple to make and it tastes good. For this little party piece, you are going to need some *organic* flaxseed oil and some organic cottage cheese (even better would be goat's milk quark or sheep's milk quark if you can find it). You can also add some berries to make it taste good, preferably berries that are in season.

Here's how you make it:

Place 6 tablespoons of organic cottage cheese in a mixing bowl.

Add 3 tablespoons good quality flaxseed oil.

(Only buy QUALITY flaxseed oil from a store that keeps it fresh in a refrigerator and always check the sell-by date.)

Add 2 tablespoons freshly ground flaxseeds

Whisk it all together with a simple immersion hand blender and you are good to go.

Optional: if you want to make it more palatable, throw in a handful of berries or ground nuts.

This breakfast is simple, filling, and unless you are dairy sensitive, it's super healthy!

BREAKFAST IDEA #5, OKAY-OATS

There are times when you may feel a need to refuel with a few carbs. Gluten-free oats are a much better option than toast. It's important to steer away from mass produced oats as they are almost certainly cross-contaminated with gluten during processing. Plain oats can be made more interesting by adding nuts, berries, or a shake of cinnamon. Buying plain oats from a health food store ensures you aren't subjecting your digestive system to added sugars.

Resist buying instant oats which usually come loaded with sugar. Instead, soak plain oats in a bowl of water overnight. In the morning simply strain them and heat them in a saucepan with a little fresh water or almond milk. Viola! They are as fast as instant oats *without* all the additives. Oats are also quick to make and a good source of fiber.

BREAKFAST IDEA # 6, MINI-MASTER

Some mornings you might not feel up to eating a big breakfast, if this is you, simply make a mini master cleanse drink (which is what I did this morning). This will not only help detoxify your liver; it will keep hunger at bay for a few hours. Generally speaking, this works best with room temperature water.

Add 3 tablespoons of fresh lemon juice to twelve ounces of water. Mix in a teaspoon (or less) of pure, dark maple syrup and a pinch of cayenne pepper. Shake and drink.

A month from now your liver will thank you. Don't be afraid to mix this up a little. In recent months I've been doing this without the maple syrup and I'm still here to tell the tale.

What did we learn from this chapter?

We are all different, what works for one person might not work for another and it's important to be open to new ideas. The breakfast options in this section are pretty basic but they will outperform cereal or toast.

Homework: for some unique nutritional insight, check out Dr. Berg on YouTube. Dr. Berg makes interesting short videos and I always come away learning something new.

Link: https://www.youtube.com/watch?v=5vloHR7J24I

Chapter 37

WHAT THE HELL DO I EAT FOR LUNCH?

The key to making any of this work is to try to plan ahead. If you are at work during lunchtime, your choices are either taking a packed lunch or eating out. For those eating out, a word of caution – remember to steer well away from fried food, which is usually cooked in bad fats, also known as trans fats, hydrogenated oils, or vegetable oils. Fast food places love to use these because they are cheap. Trust me, sooner or later those motherfatters will mess you up.

Whenever you find yourself eating out, take just a second to look around at all the other folks frequenting your local food bar. If there are lots of vibrant, healthy looking people wearing spandex you should be good to go. If not, remember Farmer Fred? When all the animals at the same watering hole look sick, what does this tell you?

Before you find yourself sitting in a new restaurant take away some of the guesswork by Googling "Trip Adviser." This is a great resource for anyone travelling or on vacation. You'll find up-to-date reviews and reading other people's experiences is a sure way to gauge what to expect. You could also look for vegan/vegetarian/gluten free/paleo places.

THE SIX P RULE

For some of us, eating out can be a luxury. If your choices are eating out or paying the rent on time, then a packed lunch is not only a great way to save money, it also helps you have more control over what you put into your mouth. The trick to making this work is, once again, preparation. Remember the rule of Ps. Proper-planning-prevents-piss-poor-performance. Leaving everything until the last minute makes for a hungry, stressful day. A packed lunch *is always best done the night before* and then left in the fridge for morning.

Again, I'm not trying to win any medals for cooking here, but I am aware that there is a new generation that may not be used to preparing their own food. The whole idea of this chapter is to get them through to dinner without having to rely on any form of fast food. For those of us caught in a bind, the ideas offered here are quick and inexpensive.

There are a million and one great cookbooks out there and I'll be recommending one of them as we move through this chapter. But when I'm out and about, here are just a few simple ideas that I use. Are they perfect? Nope, like most people, I'm sometimes caught in less than optimal circumstances and just have to do the best I can. But it *is* possible to pack a lunch without resorting to sandwiches or grains. This doesn't have to be anything fancy and dollar for dollar they are a better value than eating out.

This first part I call a "lazy salad" because it's so quick and easy to make. Great if you can afford to go all organic, but if not, don't sweat it – *any* salad has to be a better option than eating deep fried fast food, *am I right?*

The night before, pick up a boxed mixed salad and toss some of it into some kind of Tupperware box along with some thinly sliced root vegetables like carrots, celery, broccoli, onion etc. If your local store has them, throw in a handful of freshly sprouted broccoli seeds and some olives (which are loaded with good fat). Bonus points if you can source these locally. Easy now with the condiments – instead, sprinkle a little apple cider vinegar, sea salt, and MCT oil if you have some over the salad and just for good measure you can even add a little turmeric.

Tip – To make life easier, buy a $1 plastic spray bottle, remove the spray section and screw it directly onto the top of your vinegar bottle. It works like a charm and is perfect for evenly applying vinegar to salads.

So far we have invested maybe five minutes of the day preparing this. Keep coming, we are almost there. For protein you could try adding in any leftovers from the night before. If you do okay with eggs, then two boiled eggs should help keep you going. If you *really* are pressed for time, try sardines direct from the can. Hey, sardines have enough selenium to counter any mercury found in the sea. And they are a quick, easy, and good source of good fats. They are also a healthier option than eating fast food for lunch.

If you *really* want to be ahead of the game you can take a hot thermos flask filled with homemade soup. Homemade soup is super easy to make and it's something I cover in the next chapter. Note, so far *none* of these ideas have included gluten. Keep in mind when we remove gluten in the form of bread and pasta etc. we also remove an element of fiber. Some of us may need more fiber than others to help keep our bowel movements regular, again we are all unique. Fortunately, there are *other* ways of getting fiber without piling bread on your plate.

If you can tolerate it, one way is to eat more brown rice which, once cooked, can later be eaten cold. Brown rice has far more fiber than white rice. Yup, I already know about the higher arsenic content of brown rice, but remember these are your do-or-die tips for folks who may be new to preparing their own food. And these tips are a step up from eating out. Fiber is important for healthy gut bacteria because it serves as a pre-biotic. Whenever you cook rice, try adding a little pasture-raised butter. Despite what they tell you, this is a form of good fat and it will help keep hunger at bay.

For dessert, let's not go too crazy with the fruit. Maybe go with berries or, to keep things interesting, peel and slice a Granny Smith apple. Typically, Granny Smith apples have less sugar than most of those new hybrid apples. Feel free to add a squirt of lemon juice directly onto the sliced apple to stop it from going brown (nope, no need to genetically modify it).

Many people like to pack a banana for lunch, but be aware that they can be pretty high in sugar so, as always, *moderation is key.* I'm sure we have all heard that bananas are a good source of potassium but if it's potassium you are after you could also go avocado instead. Avocado ticks the good fat, good fiber box and it's lower in sugar than a banana. To boost the fat content of these desserts try whisking them up with cream of coconut – this usually comes in a can, but hey, we are in survival mode here so it all counts and adding berries to it makes it okay.

If you find yourself getting hungry between meals, try nibbling on sliced coconut or a small piece of ginger to tame that snack attack. Ginger can be peeled quickly by using the back of a spoon, try it for yourself and see. Ginger has more health benefits than you or I can shake a hairy stick at and it's a great way to stop rewarding yourself with all those unhealthy snacks.

Your absolute number one best option for a drink is always going to be natural spring water. Forget all those "healthy" fruit juices (unless you are vegetable juicing of course). Without the fiber, fruits are simply liquid sugar in a carton. If you have a problem quitting soda, don't shoot yourself in the foot by going sugar free. Additives used in those sugar free drinks are *not* your friend. If you really need that fizzy-fix you could try switching to kombucha provided you aren't dealing with an ongoing candida issue. Even then I suspect this is a much better option than soda. You can find kombucha in most health food stores and in the long run it's also better for you than all those crash and burn high caffeine energy drinks.

Tip – Wherever you live in the world you can usually find a freshwater spring that's close to you by clicking on your address at "findaspring.com." It always pays to test any new water source, however, and this is easy to do with a quick Google search.

KIDS

Kids are funny – I should know, I used to be one. Ask any kid if they would like some sliced up coconut with cucumber and carrots dipped in hummus and they will inevitably say **no.** Now, if you pay close attention you will notice that kids spend an inordinate amount of their time hanging off the fridge door complaining there is nothing to eat. Use this to your advantage.

Kids are visual; if foods are cut up and arranged in bold colors right in front of them, they will be more tempted to try them. Inside the fridge, strategically place several **open** containers of the most random healthy things you can think of and set them at kids' eye level. You can add to the visual by buying small colorful berry bowls for about a buck a piece.

Kids also like to see how far they can push you. If that's how your crew rolls, then you can even try a little reverse physiology. First, make the containers of cut of vegetables look attractive *and then tell your kids not to eat them.* It may also help to have some form of healthy dip on hand too. Once it's in front of them, sooner or later they will eat it – even if it's only to tell you how gross it is. *I know right, getting a kid to eat healthy can be like negotiating with a terrorist.*

To save on waste, don't use big containers. It could be just a few well-placed bowls that might include any of the following: sliced olives, cut ginger, purple cabbage, sliced coconut, chopped broccoli, sliced carrots, cucumber, quartered or sliced boiled egg, sugar snap peas, thinly sliced celery, radishes, sprouts, yada, yada, yada. Obviously I'm just making a few suggestions and I'm not saying to put all of these out in one day. Try rotating them and see what works best for you.
Kids are notoriously fickle eaters. It's not uncommon for them to also develop a bad habit of eating potato chips. Ideally we want to wean them off chips altogether, but for now let's not initiate a full blown mutiny. If this is you, try buying *only* plain chips. Make no mistake, plain flavored chips still have undesirable things in them but the idea is that during the transition time, kids will eat fewer of them.

Whatever you try, it helps to use a little imagination. But always remember to go easy on the fruit, especially when it's out of season. If this all seems like work, remember this is easier than being held hostage to cook meals throughout the day – and so far it's also been a pretty easy day for the dishwasher. *Now you dunnit it.*

Is it me, or is the dishwasher the only home appliance we make excuses for? Ask yourself if you are really just "rinsing" those dirty dishes before putting them in the dishwasher or have we all been hoodwinked into doing the job we've paid the dishwasher manufacturers to do?

Think about it, what if suddenly we had to rinse all our dirty socks before we put them in the washing machine? Or we had to partially iron our clothes before asking the iron to step up and do *its* job. *I know, right? People would be in the streets rioting with pitchforks – and rightly so.*

We have the technology to put a robot on Mars and yet we still have to "rinse" dirty dishes before we dare put them in the dishwasher. *Really?* I'm telling you, those damned dishwasher sales men are laughing all the way to the bank. Ask yourself, when was the last time you saw a homeless dishwasher salesman? No, you never have because they are all too busy driving around in expensive sports cars and smoking oversized, hand-rolled Cuban cigars. *But I digress.*

SPROUTING

Imagine having a vegetable garden that produces clean nutrition year round with no weeding, no back breaking digging, no bugs, no green thumb necessary, no greenhouse, and *not even any soil.* And now imagine that the crops from this garden have a *higher nutritional content than any whole food found in the supermarket!* Better still, imagine that this crop can be grown within days on your kitchen counter. It's incredibly cost effective and simple to do.

Sprouts are something you can include in your lunchtime meals and sprouting involves very little in the way of materials. It's so easy to do a child can do it – *you catching my drift?* Sprouting is a great way to get them to eat their healthy greens. This becomes easier and more fun when kids get to experiment with sprouting and see things sprout as quickly as overnight. Sprouted seeds are packed with nutrients and live enzymes. For sensitive individuals, sprouts can be a superior way to get your key nutrients rather than taking synthetic vitamins.

There really isn't too much to sprouting. Simply buy some sprouting seeds online or locally and allow them to soak in a glass jar. Usually the soaking period is twelve hours. Keep rinsing them off until they sprout. During sprouting, it's obviously important to keep everything clean. The key here is to regularly rinse the sprouted seeds to make sure they don't get any mold on them – but beyond that, there isn't much to do. **If you are just starting out, try starting with some of the *larger* seeds, it's just easier all round.** For the first couple of times, DON'T sprout more than a tablespoonful, this is a project you should *grow* into (yup, meant that pun).

Here's a simple formula for sprouting:

- Buy (LARGE) seeds from a local store or a sprouting company online
- Soak the seeds
- Pour the seeds into a strainer
- Rinse every couple of hours
- Watch for tails to sprout from the seeds
- Keep rinsing to stop them from drying out
- Always check for mold

Sprouting is good to try because:

- Anyone can do it
- It adds vital nutrients to the body
- It's inexpensive
- It doesn't involve a lot of time
- You don't need a big garden
- Sprouting even can even be done in a small apartment, caravan, or RV

There are lots of places to buy the sprouting seeds; you can buy them online or even at your local supermarket. Sproutpeople.org is an online supplier that offers decent products along with more detailed information and equipment if you need it. The bulk of the information is given freely on their site.

If your system is fragile or just out of balance, sprouting can be a good way to get key nutrients into your body. *Learning about nutrient-dense* foods, superfoods, sprouts, and juicing is a lot easier to do than learning about supplements, and can be a lot less problematic.

KICKING OLD HABITS

Whenever we change the way we eat, simple plans tend to work better than complicated ones, and no plan will work if you don't understand it. The bigger challenge is to get you to let go of old habits. I have a friend – let's call him Tom – who once asked me if I knew of a quick fix to help with his abdominal pain. It had developed over the past few months and had become a real problem whenever he ate salt and vinegar chips.

At considerable cost, his doctor had already performed an esophagogastroduodenoscopy (EGD) test to examine the lining of the esophagus, stomach, and first part of the small intestine with a camera. Nothing obvious was discovered and Tylenol was prescribed for the pain.

Over the next fifteen minutes, Tom continued to divulge the full symptoms of his stomach which now included nausea from taking the Tylenol. Finally, he stopped talking long enough to ask me what I thought. After a moment of deep thought I said that a solution was indeed available to him as the technician operating the expensive camera inside his body had missed something of critical importance.

Eagerly he listened as I motioned with my hand for him to come a little closer. As he leaned in to better hear what I had to say I gently whispered in his ear ... *"Tom, just stop eating the chips."*

A month or so passed and not a single chip passed his lips, and *as if by sorcery* his problem went away and *never* came back! Later it was declared by his doctor that his gut pain had gone into a form of spontaneous remission. Maybe the reason Tom succeeded was simply because he'd implemented that simple change.

Again, if this is all new to you, don't panic. A good rule of thumb is to simply fill 50% of every plate you serve yourself with green leafy vegetables. Do *this one thing* and you will be ahead of the pack.

I fully appreciate that sometimes all this can be a little difficult to understand, which is why I've been so keen to recommend several blogs along the way. To be fair, there simply isn't room to list *all* the good ones I've taken information from over the years and it's been a real internal struggle for me to have to leave some of them out.

The ones I'm recommending here are snapshots that represent so many others. This next one comes from a lady who makes highly informative videos covering a wide range of topics. Check her out in today's homework.

What did we learn from this chapter?

Thinking about meals ahead of time is the key to your success. Having something quick and easy that's prepared ahead of time can stop a snack attack in its tracks. If you wait until you are hungry before figuring out what snacks you are going to eat, then everything becomes hard.

Homework: Check out montrealhealthygirl.com, or search for her videos on YouTube. Brittany has an extensive understanding of the healing process and she always manages to pack a few gems into her videos. She has a genuine passion for helping people, which is very apparent and oozes through in her highly informative videos.

Link: https://www.youtube.com/watch?v=dWO5ufhPLc4

Chapter 38

WHAT THE HELL DO I EAT FOR DINNER?

Anything you decide to cook for dinner is only going to be as good as the ingredients you use. Finding local produce is my preferred option, but should supply be thin on the ground, don't panic because it's not your only option. If you know where to find it, organic produce can be delivered directly to you. And often a simple Google search will give you options in your area. These days you can even get grass-fed meat delivered direct to your door. Meat arrives fresh, sealed, and frozen via the miracle of dry ice. I've occasionally used Butcher box.com; the meat is quality and they ship for free. Once you have your materials the next step is to find a way to save on time.

Cooking a healthy meal from scratch can be time consuming which is why a pressure cooker is a useful addition to any kitchen. Pressure cookers typically cook a meal 70% faster than regular cookers. Pressure cookers are also a good way to reduce the lectin content of certain foods, which is something we covered earlier. If you have never used a pressure cooker you are in for a pleasant surprise.

OMG, THE NO PRESSURE, PRESSURE COOKER

When time is limited there can be a lot of pressure surrounding mealtimes, so here's a clever idea that's gives you control of your kitchen. Hear me out on this one because even though pressure cookers have been around for a long time, they recently went all electric. This not only made things safer, it also made cooking a whole lot easier and faster. If you only take away one tip from this chapter, then please let it be this: Google **the Instant Pot**. You can literally throw food in an Instant Pot, walk away, and come back to a hot meal in half the time! The Instant Pot has revolutionized cooking and for those who are culinary challenged like me, cooking with an Instant Pot is a game changer. The Instant Pot was the first kitchen appliance to ever go viral, and with no advertising it quickly sold out.

It's fair to say that if my wife ever decided to run off with my best friend (a) I'd sure miss him and (b) this is probably how I'd feed myself until he came to his senses.

There is an entire Instant Pot community on Facebook. I like to refer to them as potheads. Potheads offer lots of helpful recipes to get you started and the Instant Pot also comes with its own helpful cookbook. The one I have in my kitchen is sold on Amazon for around $99. It offers good value for the money because it doubles as a slow cooker with the added benefit of using a stainless steel pot. It's a win/win. As with any product I recommend, my primary affiliation is always with **you.** With that in mind, I have refrained from putting in a direct link – that way you know I am recommending this product because it works rather than trying to profit from any kind of affiliated kick back.

REGULAR SLOW COOKER

Even without a pressure cooker, another option is to use a good old *regular* slow cooker. While this option isn't quite as rock and roll as the Instant Pot, slow cookers are generally less expensive to buy and a useful tool to help get a hot meal on the table.

For those who are used to eating out of a can, here's a super easy way to make homemade chicken soup (trust me, I'm no cook and even I struggle to get this one wrong). Preparing this meal takes maybe ten minutes. Do it in the morning and you always have a healthy hot meal to come home to. This style of cooking is real back-to-basics and pretty hard to mess up. You can obviously leave out anything that you are sensitive to.

For this example, simply place a whole chicken (preferably free range, local, or organic) into a slow cooker or large cooking type stock pot. Add enough water to cover the chicken, chop up and add a couple of onions and some vegetables. These can by anything; maybe throw in some carrots, broccoli, celery, mushrooms, cabbage, potatoes, garlic etc.

Add a teaspoon of Himalayan salt and turn it up high to get it cooking and then let simmer with the bones still in for a good few hours. If you have a low enough setting you can even let it simmer overnight, which adds to the flavor. As long as you are happy that the chicken is cooked you can let it simmer for as little or as long as you like. That's it! Obviously remove all bones before serving. The more times you make this meal the easier it gets. Sometimes I'll add a little turmeric and ginger. It's really not an exact science, just practice, eat, and repeat.

Tip – You can also add a tablespoon of apple cider vinegar to the soup as it simmers. This will help leech more minerals out of the bones. Minerals are what most of us are deficient in. Cooking with pasture-raised, wild caught, and organic meats generally increases the mineral count.

Waiting until you are hungry to figure out what's for dinner is a sure recipe for frustration. Planning ahead is the key to a successful outcome. The chicken soup is a cost-effective meal that typically feeds a family of four twice over. It's the opposite of a microwave meal and your Roman ancestors probably made a similar version as they marched across Europe bossing people about.

BONE BROTH

Bone broths are a super healthy option and are easy to make. Typically, bone broth is made using the bones of pasture-raised beef, lamb, pork, chicken, or even the heads from wild caught fish. Bone broth is best left simmering for a *minimum* of eight hours – but to get the most minerals out of bones, longer is better. Beef bones can cook for up to forty-eight hours. To help flood the broth with minerals, add vinegar to the water. While the bone broth simmers, you can also add your favorite herbs or vegetables to help make the taste more palatable. Once cooked, either sip on the liquid or use it as gravy poured over meals. You can even freeze any leftovers to give flavor to a later dish. Although you can certainly cook a bone broth on the stove top using a regular large pan, I find it easier to leave it in a slow cooker.

Tip – Given that minerals are essential for the absorption of vitamins, think of bone broth as a daily multi-mineral alternative. Bone broths are a great way to safely increase mineral intake, this can be a particularly useful way for sensitive individuals to get their minerals. It's worth noting that without minerals, vitamins cannot be absorbed properly.

The amount of minerals found in bone broth is largely dependent on the quality of the bones. Finding bones from grass- or pasture-raised animals in your area is easy to do with a quick Google search.

Bone broth is a solid staple of the paleo diet because it contains an abundance of the amino acids arginine, glycine, glutamine, and proline. All of these amino acids have powerful healing properties, *especially for the lining of the gut.* Some digestive issues can be helped with a bone broth fast; some believe a three-day bone broth fast can help heal the damaged lining of the gut. Bone broth can help alleviate joint pain and boost your immune system. Bone broth is collagen-rich and collagen is known to tighten the skin and even make your hair shiny.

If you don't have the time or resources to make bone broth for yourself, Dr. Axe has just brought out an instant powdered bone broth that literally takes 5 minutes to make. I haven't tried it yet, but I suspect that any bone broth Dr. Axe puts his name on will be a decent quality product.

Recommended reading – *The Keto Diet* by Leanne Vogel. I'm currently halfway through reading this and I can tell it's going to be one of my go-to books. It's beautifully designed, well written, and all her recipes are easy to follow.

What did we learn from this chapter?

Cooking at home gives you greater control over what you eat. This is helpful for anyone with food sensitivities. Bone broths come loaded with minerals and amino acids which can help heal the gut.

Homework: to help keep this information balanced, here's a wonderful short video by Christa Orecchio. Christa always puts a smile on my face with her clear, easy to understand style.
https://thewholejourney.com/is-a-ketogenic-diet-good-or-bad/

Chapter 39

FREESTYLING

One of the problems with blindly taking supplements is that so many health problems today link back to an immune system that's been spooked. With over a hundred autoimmune conditions to choose from, it's plausible that many patients are undiagnosed or even misdiagnosed. This is important because many supplements are capable of tipping the Th1 Th2 balance too far in one direction. If you have been down the pill-popping road *and felt worse for it,* then perhaps consider autoimmunity as an option.

There are a lot of variables surrounding supplementation and they can at times be incalculable. You may recall that we first talked about this back in Chapter 13. What works well for one person might not bring the same results in another.

While there could be many reasons for such differences, I suspect that in illness, the liver and kidneys are usually pulling a double shift and, as you can imagine, taxing an already overloaded system with handfuls of supplements rarely bodes well. Keep in mind that the liver performs a wide range of bodily functions; some estimates suggest that the liver is involved in more than 500 hundred different functions! It's imperative we show it some respect.

Still, there are times when genuine deficiencies need to be addressed in the body and that, my friend, *is the aim of this chapter!* The fact that this subject is so late in the book highlights my reluctance to lead you down a pill-popping path. The problem is that many of us have become quick to think of pill-popping as an effective solution. It is not.

So why do we need supplements?
In a perfect world we wouldn't need them at all and no doubt there *was* a time when we could have gotten all our vitamins and minerals from the foods we ate. If your body could talk to you, *this would be the preferable way.* However, modern farming practices are quick to bring crops to

market and slow to allow the soil time to recover. This really means that anyone eating standard supermarket food will at some point usually need to plug a few nutrient gaps.

So let's back up and ask how our early ancestors managed to survive *without* pockets full of pills? The short answer is right under your feet. Today, as never before, our soils are in a state of exhaustion.

To compensate for their lack of trace minerals, farmers have learned to prop up the soil with chemical additives. Doing this only serves to compound the problem because it causes an *imbalance* of trace minerals and disrupts the life cycle of important microorganisms found in the soil.

SOIL

We should first think of soil as a bank account. If you take too much out, you have to deposit some back in or the soil simply becomes bankrupt – and this is where we are today. Our ancestors had the good sense to rotate crops and give the soil time to recover. Today we feed our crops harsh chemicals and fertilizers in an attempt to *force* them grow quicker. Make no mistake, the result is more profitable crops for the farmer, but for your body's cells, those missing minerals soon add up to have a negative effect on your health.

Side by side, crops grown this way may look the same, but vegetables absorb these important trace minerals through their roots – which you then eat. Your trillions of tiny cells require a wide range of trace minerals to keep your body running optimally.
Let's be clear, whenever food is grown for profit, it arrives on your kitchen table devoid of important minerals. When the soil becomes mineral deficient *you* become mineral deficient!

Whatever minerals were found in farm soil 100, fifty or even twenty-five years ago are almost certainly not found in the soil today. Today, commercially grown, nutrient *deficient* crops are really imposters of the real thing. They may look the same as regular crops, but they are weaker than their clean cousins and as such are more susceptible to bug infestations. Man's solution? Spray the crops with more poisons! *I know, right? You couldn't make this stuff up.*

Think of it this way:

> *Man owes his existence to a six-inch layer of topsoil—*
> *and the fact that it rains.*
> – Anonymous

Our great grandparents had a solution to solve this mineral depletion and it wasn't at all complicated. They knew that if they placed old food scraps in a small garden pile, the scraps would gradually decompose. This decomposed matter could then be added back into the soil as compost creating a *perfect* cycle. A compost pile costs zero money to build and yet it's incredibly beneficial to the soil. This process is really nothing more than putting the nutrients back into the soil the old fashioned way.

Many of our small, *local* farmers today still work this way, and as I mentioned earlier, many of these small farmers *may or may not have* the organic seal and that's okay too. For my money, knowing a small farmer who understands soil by name is of equal importance.

The answer to nutrient-poor foods that society has come up with is to sell you synthetic multivitamins. Often these types of low-end vitamins are sold in large discount stores and do more harm than good. Quality is key with any supplement, and there is some merit to occasionally taking a food-based multivitamin, but even this can have drawbacks.

Given that we are each unique it can be a real challenge to find a single pill to fit all our needs. Running parallel with this problem is the current upsurge in thyroid and autoimmune diseases and the fact that many of the ingredients in the pills can even make you feel worse. So what's the answer? First, know that **you simply cannot supplement your way out of a bad diet and with a good diet most people don't need supplements.** Second, perhaps adopt a more targeted approach to occasionally using supplements. When we are trying to hit a nutritional target, we could think of the standard multivitamin as a shotgun approach, i.e., as hitting a

435

broad number of targets. A more targeted approach would be like using a sniper rifle with a telescopic lens.

The easy way to ensure your food has the vital minerals you need is to bring this full circle and grow some of your own food. This is something you can do even with a single raised bed measuring just 4ft x 8ft. As any simple soil test demonstrates, foods grown in *nutrient dense soils* have more minerals. When you run the cost side by side, home grown food simply outperforms all other options. As soon as I am settled again, planting a garden will be my number one priority. For now, I'm still trying to adjust to my new living environment and like millions of others my diet has become less than ideal.

With that in mind, here are some of the supplements I *occasionally* take myself and why. Unless you know **why** you are taking a supplement, then really you have no business putting it in your mouth. I also make a point of tracking everything I take in a day planner to monitor results. I strongly urge you to do the same. Keeping your notes simple makes this process so much easier to do.

Over the years I've tried literally hundreds of different supplements. And some of them worked better than others. For me, rather than being brand loyal or tied to any one supplement long term, I respond better when I switch it up from time to time. I refer to this style of supplementing as "freestyling."

As long as I feel a benefit from taking a supplement I'll stick with it, but as soon as I feel the benefits begin to plateau, I'll drop it like a hot potato and rotate to the next supplement. At some point I'll eventually cycle back around to the same supplement. This style of rotating my supplements seems to works for me, perhaps because over time I'm covering more bases, or perhaps because I've simply become better at trusting my own intuition. Unfortunately, the downside of this means I'm sometimes left with a graveyard of half-used supplement bottles.

But remember, although there are many beneficial supplements on the market, the least complicated route is to get the lion's share of your minerals and vitamins from clean nutrition, bone broths, foods grown in nutrient dense soils, and pasture-raised meats. All these are much easier to get right than are supplements.

As our time is now quickly running out, I guess I'm forced to narrow this down a little. Obviously, all minerals and vitamins play an important role in the body but if I were about to be stranded on a desert island I would hope to have with me the following: a good probiotic, magnesium, a form of krill oil, and good old vitamin C. If you are wondering why I didn't mention the all-important **vitamin D** it's because on this desert island I'd imagine there would be plenty of sunshine – so perhaps I'll go with a B complex instead.

Trying to narrow so many supplements down to just five is a difficult challenge because there are so many *other* compounds that play an important role in good health. Hence the reason I tend to "cycle" often which typically means I'm hitting more bases over time. Is this a perfect system? Nope, but to be honest, when it comes to taking supplements I've yet to see a system that is. Either way, let's first take a look at probiotics.

PROBIOTICS help increase the amount of good bacteria found inside the gut and are typically taken orally. It's debatable, but for my money I highly rate probiotic supplements simply because it's estimated that the bacteria in your body outnumber your cells by about ten to one. That could be as many as 100 trillion bacteria living inside you! If you think about it, you are actually more bacteria than you are human. *I know, right? All that antibacterial soap is slowly killing you!*

Typically, the majority of these bacteria live in the intestinal system which we now know is heavily involved with the immune system and even serotonin production. Given the significance of this, it's important to *optimize* the health of the bacteria in the gut in any way we can and probiotic supplementation is one way. There is some debate surrounding which probiotics work best, but it really doesn't matter how good your probiotic is if the bad bacteria in your gut are being fed excessive amounts of sugar.

Keep in mind there are things that nourish the good bacteria and there are things that can accelerate the growth of bad bacteria. One of the fastest ways to upset this balance is to take antibiotics. Obviously there are times when this is unavoidable which makes the topic of probiotics all the more valid because probiotics help repopulate the gut bacteria. It's probably worth mentioning that approximately 70% of all the antibiotics being manufactured today are used in the food supply. *I know, right? Ever wonder what happens when we eat the animal that eats antibiotics?*

Where we choose to buy the foods we eat will have a profound effect on the delicate balance of good and bad bacteria in our gut. One of the most effective ways to help *suppress* the *bad* bacteria is to limit your sugar intake. Sugar feeds bad bacteria and let's not forget that fruit, and fruit juices in particular, are also loaded with sugar – some more than others.

On the flip side, clean, whole vegetables help feed the good bacteria. The fiber in these foods can be thought of as pre-biotics. You can also eat foods that are high in natural probiotics such as fermented vegetables like sauerkraut, kimchi, and certain pickled vegetables – preferably organic when possible because most non-organic produce is sprayed with harsh chemicals that may affect those trillions of good bacteria that live inside you.

Be aware that store-bought yogurt and kefir is typically loaded with sugars and additives *despite what the marketing on the label says.* Also, if your water is chlorinated it's going to affect your good bacteria. Knowing that our tiny gut bugs make up 90% of who we are, some estimates suggest those tiny gut bugs outnumber our cells by 10 to 1. Perhaps we should be showing them a little more respect. Dump the junk water and go with natural spring water whenever possible.

Whenever you make bold moves to change the good bugs in your stomach it's best to start small and go slow. An ideal starting point is to gradually introduce fermented foods into your diet, especially if you are dealing with candida. When it comes to supplementing with probiotics some are best taken on an empty stomach and others require food, so always read the label. There are lots of good probiotics on the market.

Given that we are all so different a little trial and error can be expected. When you hit the right probiotic you may *feel* your overall mood improves, the time to switch is when that feeling plateaus.

As a rule of thumb, try to steer clear of bargain priced probiotics. In my opinion you are better off paying a little extra and getting a quality probiotic. Here are three suggestions, but there are plenty of other good probiotics on the market. Prescript-Assist sells a probiotic that is made up of SBOs (soil based organisms). Whenever I look to switch things around a little, I also seem to do well with a probiotic made by Elixa Probiotic, although at the time of writing they are currently sold out in the U.S.

Dr. Mercola also sells a good probiotic as does Standard Process which is their prosynbiotic probiotic. These aren't the only four options out there; I'm just trying to save you a little time. Ultimately it's important to find one that works for *you*.

MAGNESIUM makes it to the list *not* because it's an essential mineral but because it covers so many bases. From head to toe magnesium is involved in more than 300 metabolic reactions. It can help with everything from normalizing blood pressure to keeping a steady heart rhythm. A lack of magnesium can play a key role in anxiety and fatigue and it may surprise some to know that magnesium even plays a key role in the skeletal system. For sure, it's just as important to the health of your bones as calcium is. Magnesium also made it to the list because a deficiency can be caused as a result of parasitic infection, candida overgrowth, or as a result of a poor diet such as the Standard American Diet. However, before you rush out to add it to your routine you should know there is a little more to magnesium supplementation than meets the eye.

Magnesium is not easily absorbed in pill form. Its ability to be utilized in the body is co-dependent on several other compounds such as calcium and vitamins D and K2. This tight group is commonly found together in certain foods such as spinach and other dark leafy greens, also in fish in the form of mackerel – hence the reason I keep harping that plate in front of you contain 50% dark green leafy veggies and that diet is so important.

Also, keep in mind there are nine common types of magnesium, all of which differ slightly in the benefits they offer. Perhaps this is another reason I find it helpful to switch things around from time to time. If you are just starting out, try applying magnesium transdermally, which simply means applying it to the skin. Doing it this way helps with absorption issues. Transdermal magnesium can be bought in lotion form and is ideal for sensitive individuals or children. Ancient Minerals is a decent enough product and a simple Google search will take you to it.

Another way to load magnesium is by adding magnesium bath salts to your bath and soaking in them. Ideally, steer clear of any product with added perfume in the ingredients. Ultimately, let yourself be guided by how each makes you feel. For those attempting oral supplementation, it may prove helpful to try alternating with either magnesium citrate or magnesium orotate. If you find yourself drawn to cycling either of these forms, always take them in sensible moderation rather than trying too much all at once.

KRILL OIL is loaded with the omega-3 polyunsaturated fatty acids **DHA** (docosahexaenoic) and **EPA** (eicosapentaenoic acid). Both of these help keep the brain firing on all four cylinders. Krill oil is unique because unlike regular fish oils it can be absorbed directly by the brain with very little processing. It may also help support better concentration, memory, and learning. Krill oil also has more antioxidants than regular fish oil and is generally considered safer because of its lower levels of contaminants such as mercury. Mercury can be a problem, especially in tuna, marlin, and swordfish.
Krill oil also contains astaxanthin which can be helpful to the eyes. Given that the eyes have a high density of mitochondria, some reports suggest astaxanthin helps protect mitochondria from oxidative stress. Just for good measure, krill oil is thought to support a healthy heart, the brain, and the nervous system as well as keep cholesterol and blood lipids in the normal range. It also helps maintain healthy blood sugar levels, keeps joints healthy, supports liver function, and even supports the immune system.

VITAMIN C is a water-soluble vitamin, which means your body doesn't store it. Humans do not have the ability to make vitamin C as many animals do, which means you need to consume it via your diet. This is one reason vitamin C made it to the list but also because it covers so many bases.

Vitamin C is my go-to supplement whenever I feel a cold coming on, but the benefits of vitamin C can be used to treat a much wider range of health problems. It's also known to be useful in wound healing and skin health. It can be used to treat joint and muscle problems and it plays a role in a healthy heart. *Yup, you heard me right on that last one.*

When it comes to the heart, vitamin C is right up there with healthy exercise. Vitamin C is a powerful antioxidant, known to block some of the damage caused by DNA-damaging free radicals. Over time, free radical damage may accelerate aging and contribute to the development of heart disease. Vitamin C also benefits the eyes and is thought to lower your risk of cataracts. Vitamin C supports the immune system and is important for respiratory health. Larger doses can be useful for allergies and asthma due to its antioxidant and anti-inflammatory effect.

The brain and nervous system also have a need for vitamin C. Some sources suggest deficiencies can lead to a degeneration of the nervous system with possible links to neurological based diseases such as ALS, Parkinson's, and Alzheimer's. Vitamin C is needed to help keep the tissue in the digestive tract healthy and has been shown to be useful for stomach ulcers, gastritis, and H. Pylori, which is a bacterium known to cause chronic inflammation/infection in the stomach and duodenum.

The recommended daily allowance (RDA) for vitamin C has been established at 40 to 60 mg per day although some might suggest this is on the *low* end. According to Nobel Prize winning scientist Linus Pauling, elevated doses of vitamin C may have a role to play in the fight against cancer. Pauling spent his life advocating amounts of 1,000 mg or even higher until he died at the age of ninety-three. High doses of Vitamin C are sometimes administered by IV.

Most take Vitamin C orally. The brand I personally use is sold by Beyond-Health. It's a little pricey but compared to buying all those cold and flu remedies from the pharmacy it evens out in the long run. An ounce of prevention is always better than a pound of cure. This brand of vitamin C is a buffered powder and contains trace amounts of potassium, calcium magnesium, and zinc.

You can also increase your vitamin C level by squeezing a fresh lemon or lime into water and drinking it. It might surprise some to know that red peppers are high in vitamin C and compared to oranges they obviously have less sugar. For anyone with an iron deficiency, pairing Vitamin C with iron has been shown to improve absorption, although another option would be to eat more beef liver. Pairing Vitamin C with the amino acid N-acetylcysteine (NAC) is an inexpensive way to help the body build glutathione, which is considered the body's master antioxidant.

Another option to increase glutathione is to use a liposomal glutathione supplement which helps the glutathione be better absorbed through the GI tract. If you can afford it, a more efficient way to increase glutathione is by IV, although this option is not only more expensive it also requires a qualified doctor to be in the loop. Glutathione administered via an IV has been shown to be helpful in the fight against Parkinson's disease. *But I digress.*

Not all **B-COMPLEX** supplements are made equal and again you are better off steering well clear of bargain basement supplements. A *whole foods-based* B-complex is the preferred way to go and there are plenty of good ones on the market. B vitamins play an important role in keeping the body energized throughout the day as well as helping convert our food into fuel. The idea of taking a good quality B-complex is that it has eight B vitamins added which include, B1, B2, B3, B5, B6, B7, B9 and sometimes B12.

B12 is a big one as it does so much in the body. It can also be purchased on its own. A B12 deficiency can sometimes leave a person feeling tired or unfocused and can also sometimes be coupled with a dizzy feeling or even heart palpitations. With so many overlapping symptoms, getting an accurate diagnosis can be particularly problematic. Typically, a B12 deficiency is measured based on the serum vitamin B12 levels within the blood. As we all know, standard blood tests are not infallible and there are times when some patients will fall through the cracks. A more precise screening might be one that checks for high homocysteine levels. Unfortunately, this test is usually only given to patients who have a known case of anemia or heart disease-related symptoms.

Sometimes doing things the old school way by cross-checking a list of symptoms can prove just as helpful. Things to be on the lookout for might include an inability to concentrate, chronic fatigue, muscle weakness, joint pain, shortness of breath, dizziness, poor memory, heart palpitations, bleeding gums, a poor appetite, digestive problems, and even mood changes such as depression and anxiety.

While there could be any number of reasons for the above symptoms, it's important to note that a deficiency in B12 is more likely to occur in someone who has absorption issues in the gut (hello again cheeky-leaky). Some vegans may also lean toward a B12 deficiency. The elderly are particularly prone to B12 deficiency and for anyone with a relative showing signs of early dementia, adding a B-complex supplement will prove beneficial. Foods high in B12 are beef, chicken, liver, and fish such as wild caught salmon, herring, mackerel, and sardines.

When supplementing, keep in mind that the body strives to remain in balance and sometimes this challenge is best tackled with herbs. Herbs have been used in medicine since the beginning of time and some are far more potent than others. It's worth noting that herbs such as Echinacea, astragalus, olive leaf, cat's claw, elderberry, and goldenseal all have the potential to crank up the immune system.

While this may be the desired effect for many, for the autoimmune patient this can be a double-edged sword. However, all is not lost. There is a subcategory of herbs known as adaptogenic herbs. Put simply, these herbs help the body adapt. Rather than stimulate, they are known to soothe the immune system, hence the name *adapt*ogenic. For some, adaptogens may prove to be the missing link.

When used in conjunction with a clean diet, think of adaptogenic herbs as a natural substance which assist the body in adapting to stress and to help bring a normalizing effect upon bodily processes. Adaptogens are highly versatile which can be especially useful when trying to balance out either Th1 or Th2 dominance of the immune system.

Adaptogens can help increase the body's resistance to mental, physical, and environmental stress, although results will be hindered if the original stressor (i.e. food allergy) remains a constant. We briefly mentioned Cordyceps earlier which are not adaptogens in the classic sense, but they do have adaptogenic qualities, hence they get a quick mentioned again here.

What follows is a very basic summary of some widely used adaptogens. If this is all new to you, try to find an experienced herbalist to work with.

Ashwagandha has been used in Ayurvedic medicine for over 2000 years. Its immuno-modulating effects help the body adapt to stress. It can also be helpful in treating anxiety.

Ginseng is probably one of the more well-used adaptogens among herbalists. Asian ginseng is used most often because it is the most potent of the ginseng family. Studies show that Asian ginseng has great antioxidant effects, as well as helping your body adapt to stress. In some people it can be helpful in lowering blood pressure.

I've put **Chaste Tree Berry** (vitex agnus-castus) on the list especially for the ladies. Chase tree mimics the master hormone, progesterone. *So what does that mean?* Well for starters, better balanced hormones =less stress, less PMS, and less difficulty transitioning into menopause! Although it may take up to eight weeks to feel the full effect, Chaste Tree can be a total game changer for many women. Give it time and it may just be your silver bullet.

Holy Basil helps fight fatigue and stabilize your immune system. It can also be used to regulate blood sugar and hormone levels.

Rhodiola is another potent adaptogen that has had many research studies done on it. Rhodiola helps the body adapt to stress-induced mental and physical fatigue. Studies found that Rhodiola restores normal patterns of eating and sleeping after long-term stress. It also helps combat mental and physical fatigue, protects against oxidative stress, heat stress, radiation, and exposure to toxic chemicals. Rhodiola also protects the heart and liver, increases use of oxygen, and improves memory.

Gynostemma (or jiaogulan, as it's sometimes called) is another adaptogenic herb and a potent health tonic made as a tea. In addition to helping balance the immune system, it also increases stamina and helps reduce stress. Gynostemma has a slightly woody taste which, given its health benefits, doesn't faze me in the slightest.

The 2nd HEALING TRIANGLE

Okay, I know the sands of time are quickly running out on us, so a more serious illness may call for a more a direct approach. So before we leave this section, I'd like to quickly mention the idea of a 2nd healing triangle. As mentioned earlier, your liver plays a key role in your recovery. If you are smart, treat your liver like your new BF and it will become a formidable ally to have on your team. Right now, even as we talk, your liver is busy doing everything it can to protect you from a daily assault of toxic chemicals. It's currently performing a wide range of tasks just to keep you alive. For this reason, the liver forms the *first* part of this triangle.

Hear this: every year we change the oil in our cars, perhaps you change your own oil or perhaps you pay someone to do it for you. Every time you take your car in for an oil change, did you ever stop and think about your liver? Occasionally it needs to be cleaned too.

There are many ways to do this and by now I hope you have a basic grasp on *how* to do this. If all else fails, find someone to help you the same way you would pay someone to change your oil. If money is tight, this book is full of people and places where you can find more answers. Earthclinic.com often has interesting information to offer.

Next, we should by now also know that sugar has become a thorn in the side of all humankind. It's everywhere and anywhere; it's plastered on billboards and even sold to our kids in schools. So much illness has its roots firmly planted in sugar. A reduction of sugar may prove helpful, but as we know sugar can be an additive. If you currently face a *serious* health challenge, simply reducing your *known* sugar intake may not be enough.

Fortunately, the second part of this triangle deals with this problem quite well. The ketogenic diet comes in many forms. Find a nutritionist who *understands* the importance of cutting sugar to a wellness level *based on your individual needs.* Starving the body of sugar is the second part of our triangle, but this doesn't mean you have to starve yourself. As we mentioned earlier, the body *already* knows how to burn ketones and does so efficiently without sugar.

With a liver that's firing on all four cylinders and a body that's burning ketones (optimally) you only need one more part to the puzzle. That final part is oxygen. With the liver working, starve the body of sugar, flood it with oxygen and good health can be yours for the taking! If you have the funds, flooding the body with oxygen is easy but I suspect not everyone who comes to this book has the means to pay for ozone therapy or a hyperbaric chamber (although I believe there are now companies online that rent chambers). Either way, in this internet savvy world, your options for increasing oxygen are plentiful.

While for legal reasons I cannot give you specific doses, I can at least suggest taking in an abundance of fresh air as a good starting point. Yup, there are a few other more controversial ways out there, but you should first consult with your doctor before attempting anything new.

A WHOLE NEW YOU

Give the body what it needs and it will find a way to renew itself. It's sometimes said that every seven years or so we grow ourselves a whole new body. While there is some truth to this concept, our cells are constantly replacing themselves at varying rates. The lining of the stomach, for example, is replaced about every three days, while it's estimated that bones turn over every seven to ten years. On average, the entire outer skin is replaced about every two weeks and the liver regrows itself every couple of years.

This cycle of events is not only remarkable it's a little freaky. Physically you are not the same person you were seven years ago. This presents a window of opportunity for anyone willing to make changes. How your body reacts tomorrow is closely tied to the raw materials being used today.

Even parts of your brain will regenerate, although not all. Some of us might warm to the idea of having a whole new brain; others will take comfort in knowing that essentially our memories remain the same.

As our time now draws closer to the end, I'm actually quite shocked at how much work goes into writing a book. Over the past year I've lost count of how many times I've had to dismantle this whole book and then rewrite it from scratch. When the madness of self-imposed standards met devotion, each and every paragraph became a bargaining chip for just a quiet moment alone with my own thoughts. To some degree, it's a relief to be almost at the finish line, but I'll also miss the process of writing for you *as there was so much more I wanted to share.*

So from here, I'm really not sure where I go next with my life. While construction work pays my rent, it really doesn't get any easier on the body. I guess a lot depends on whether this book strikes a chord with people. Unfortunately, the world has no shortage of struggling unknown authors. Perhaps I'll take out an ad in the local paper that reads, **"Handyman – will write for food"** lol.

What did we learn from this chapter?

Supermarket food is grown for profit. Those who eat it daily may at some point develop a mineral deficiency somewhere within the body.

Rapidly changing the gut biome can bring unwanted side effects. As always, go slow with a small test dose first rather than subjecting yourself to a mega dose. BEFORE moving into oral supplementation, try to gradually increase your probiotic intake through fermented foods.

Homework: check out a website by the name of earthclinic.com. It is full of helpful tips, all presented in an easy to understand format. It also covers supplements and a wide range of ailments. I use it often.

Link: https://www.earthclinic.com/

P.S. Given that you are now *almost* done reading this book, I'd be real interested to know how this information is being perceived. If you are enjoying it, a book review from you would be awesome. If you think this book sucks, please feel free to tell me **why.** Perhaps together you and I can make a much *better* version.

Chapter 40

95% HOPE

Congratulations, by making it this far you now have a set of tools capable of bringing about a positive change for you. And given the correct raw materials you also have a body that knows how to heal. Preventing things of a toxic nature from entering your body is the essence of good health. Had I known this information *before* I became ill, I believe I could have sidestepped my illness completely or at least shaved years off my recovery time. Keeping an open mind is also a smart step in the right direction.

As your new journey begins, treat these chapters as simple stepping stones and always be on the lookout for new and insightful information. These are exciting times we live in with fresh data constantly streaming in from every direction. The day you become the smartest person at the table is the day you know you are sitting at the wrong table. Throughout this book I've always tried to keep things real. I've never pretended to have *all* the answers. I'm not sure anybody does. At best, discovery is a collective effort and a great starting point is to check out all those people mentioned by name in this book.

As we now begin our final descent I'm reflecting on the time we have spent together. For a book written primarily about health it sure seems to have rendered its fair share of twists and digressions, and there are still a few more to come. At the beginning of this story you found me trapped inside a sickly body and unable to work. It's now been six years since I first became ill and seriously, as it happens and as I type this, it's actually six years *to the day*!

While I'm thankful for all the things I have learned, it might surprise you to know that I'd trade them all in a heartbeat *not* to have gone through what I did. Forgive me if I appear ungrateful, but clawing back 95% of my health *isn't* something I choose to celebrate. Nope, today's ironic anniversary is all about the 5% that's stubbornly remains, and how nobody has ever said "sorry."

Don't get me wrong, I'll take a *partial* recovery over no recovery any day of the week, but I'm also very aware that a problem left 5% unresolved is still a foot in the door to serious illness. I've worked so hard to get to this point and yet there are days when trying to keep an annoying subset of rogue symptoms under control feels as if I'm trying to hold a giant beach ball underwater.

Before I took my seat in that fateful doctor's office, running was something I took pleasure in. I could actually go quite a few miles without breaking a sweat. But once those unfortunate wheels were set in motion, things have never quite been the same and any attempt to run even a short distance still leaves my legs feeling heavy and tight, so I walk instead.

This stubborn problem continues to challenge me and keeping a lid on it isn't always easy. Given everything I was forced to learn and then apply, it's quite remarkable that this 5% still remains. I often wonder what would have become of me had I not been so persistent? What I do know for sure is this: whenever an illness is "triggered" the more you know the more you wish you didn't know. Whatever it was they introduced into my bloodstream in 2011, it still lurks inside me, albeit to a lesser degree.

Perhaps in this moment I'm seeing my glass as 5% empty, but so far I've narrowed it down to one of two things: either my own understanding of the problem has reached its limit, or the problem was intentionally made difficult to understand. If you choose to believe the latter, then it should also serve as a dark reminder that there are times when a routine doctor's visit can have destructive consequences. As a direct result of that 2011 encounter, I believe my life has not only been made more difficult but it may also have been made shorter than even God intended. *I guess we will see.*

Those times I've used the term God in this book have been my feeble attempt to describe whatever entity governs this vast universe. I guess I find *this* concept more plausible that accepting we all somehow grew legs and walked ourselves out of the sea.

I'm really *not* a religious person as such, but the day I felt the coldness of death moving through my bones I happened to come across a small piece of scripture that gave me a glimmer of **hope.** I'd like to share it with you because back then I really couldn't see it.

> *"For I know the plans I have for you," declares the Lord,*
> *"plans to prosper you and not to harm you,*
> *plans to give you hope and a future."*
> – Jeremiah 29:11

When we are forced to accept our own mortality, what we choose to think has the power to enslave or liberate us on the turn of a single thought. Perhaps my eyes now see things differently. *How so?*

As someone who likes to be productive, the time I spent confined to a sick bed often left me feeling unproductive and isolated. In some ways, being trapped by illness gave me a rare insight as to how an inmate might cope when forced to endure a lifetime of incarceration. Sometimes the only places I got to visit were inside my head – barren destinations that frequently passed through my mind like tumbleweeds rolling across an open plain.

However, one place I visited was quite different, and to this day it's held a lasting impression. In the middle of enduring much suffering it was as if a gateway opened up deep in my subconscious. I can still recall in quite vivid detail standing barefoot inside a small stone cottage located somewhere on a grassy hill. The smooth stone floor warmed with the amber glow of sunshine which filtered through a stained glass window. I've never lived in such a place but it immediately felt like home and everything I touched had a distinct natural feel to it, almost as if plastic and paint had never been invented.

Within that fleeting moment of peace and simplicity it actually crossed my mind that perhaps my sickly body had given up and died. And to be honest, wherever it was that I'd found myself, I was in no rush to leave. Snapping back to reality left me reluctantly pondering the meaning of such a detailed image. Maybe I'd caught a glimpse of how we were supposed to live – in the moment, simply, and free of worry rather than chasing every dollar. I guess some parts of this book were inspired by that blissful feeling, others were written to address the inadequacies of a medical establishment that left me out to dry.

I know a solution is out there somewhere, but here I am still relying on persistence to find it. Persistence is believing that problems have solutions, just as doors have keys. It's the noble art of being knocked down ten times and getting up eleven.

Over the years I suspect you have had your fair share of troubles and I've had mine too. That ugly wheel of *mis*fortune can be such an unpredictable part of life. We all have "character building" days – you know the ones I'm talking about, those days when you lose your job and your car keys in the same afternoon. Unfortunately, bad days aren't limited to losing replaceable things, although that sucks too.
Bad things happen to good people daily and *none* of us are immune. Maybe you already know what it's like to lose someone close to you, or perhaps you know what it's like to suffer from medical injury or be a victim of a crime. While our past certainly shapes us, it doesn't have to define who we are. For just a moment, I'd like to ask you to pause here, set down the book, and let your mind *briefly* drift back to one of those more challenging days.

I can only imagine where your mind went to and how that unfortunate day might have affected your life. I wonder, if you again had the opportunity to travel backward in time and were somehow able to stand next to yourself, *what words of wisdom would you whisper in your ear?*

If I could go back in time, I'd tell myself, *be still and know that in the end it's going to be okay. Just don't lose hope.* In that hour of dark desperation, when a storm of shit rains down on us, we don't always need to know the reason; we just need to know it's going to be okay. It's as if our earthly soul needs something tangible to hold onto, perhaps just a small flicker of hope to reignite our human spirit. When we are deprived of such hope the world becomes a daunting place.

Understand that the vast majority of people on this planet all want the same things that you do, meaningful work, someone who believes in them, and *hope*. Nobody wakes up and asks, "How can I make my life more difficult today?" They really don't. No, that circumstance is usually imposed on us by the powers that be – but it doesn't have to be that way.

Look beyond those daily news headlines and you will notice that most of us are simply just trying to get by. Not everyone is an axe-wielding maniac, although there are some that are. Not everyone is out to deceive you, although there are some that will. It's my humble assumption that those who are exposed to a toxic environment are the ones mostly likely to make toxic choices.

Put your humanitarian goggles on for just a second and you will see that people are a product of their environment. You and I were not made to be dumb creatures. In case it escaped your attention, we are the only mammals on this planet driving around in cars, yet when the human brain is flooded with toxins we all have a tendency to make really dumb choices. Having seen a very different world, albeit briefly, I believe that simplicity is a greatly undervalued commodity and our world was never meant to be this toxic.

Alas, the darkness created in this life has always been rooted in greed and arrogance and yet it is this same darkness that helps us see the brightness of light. Come my friend and let us travel down one last road together.

You may have noticed how in recent times the word "hope" became part of a political slogan. The word was hyped up and bandied around with broad smiles and a promise that we all wanted to believe in. You may have also noticed *political* hope rarely reaches the bottomless pit of human despair. Stay with me here, because even though those damned spin doctors hijacked the word hope, it's vitally important they aren't allowed to keep it.

It's often said that gratitude can have a profound effect on the human soul. Gratitude has been shown to turn off stress, blast away critical thinking, wipe away selfishness, and even overturn that most destructive of all human conditions – victim mentality.

However, if you *really* want to take your health to a whole different level, *learn to give and be grateful for the experience.* I know what you are thinking because I thought it too – *how much is this going to cost me, right?* If counting your money with fingerless gloves on is your thang, then you can just go ahead and relax, *this final tip works with or without your money.*

> *To be truly radical is to make **hope** possible*
> *rather than despair convincing.*
> – Raymond Williams

As rational thinkers, it can be difficult to understand how we can benefit ourselves by helping others. I wouldn't be wasting your time or mine if I hadn't experienced the *value* of this firsthand. Make no mistake, giving something back is a powerful tool to have under your belt. This can be as profound as saving a life or as simple as helping someone across the road. At this point, it's important not to let the simplicity of this concept undermine your perception.

Let's take a step back and look at this from a fresh angle. You can take it to the bank that right now there is someone out there who is experiencing a soul-crushing day, the depths of which you and I can only imagine. How would *you* like to become an intrinsic part of *their* story and in the process *reap the reward?* The trick to doing this *is to expect nothing in return.* Once you get to that level, something freaky happens. **Giving freely opens the path to receiving.** *I know, right? But stay with me, I promise this final tool has a great deal of merit.*

Back when I was too ill to work there were people in my local community who pitched in and left prepaid grocery and gas cards in my mailbox. Generosity came with no strings attached at a time when I felt had no value, although the money quickly came and went, those envelopes represented more than just food and gas, they also gave me hope. I later learned that some of those people who gave had never met me and yet

454

they still chose to help. The fact that random people chose to step in **without expecting anything** in return kinda blew me away. Six years later those random acts of kindness remain firmly rooted inside me.

So where does all this fit in? Let's go back to that bad day **you** were having, maybe you *did* lose your car keys and your job in the same afternoon. On that lousy bus ride home how would you feel if suddenly you found an envelope on your seat. Inside that envelope there was no note, just a few dollars, perhaps only enough to buy yourself dinner at the end of a long miserable day. *I know, right? WTF? (Who's-This-From?)*

In the absence of any note you'd be forced to ponder the meaning of it all. Suddenly in the middle of a shit storm this would become an almost surreal single ray of sunshine. But how the heck did that envelope find you on that bus, and why?

Here's how.

Whenever people stop what they are doing and take the trouble to look up, it becomes pretty easy to spot those around us who are having a really bad day — perhaps even struggling to keep their heads above water as I once was. To see someone who's *genuinely* in need and then, *without drawing attention to yourself*, be prepared to step in and help is really a beautiful thing. To anonymously put a few bucks in an envelope and find a way to discretely slip it to them becomes more than just a goodwill gesture, it's a symbol of **hope**.

Okay, where am I heading with all this?

There's a whole mountain of published scientific data that points to how we can lift ourselves by lifting others. No, seriously, this is sometimes referred to as "Helper's-High." One study showed that helping others led to a measureable increase in longevity (think of Edie Simms, that remarkable 102-year old lady who spends her days helping younger members of the nursing home!) Another study showed a measureable decrease in pain. With equal importance, it was also shown that people who observe feats of generosity are more likely to do the same, thus causing a ripple effect throughout an entire community. *Wait a second, are you getting this? When one person performs a good deed, it literally causes a chain reaction of other altruistic acts!*

The volume of data relating to this subject is incredibly vast, although it pains me to say I'm actually not a huge fan of citing scientific data. *Why?* Over the years I've lost count of how many times I've read something that was "cited" only to learn somewhere down the road that the data was skewed in favor of the person collecting it. But in this case there is no financial incentive behind the concept of giving freely, so the data is as pure as it can be! Don't take my word for it – if you like we can pause here while you go check it out even on sites such as PubMed.

Think about it, this world has become a breeding ground for habitual greed, egotism, and materialism and these are the very things that steal our inner peace. And most people don't even know it. The *opposite* end of that spectrum is to help someone and expect nothing in return.

To help you tap into the health benefits of this for yourself, it really doesn't matter what you do so long as you do it. Even if you don't have a spare dime, you can still get in the game by starting small, perhaps holding a door open for someone or simply making a conscious effort to let a few extra cars out in traffic. Over time you'll obviously want to step up your game, but for now it's all good. Notice that so far *none of these ideas require large amounts of time or money.*

If the secret to living is giving, then your mission from today on is a simple one: **be a symbol of hope.** Help someone, even in a small way, and in the process boost your own health!

PERSISTENCE

So as my story now draws to a close, *know that yours is just beginning.* Over the course of this book we have crammed quite a few tools into our proverbial toolbox, and it seems that our old friend persistence remains a firm favorite, if for no other reason than it displays total disobedience in the face of adversity. Persistence lives deep inside each and every one of us, the trick is to bring it to the surface where it can be of most use to us.

Persistence requires no skill. It is nothing more than finding ways to move sideways when there appears to be no way forward. Persistence is simply about exhausting all options and then somehow finding a way to try just one more. It should come as no surprise that persistence is a close cousin of defiance. Once you have a handle on defiance you are rich for all that you need in *this* life.

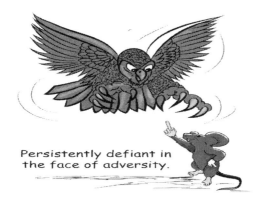

Persistently defiant in the face of adversity.

Both persistence and defiance are such important qualities that I personally plan on taking them both with me to the afterlife. Prior to taking that great elevator to the sky, my last desperate breath on this earth will be spent trying to hold my middle finger in position. Why? "Victory belongs to the most persevering." - Napoleon Bonaparte. Besides, once rigor mortis sets in good luck to anyone attempting to straighten the finger out again!

Until then, I'll continue looking at my own health riddle objectively morning, noon, and night as I have done every day for the past six years. If you are the type to keep score that translates into at least 6570 (and counting) different ways a persistent person can look at a problem. I trust you have enjoyed reading this book as much as I have enjoyed writing it for you. Offering something safe and middle of the road was never my intention, and anything in between will surely have been a wasted effort. Maybe with more time, additional information could have been added but offering more would have also seen me teetering on the edge of procrastination and our paths might never have crossed.

At last count there were at more than 140,000 words in this book. I'm human, if any typos slipped through I hope my passion for the subject outshines my punctuation. Lord knows, trying to write out of a suitcase wasn't always easy, yet here we both are at the finish line. Creating something *worthy* of sharing was always my intended goal and it is my deepest hope that I have achieved that standard for you.

As I write this final page I'm also aware of how fickle the outside world can be, and perhaps I now set myself up for a few scathing reviews and even ridicule. I am at peace with this arrangement knowing that silence is a luxury best reserved for those unaffected by adversity. Fear of criticism is a poor excuse for *not* doing something. With that in mind, I find the words of Elbert Hubbard a comfort: *"To avoid criticism, do nothing, say nothing, and be nothing."*

If you've read this book as a paperback version, then I'd like to now challenge you to set it free. Leave a copy in the most random place you can think of, perhaps with a five-dollar bill left inside as a bookmark. Let the finder experience a totally random act of kindness, and perhaps in turn they will do the same.

So before I crawl back under my rock, may I ask for a small favor of you? With no slick, million-dollar marketing team behind me, good old fashioned word of mouth has always been my preferred way to advertise. If you enjoyed this book, would you please recommend it to a friend? *Your voice is my lifeline.* As you probably guessed, social media really isn't my thing, so I'll take all the help I can get. A plug from you on any one the following platforms would be totally awesome.

☐ AMAZON
☐ GOODREADS
☐ FACEBOOK
☐ INSTAGRAM

As someone who prefers to blend into the background, I find this shameless request for self-promotion *painfully* awkward. However, for Amazon to even notice this book, it desperately needs fresh reviews. As an unknown author, this presents a real challenge for me. Having just busted my ass writing this book, it would be a real shame if people couldn't find it. **Your review makes this book visible,** and *a simple one-line review beats no review at all.*

Thank you in advance.

If I'm given the opportunity to pick up my pen again, perhaps next time I'll write less about physical health, and more about mental conflict. I find depression and anxiety such fascinating topics and yet they are made so difficult for people to understand. Maybe I'll call that book, *The Noble Art of Taming the Mind* or *Who Knew What the Handyman Knew, WTF?*

The challenge with this book *wasn't* finding things to write about, it was trying to gauge when to stop, and here seems a good a place as any. So for now, I guess that's it, except to say *thank you* for your valued support and good luck on your own journey.

Oh yeah, one last thing, **Dad, if you can somehow see me, I miss your face and I dedicate this book to you.**

Author gently sets down the pen and quietly leaves the room.
I know, right? Dropping the mic would have been a tad pretentious.

Kindest Regards
James

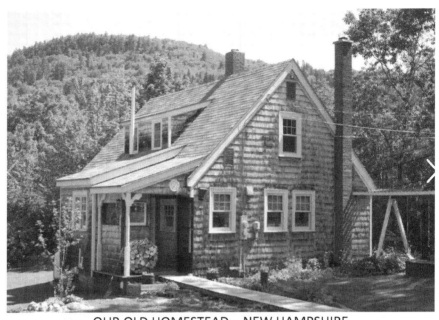

OUR OLD HOMESTEAD – NEW HAMPSHIRE

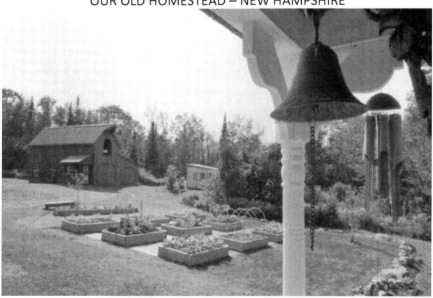

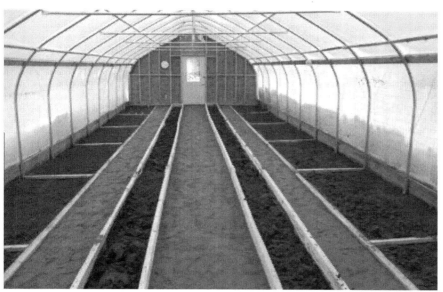

OUR OLD HOMESTEAD – NEW HAMPSHIRE

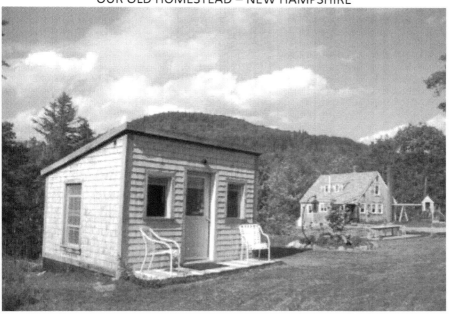

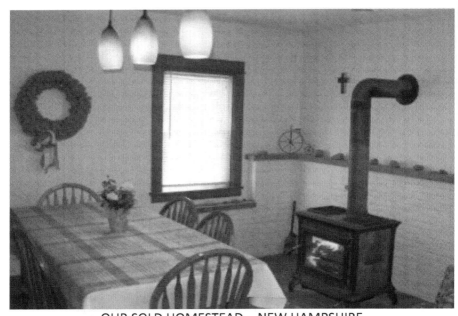

OUR SOLD HOMESTEAD – NEW HAMPSHIRE

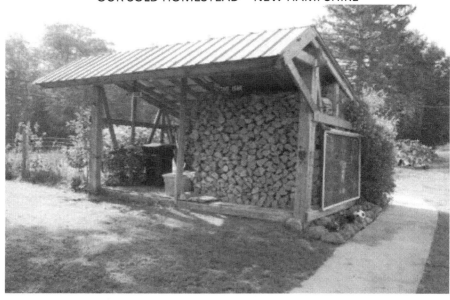

Looking for a new place to call home.

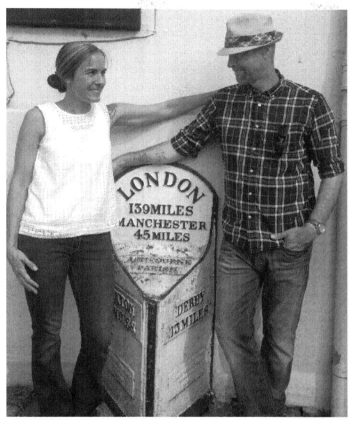

For updates (and fresh health tips) here's my Facebook link.
https://www.facebook.com/james.lilley.393950

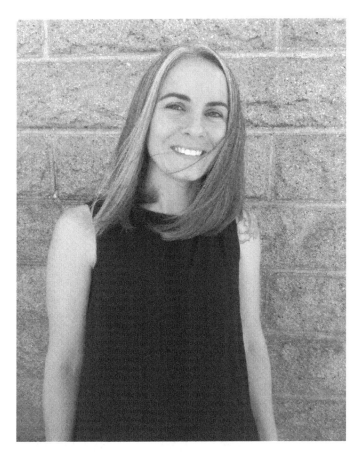

My wife, Amanda, you can check out her many beautiful knitting patterns on Ravelry.com

Thanks for supporting an indie author,

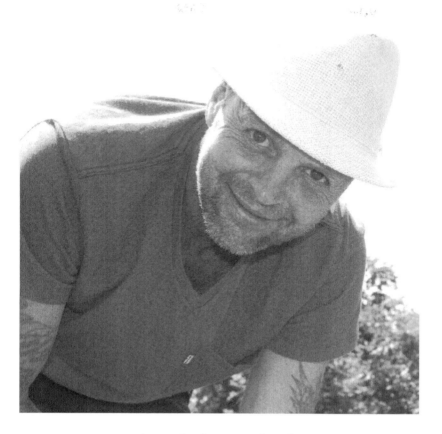

I genuinely appreciate it.

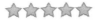

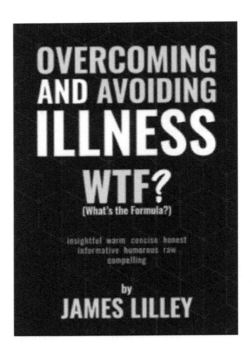

S.O.S

Without fresh reviews this book quickly becomes invisible on Amazon, whether you loved or loathed it, your voice is powerful, so please use it.

Amazon
Top customer reviews

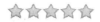

Feel better/get better – the way to do it is in this book!

This is one of those books that will quite literally change your life. Not every single thing in here is going to apply to you, but my bet is a whole lot of it will, and what doesn't will probably be something that applies to someone you know. This author, like so many people, suffered through a debilitating set of symptoms that were (as far as I can tell) never diagnosed and for which he didn't get much help from the medical profession. (I know several people in this situation and I bet you know some, too - or have had the same experience yourself.) Anyway, he set out to cure himself and succeeded (at least "95%") and this book is everything he learned along the way. It's chock full of information about foods, allergies, supplements (and what to do and NOT do with them), and even cleanses, and all this information is offered up in a way that's meant to get you to focus on those things that are most relevant to your situation and the best way to pursue your own study and research.

It's well-written and personable - he's not trying to be an expert or pose as any kind of healthcare worker, he's gifting to others all the work he's done over the last several years. Some of what's in here you'll already know and some of what you'll learn will surprise - even startle - you and I guarantee you will make changes in your life that are going to dramatically benefit you starting almost immediately. This has been true for me.

For people who read from the back,
hello to you, here's what you missed.

Based on six years of meticulous research, this remarkable story unfolds into a step-by-step, problem-solving tool. It's your shortcut to a less stressed, more energized, healthier version of you. Tightly crafted, yet flowing with genuine compassion, a rich vein of insight comes to the table via the author's own battle with serious illness. It's all in here waiting for you, peppered with a delicate hint of British humor.

Here's what we know for sure. Sooner or later most will face a health problem. In a perfect world a solution is found and once again life is good, but I'm guessing you already know the world we live in is far from perfect. What becomes of those who leave the doctor's office with a set of lingering symptoms, or a treatment plan that makes things worse? What's your next move if you are told your illness has no solution?

Do you have a plan?

Come inside and discover the elusive answers you crave, together we will set about rebuilding your health brick by brick. Let the route to wellness take you down some beautiful winding roads. Unshackled from a conventional publisher, there is nothing to fear from telling it like it is.

It's actually quite remarkable that you even found this unusual book, *or perhaps this book found you.*

Amazon
Top customer reviews

Chronic illness? Read this

Up until I developed several chronic illnesses, I was a firm believer in conventional medicine. It was my profession for decades. Now though, conventional medicine has little to offer me, and I am ill. Chronically ill. I have been researching alternative medicine for a while now, perhaps due to my long standing bias against alternative medicine due to being so pro conventional medicine for so long, it took me a long time to appreciate different ways of getting better.

The author has done a tremendous amount of research for us all in this book. As I read, I was reminded of much I had discovered myself. This book puts much of what I had already learned plus more into a wonderful format that is approachable and easy to digest. I wish this gentleman well and would like him to know that I have already taken some of the steps on the path, some of the hard ones for me, thanks to this book. Thank you

SPECIAL THANKS TO

My wife, I know this past year hasn't always been easy. Dealing with the madness of my new writing obsession while living on a shoestring budget was at times challenging I know, but once again we kinda made it. Thanks for always showing me what a PDF file is and for loaning me your computer. Perhaps now that the ink is dry you can see why this project was so important for me to finish. P.S. I love you.

To my old friend Steve Shaw, whom I've always trusted to always tell me like it is. To my old army buddy Howie who gave me the same level of honesty. To Dalton Lawrence, thank you, sir, for your support and input. Thanks to to Kaylia Dunstan, for helping to keep my thoughts on track. To Lesley Dahl, what an insightful breath of fresh air you helped bring to this book.

To my dear old mum, who has been through so much and yet remains my rock. To both my sisters, your valuable feedback was always helpful and I know I probably drive you both bonkers. To Jade, thank you for *always* bigging me up. To Cortney, I still miss you and I hope you are okay. To Miss Emma, thank you for your wonderful contribution to this book, your letter was quite moving. To the one and only Miss Abigail, thank you for always being you. For sure, Grandad would be proud of you all.

To all the many health gurus featured in the pages of this book, over the years I've learned so much from each and every one of you. I'm truly grateful for the good work that you do and for taking the trouble to post such informative books and videos. For every health guru mentioned in this book there must have been at least a hundred others that I didn't get a chance to mention because there simply wasn't room. These are my true unsung heroes as I learned so much from so many.

And finally, James, who *really* dislikes having his photo taken, but agreed to take a hit for the team as a way of saying **thank you**, especially to those who took time out of their busy day to leave a review. I truly appreciate it

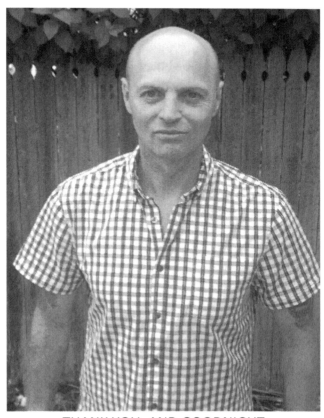

THANK YOU, AND GOODNIGHT

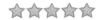
This is a must read! Recommending this to all my clients!!!

I have sat with this masterpiece, reading it from cover to cover in its entirety, twice now. I have not been able to put it down, between the warm delivery of this work, and the endless re-invigoration of information offered. This book does what others have yet to do, and that is to break down a most complicated issue of acute to chronic illness into an easily read, yet impeccably researched guide to the foundation of health and HOW to be the picture of health. With drug companies lining the pockets of the medial world, and doctors in patient's purses, James has stripped away he fog blinding us, while revealing through well documents accounts of a personal, treacherous, endured course of what was once, and could have been, a slow an arduous death. James delivers a wealth of knowledge through a conversation that feels like an invitation to tea, while he reveals the meaning of health and how to achieve your optimal state.

What is more, is that there are no products, supplements, programs, or additional books being pushed or offered; but an empowering and comprehensive roadmap placing you in the driver's seat of your own body. From cellular foundations of health and disease, to home testing of organ functions, nutrition, and rebalancing what has been off kilter, these short chapters are easy to navigate with interactive invitations to help you become your own expert and take charge of your health. This will literally be the only book you will ever need for staying healthy and disease free the rest of your life.

Printed in Poland
by Amazon Fulfillment
Poland Sp. z o.o., Wrocław